MOSBY'S
FIRST RESPONDER
TEXTBOOK

MOSBY'S FIRST RESPONDER TEXTBOOK

Walt A. Stoy, PhD
and the
Center for Emergency Medicine

with 345 *illustrations*

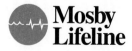
Mosby Lifeline

St. Louis Baltimore Boston Carlsbad Chicago Naples New York Philadelphia Portland
London Madrid Mexico City Singapore Sydney Tokyo Toronto Wiesbaden

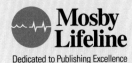

Mosby Lifeline

Dedicated to Publishing Excellence

A Times Mirror Company

Publisher: David Dusthimer
Editor: Claire Merrick
Senior Assistant Editor: Melissa Blair
Developmental Editor: Debra Lejeune
Project Manager: Chris Baumle
Production Editor: Anthony Trioli
Art Director: Max Brinkman
Composition Specialists: Kevin D. Dodds and Christopher D. Six
Design Manager: Nancy McDonald
Cover Designers: Diane Buric and Ron Zinn
Manufacturing Manager: William A. Winneberger, Jr.

Printed in the United States of America
Composition by Mosby Electronic Publishing
Printing and binding by Von Hoffmann Press, Inc.

Mosby–Year Book, Inc.
11830 Westline Industrial Drive
St. Louis, Missouri 63146

Library of Congress Card Catalog Number   96-79893

97 98 99 00 01 / 9 8 7 6 5 4 3 2 1

*This textbook is dedicated to those of you
who are accepting the challenge
of being first on the scene.*

The author and publisher have made every attempt to ensure that the patient care procedures presented in this text are accurate and represent accepted practices in the United States. They are not provided as a standard of care. It is the First Responder's responsibility to follow patient care protocols established by a medical direction physician and to remain current in the delivery of emergency care.

Infection control practices may vary from agency to agency and may be updated periodically. It is the First Responder's responsibility to follow their local protocols regarding infection control and personal protective equipment.

The scene photographs in this text were taken during past emergency responses. They may depict some patient care activities that do not accurately represent the current practice in pre-hospital emergency care.

Primary Author and Editor
WALT ALAN STOY, PHD, EMT-P

Walt Stoy, Director of the Office of Education at the Center for Emergency Medicine, has more than 20 years experience in prehospital emergency medicine and is internationally known for his expertise in prehospital education. Dr. Stoy is also a Research Associate Professor of Emergency Medicine, Department of Emergency Medicine at the University of Pittsburgh School of Medicine. Dr. Stoy is currently the Project Director of the Paramedic and EMT-Intermediate: National Standard Curricula Revision Project. Dr. Stoy served as the Principal Investigator for the 1994 EMT-Basic: National Standard Curriculum and as Project Director of the 1995 First Responder: National Standard Curriculum.

As the Director of the Office of Education at the Center for Emergency Medicine, Dr. Stoy is responsible for all the education programs offered by the Center including education for EMTs, paramedics, and continuing education in cardiac and trauma life support for all levels of healthcare professionals and the lay public.

Dr. Stoy is also the author of many instructional video guides for American Safety Video Publishers. These videos are used in educating prehospital professionals across the country. In addition, Dr. Stoy has lectured extensively on prehospital patient care at professional meetings across the United States. He serves on committees of numerous organizations committed to excellence in the practice and education of prehospital emergency medicine. Dr. Stoy has conducted research and has been published in professional emergency medicine journals.

Author and Developmental Editor
DEBRA A. LEJEUNE, BS, NREMT-P

Debra Lejeune is the Coordinator of Publishing at the Center for Emergency Medicine and oversees all aspects of publishing including textbooks, videos, and other productions. Ms. Lejeune joined the Center for Emergency Medicine in 1991.

Ms. Lejeune received her Bachelor of Science degree from the University of Pittsburgh, and is currently pursuing her Master of Education degree from the University of Pittsburgh's School of Education. She is also a flight paramedic for the STAT MedEvac flight program.

Authors
GREGG S. MARGOLIS, MS, NREMT-P

Gregg Margolis is the Associate Director of Education at the Center for Emergency Medicine. He is responsible for the development, coordination, management, and supervision of all levels of emergency medical education. Mr. Margolis served as the Co-Principal Investigator for the revision of the First Responder: National Standard Curriculum, and as the Principal Investigator for the revision of the Paramedic and EMT-Intermediate: National Standard Curricula.

Mr. Margolis obtained his Bachelor of Science in Physiology and his Masters Degree in Healthcare Management and Supervision with an emphasis in Education from the University of Pittsburgh. He is currently pursuing his Doctorate in Education. Mr. Margolis is a flight paramedic with the STAT MedEvac flight program.

THOMAS E. PLATT, BA, NREMT-P

Thomas Platt is the Assistant Director of Education at the Center for Emergency Medicine. He is responsible for the development and implementation of basic life support training. In addition, Mr. Platt has worked on the 1994 EMT-Basic: National Standard Curriculum. Mr. Platt also served as Co-Principal Investigator for the revision of the First Responder: National Standard Curriculum.

Mr. Platt received his Bachelor of Arts degree in Public Administration at the University of Pittsburgh, and is currently pursuing his Master of Education degree from Pennsylvania State University. He is an active volunteer paramedic with a community ambulance service, and he works part time as a flight paramedic with the STAT MedEvac flight program.

AMY M. TREMEL, BS, NREMT-P

Amy Tremel is the Coordinator of EMS Education at the Center for Emergency Medicine, which she joined in 1989. Ms. Tremel oversees paramedic education at the Center.

Ms. Tremel obtained her Bachelor of Science degree in Biology in 1989 from the University of Pittsburgh and received her secondary teaching certificate in 1990. She is currently pursuing her Master of Science degree in Health Supervision and Management at the University of Pittsburgh. She currently is an active volunteer paramedic at a local EMS agency.

PAUL M. PARIS, MD, FACEP

Paul M. Paris, MD, is the Medical Director at the Center for Emergency Medicine and acted as advisor for this textbook.

The Center for Emergency Medicine is a multi-hospital consortium dedicated to the advancement of emergency medicine through research, education, air medical transport, and quality care.

Office of Education

The Center's Office of Education provides educational programs to thousands of students each year, including EMTs, paramedics, nurses, physicians, medical students, and the lay public. Courses include Cardiopulmonary Resuscitation (CPR); Advanced Cardiac Life Support (ACLS); First Responder; Basic Trauma Life Support (BTLS); Emergency Medical Technician—Basic, Emergency Medical Technician—Paramedic; EMS Computer Learning Center; First Aid; and Wilderness Emergency Medicine. Working with the U.S. Department of Transportation National Highway Traffic Safety Administration, the Office of Education staff revised the EMT-Basic: National Standard Curriculum in 1994, the First Responder curriculum in 1995, and is revising the Paramedic and Intermediate Curricula to be completed in 1997.

Office of Research

The Center is known internationally for its research in emergency medicine. The Center researchers have helped to shape current emergency medicine protocols through ground-breaking studies in many important areas, including resuscitation from cardiac arrest, airway control, automated external defibrillation, pediatric emergencies, and pain management. The Center and its research affiliates have been responsible for more published studies in emergency medicine than any other facility in the world.

STAT MedEvac

STAT MedEvac is the region's leader in air medical transport and is accredited by the Commission of Accreditation for Air Medical Services (CAAMS). The program provides medical transport of critically ill or injured patients regionally and nationally. The program transports nearly 4400 patients annually, making it one of the busiest air medical programs in the country. The fleet now includes seven helicopters, one dedicated medically-configured turbo prop airplane, and a Learjet. An instrument-rated Dauphin AS-365N helicopter and two instrument rated BK117 helicopters make flying in adverse weather conditions possible. STAT MedEvac is the only provider in the region for international medevac missions.

Residency Programs

The Center is also home to the University of Pittsburgh Affiliated Residency in Emergency Medicine. This is one of the leading emergency medicine residency programs in the nation. The residency is a joint effort between several of the Center for Emergency Medicine's member hospitals.

National Association of EMS Physicians (NAEMSP)

The National Association of EMS Physicians is based at the Center for Emergency Medicine. With a membership of more than 1500 EMS professionals, this organization fosters excellence and provides medical leadership with the goal that all individuals and communities receive high quality prehospital emergency medical care.

National Association of EMS Educators

The National Association of EMS Educators is based at the Center for Emergency Medicine. With 900 members, this organization is designed to enhance the educational effectiveness of EMS programs.

The 1990s have ushered in a period of change in EMS and health care the likes of which we have never witnessed before. For various reasons, the way we prepare for and deliver our services will never be the same. EMS education, as much as any other component of the EMS system, has witnessed many events that have significantly effected the way we deliver our educational services. Major milestones include: the 1990 National Highway Traffic Safety Administration (NHTSA) sponsorship of the National Workshop on EMS Training; the 1994 EMS Education and Practice Blueprint; also in 1994 the release of Revised EMT-Basic National Standard Curriculum; the 1995 founding of the National Association of EMS Educators; and the 1996 EMS Agenda for the Future. These and other events demonstrate both a need and a desire by many to improve the way we prepare for our profession and provide our services. Each of these activities represents quantum leaps, and all make the profound statement that we can do much better both in our educational process and in our outcomes.

This text, **Mosby's First Responder Textbook**, represents the fruits of those events. Of significance is that the authors, Dr. Walt Stoy and the Center for Emergency Medicine, were principles in each of those major milestones. Dr. Stoy was the Principal Investigator for the DOT EMT-Basic National Standard Curriculum that set new standards for curriculum development and design. This revision provided the template for all future National Standard Curricula including the First Responder: National Standard Curriculum, and later the EMT-Intermediate and Paramedic: National Standard Curriculum. These National Standard Curricula include sound educational principles and establish a format for teaching that we have never seen before.

We have now learned that it takes more than a list of knowledge and skills to teach and to learn. There is a process and there are principles that are critical to learning. A curriculum includes material both for the educator and the student. This student text is the first for First Responders that embraces sound educational principles and follows the format developed for all DOT National Standard Curricula. After all, it was written by the very educators that developed the standard.

You will find that this text is organized in a logical format for you, the student. It makes learning fun. We have chosen emergency services for our careers because we believe it to be interesting and rewarding, even in light of the fact that it can also be stressful. This text helps you realize the fun and rewarding aspects, prepare for difficult aspects, and sort through and deal with the stressors. It is the complete text. You will notice liberal use of key terms, scenarios, alerts, and review questions, and the reoccurring call to measure your new knowledge against the cognitive, affective and psychomotor objectives established by the DOT National Standard Curriculum.

As First Responders, you will often be the first EMS professional that your patients contact. Your actions will have a profound effect on the outcome of that patient, whatever the level of sophisticated care to follow. This text will help establish a sound foundation that will serve you for the rest of your career, whether you use this as a your first step to more advanced levels of care or as a First Responder providing critical services to patients entering the EMS system.

John L. Chew, Jr.
President
The EMSSTAR Group LLC

Welcome to the beginning of your study to become a First Responder!

This textbook is an instrument for your use along with the classroom study of the 1995 First Responder: National Standard Curriculum.

The goal of the authors and reviewers involved in this project is to provide you with a basic textbook for easy and quick reference to the information necessary to succeed in your First Responder program. As EMS educators, we wanted to provide a text to meet the needs of both instructors and students with different learning styles. Using many illustrations, we wanted to provide a visually appealing book complete with easy-to-read text and graphically displayed information. We also planned this textbook to offer flexibility for students and instructors as EMS education and the EMS community continue to evolve.

The Approach

This text focuses, quite simply, on what First Responders *need to know*. One of the problems in providing too much information is that students are forced to determine what content is really important—where to focus attention. Therefore, the topics covered in this text are more concise and focused than that of similar texts. Nonetheless, all of the information in the National Curriculum and all that First Responders must know in order to provide quality emergency medical care is covered with as much background information and explanation as necessary for students to learn and become excellent prehospital providers. Information that some First Responders may need to know is covered in the Appendices. This material is not part of the First Responder National Standard Curriculum.

The Author–Reviewer Team

This textbook is the result of many individuals contributing their time and energy to see it through to successful completion. In addition to the principal writers, countless reviewers, outside consultants, and treatment specialists contributed to this project in numerous ways to ensure not only its technical accuracy and completeness, but also its effectiveness as a teaching and learning tool.

The National Standard Curriculum

In 1995, the United States Department of Transportation National Highway Traffic Safety Administration released the First Responder: National Standard Curriculum. Walt A. Stoy, PhD, of the Center of Emergency Medicine, was the Project Director for this new curriculum. Gregg S. Margolis, MS, NREMT-P and Tom Platt, BA, NREMT-P were the principal investigators for this project.

The goal of this textbook is to teach First Responders to assess and care for ill and injured patients with minimal equipment. Appendices have been included at the end of some chapters to teach students who have access to some emergency medical equipment how to properly use this equipment for patient care.

Organization of Content

This textbook, like the National Curriculum, is divided into seven divisions. Division One, Preparatory, is designed to help students understand emergency medical services and how the First Responder fits into this system. It also includes material on the well-being of the First Responder; legal and ethical issues; the human body; and lifting and moving patients. Division Two focuses on the airway and basic airway skills. Appendices A and B cover information on oxygen delivery and other ventilation devices. Division Three describes the patient assessment process, including the scene size-up, initial assessment, First Responder physical exam, and the ongoing assessment. Appendix C includes information on assessing vital signs. Chapter Four covers circulation and the steps of cardiopulmonary resuscitation for adults, infants, and children. Appendix D contains the information First Responders will need to know to use an AED. Division Five includes information on dealing with ill or injured patients. Appendix E has the information needed to apply simple splints. Division Six covers information about childbirth and caring for infants and children. Division Seven focuses on EMS operations.

Chapter Outline

Each chapter begins with an outline of the material included within. This affords the student an opportunity to see how the information fits together at a glance. This outline is also useful for reviewing material later.

First Response Scenario

Each chapter opens with a short story of First Responder patient care in a realistic prehospital situation. The patient's problem described in the scenarios relates to the chapter topic. These scenarios help you focus on the material covered in the chapter and on the real-life context in which you will use your First Responder skills.

Introductory Paragraph
A brief chapter introduction sets the stage for the chapter's topics and provides backround information as the context for the overall meaning of the chapter.

Text
The text of each chapter is broken into small sections of information to allow you to proceed through your reading and learning in a flexible but organized manner.

Information Boxes and Tables
Information boxes and tables are placed throughout the text to highlight special information, making it easier to learn and review. These special displays include "First Responder Alerts" that call attention to critical information or safety warnings. Technique boxes outline step-by-step skills and performance. Principle boxes highlight essential information and procedures.

Review Questions
At the end of each major section of the chapter are review questions to test your comprehension of the material thus far. If you have difficulty answering any of these questions, go back and review the material before proceeding to the next section.

Illustrations
The textbook is heavily illustrated with full-color photographs and drawings. The important aspects of all essential skills are illustrated to help you see the correct steps laid out before you begin practicing them.

Chapter Summary
At the end of each chapter is a summary organized around the key topics in the chapter. This allows the student to integrate all of the key information in the chapter, as well as to return to the chapter later for a quick content review.

United States Department of Transportation National Highway Traffic Safety Administration First Responder Objectives
The objectives found at the end of each chapter parallel those of the National Standard Curriculum. Cognitive objectives include what you should know after reading and studying the chapter; affective objectives focus on attitude: what you should understand and feel about patients and family members in relation to the chapter content; and psychomotor objectives list what you should be able to do after studying the chapter and practicing the skills in your course.

At the end of each appendix the DOT Objectives for EMT-Basic level are listed. Appendices cover advanced First Responder skills and the Objectives are provided as a guide for learning these skills.

Glossary
At the end of the text is a glossary that defines the medical and First Responder terms used throught the book. It includes all the key terms as well so that you do not need to hunt through individual chapters for definitions.

AUTHOR ACKNOWLEDGMENTS

The authors would like to thank the following individuals and organizations for their contributions to this book:

David Culverwell, David Dusthimer, Claire Merrick, Rina Steinhauer, and Melissa Blair of Mosby Lifeline for their desire to see this project through to completion. We appreciate their continued faith in us.

Vincent Knaus and William Hrovoski for their excellent photography.

Kimberly Battista, Stacy Lund, and Duckwall Productions for their beautiful illustrations.

The University of Pittsburgh Medical Center, Pittsburgh EMS, Peters Township Ambulance Service; Peters Township Fire Department, and STAT MedEvac for their contributions to the artwork and development of the rescue photographs.

Parr Emergency Product sales and Laerdal for their generous contribution of medical equipment and supplies for the illustrations.

The staff and students of the Center for Emergency Medicine for being available at a moment's notice to offer advice, opinions, and participate in a number of ways too numerous to mention.

All of our families and loved ones for their support and encouragement.

Special thanks to Neal Hannan, EMT-P for his help in completing this textbook.

The publisher and the editors wish to thank the reviewers of this book who dedicated countless hours to intensive review. Their feedback and comments were invaluable in developing and fine-tuning this text.

Edgar Batsford
Training Coordinator
Rhode Island Department of Health
Division of Emergency Medical Services
Providence, Rhode Island

Dave Busse
Program Director
Basic Programs
Paramedic Academy
Justice Institute of British Columbia
New Westminister, British Columbia

Stephen Stuart Carter
Manager
Special Programs Section
Maryland Fire and Rescue Institute
University of Maryland at College Park
College Park, Maryland

John L. Chew, Jr.
President
The EMSSTAR Group LLC
Annapolis, Maryland

Tom Ferrell, MS, EMT-P
EMS Instructor/Coordinator
Sandhills Community College
Pinehurst, North Carolina

Joseph A. Grafft, MS
EMS Manager
Metropolitan State University
FIRE/EMS Center
St. Paul, Minnesota

Edward J. Kalinowski, BSN, MEd
Associate Professor
Chairman, Department of Emergency Medical Services
Kapiolani Community College
Honolulu, Hawaii

Sergeant E. C. Maness
EMS Coordinator
North Carolina Highway Patrol
Raleigh, North Carolina

Dan Manz
Vermont EMS
Burlington, Vermont

Bruce J. Walz, PhD, NREMT-P
Associate Professor and Chair
Department of Emergency Health Services
University of Maryland Baltimore County
Baltimore, Maryland

We also gratefully acknowledge the important contributions of those who posed as models in this text:

Eugene Adams, Sty Adelsperger, Hector Alonso-Serra, Wade Amick, Brandy Banks, Edward Batles, Andrew Bell, Eleanor May Berwick, Brenda Biringer, Barbara Blachley, Melissa Blair, Richard Boland, Jim Bothwell, Nicole Bryner, Dr. John Burton, Brian Check, Cynthia Lisa Cole, Nathan Cosgrove, Pamela Cosgrove, Raymond Cosgrove, Wayne Cosgrove, James Crecraft, David Czurko, Terry Dawson, Ramon DeCampo, John Dougherty, Lillian Douglass, William Duerr, Scott Eckles, Lisa Esposito, Raymond Everitt, Nicole Federico, Jonathan Fischer, Susan Follet, Maureen Foster, Matthew Fox, Susan Frankenberry, Shiloh Fry, John Gobbles, Donald Goodman, Dorothy Gregor, Tim Hagerty, Heather Hales, Attila Hertelendy, Dennis Hohl, T. Chris Hoy, William Hrovoski, Rob Hruska, Rebecca Humes, Steve Jensen, Theresa Jones, Barry Judy, Kenneth Jurick, Linda Jurick, Chad Kauffman, David Keller, Jacob Keller, Kevin Kelly, Vincent Knaus, Jeff Kramer, Timothy Krug, Michelle Kubala, Terry Lane, Julia LaSalle, Debra Lejeune, Jeffery Lejeune, Kate Levdansky, Deidre Levdansky-Kuban, Jriullus Lewis, Scott Lewis, John Linden, Jacqueline Jones Lynch, Monica Lyon, Norman Lyons, John Mann, Edward Margolis, Carolyn Margolis, Mary Kay Margolis, Gregg Margolis, Scott Marshall, Dave Maughn, Richard McClelland, Pamela McCready, Linda McDaid, Red Mac McKelvey, Noel McMullen,

Sandra McMurray, Cindy McQuillis, Daniel Mitchell, Dr. Harold Moss, Michael Nagt, David Naples, Clifton Neff, Philip Neff, Ronald Nelson, Elizabeth Newton, H. Brian Nickerson, Alana Osman, Frances Pasternack, Amanda Lee Platt, Christine Marie Platt, Donna Platt, Tom Platt, Robin Pointdexter, Marie Pomorski, Alison Poole, Michelle Proctor, Janan Raouf, Tracy Reed, Jeff Reim, Victoria Reiniger, Eric Rhodes, Myron Rickens, Trevor Robinson, Kenyatta Rogers, Tammy Romero, Steve Rudic, Jeffrey Ruffing, Tahnee Rygielski, Ritu Sahni, Terresa Salatino, Elizabeth Salvador, Aaron Smith, Renee Schneider, Valerie Schreiber, Scott Seger, Bob Simak, William Snodgrass, Jr., Jason Spade, Charlie Stengel, Christopher N. Stevens, Dr. J.E. Stevens, Jacob Stoy, Joseph Stoy, Rebecca Stoy, Walt Stoy, Nancy Succop, Amy Lee Taylor, Amy Tremel, Hannah Tremel, Jeff Tremel, Ronald Vezzani, Drummond Vogan, Diana Ward, Bob Weekman, Wayne Westfall, Sheldon Williams, Sheldon Williams, Jr., Shelona Williams, Sheltaya Williams, Matthew Wlodarczyk.

CONTENTS

EMCoach

CEMA course

EMAC

1°

HAZMAT ← Awen

Negligence

Preparatory

IN THIS DIVISION

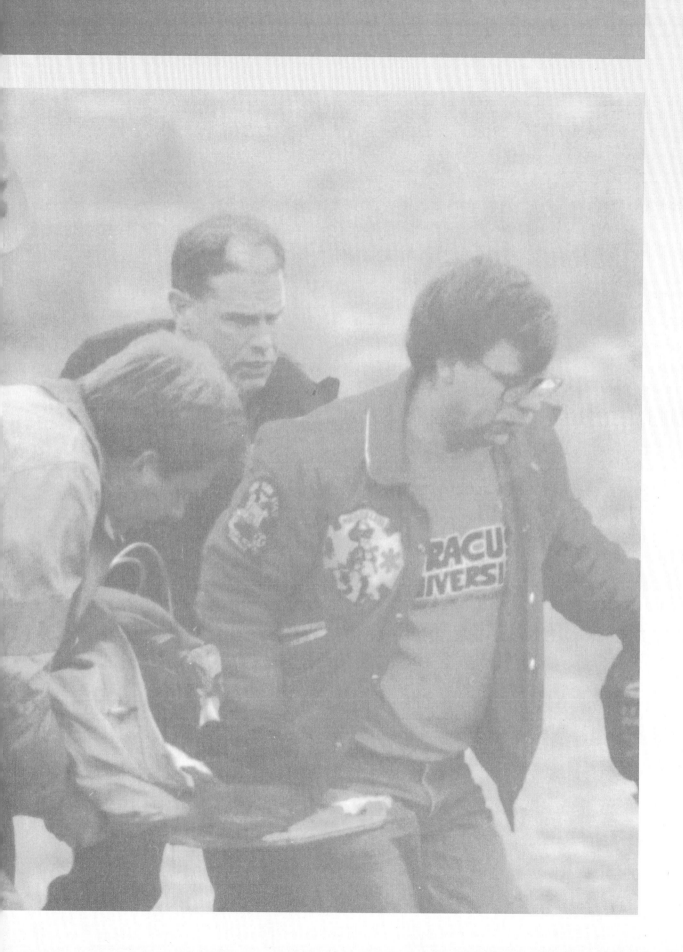

Introduction to EMS Systems

I. The Emergency Medical Services System
  A. The National Highway Traffic Safety Administration Technical Assistance Program
  B. Access to the Emergency Medical Services System
  C. Levels of Education
  D. The Healthcare System
II. Roles and Responsibilities of the First Responder

A. Personal Safety
B. Safety of the Crew, Patient, and Bystanders
C. Patient Assessment and Care
D. Transport and Transfer of Care
E. Professional Attributes
III. Medical Direction
  A. Direct Medical Direction
  B. Indirect Medical Direction

KEY TERMS

Direct medical direction   Medical direction in which the physician speaks directly with the provider in the field; also referred to as on-line medical direction.

Emergency medical dispatcher   An EMS dispatcher who has received special training in providing pre-arrival instructions to patients or others over the phone before the EMS response arrives.

Emergency Medical Services (EMS) system   A system of many agencies, personnel and institutions involved in planning, providing, and monitoring emergency care.

EMT-Basic   A prehospital care provider trained to provide basic level care for ill and injured patients.

EMT-Intermediate   An emergency care provider with education above the level of EMT-Basic in one or more advanced techniques, such as vascular access or advanced airway management.

EMT-Paramedic   An emergency provider with education above the level of EMT-Basic to the level of full advanced life support.

First Responder   An EMS provider who utilizes a minimum amount of equipment to perform initial assessment and intervention, and who is trained to assist other EMS providers.

Indirect medical direction   Any direction provided by physicians that does not involve speaking with providers in the field, including but not limited to, system design, protocol development, education, and quality improvement; also referred to as off-line medical direction.

Medical direction   The process (usually by a physician) of ensuring that the care given to patients by prehospital providers is medically appropriate; also called medical oversight or medical control.

National EMS Education and Practice Blueprint   A consensus document that establishes a core content for the scope of practice for the four levels of prehospital care providers.

Quality improvement   A system for continually evaluating and making necessary adjustments to the care provided within an EMS system.

FIRST RESPONSE

It was the fifth week of police recruit training and Carlos was very concerned about the upcoming First Responder course. He knew that police officers were supposed to help people, but he did not choose to become a police officer to be a doctor. During a break he decided to discuss this with a veteran officer, Wess. Wess told him that being a First Responder was nothing like being a doctor. He explained the Emergency Medical Services (EMS) system to Carlos, and told him how important and what an integral part of that system First Responders were. Wess explained to Carlos that, as a police officer, this information would be extremely valuable. It was highly likely that Carlos would respond to many medical emergencies and motor vehicle crashes during his career. The people that he would provide care to could be the citizens of his community, his fellow officers, and possibly his family.

Wess further explained that police officers weren't the only ones serving in this vital capacity. He told Carlos about the firefighters who became First Responders as part of their training. He also talked about some industrial response teams in which businesses and industry use First Responders to provide emergency care in their facilities before EMS arrival. He also provided some examples of other people who serve as First Responders, such as public works employees, school teachers, athletic trainers, life guards, and many other professional people, who become First Responders as part of their jobs.

Wess recalled the time that he responded to a motor vehicle crash and found an unresponsive patient. He opened the man's airway, monitored his breathing, and stopped some bleeding. The EMS crew told Wess that his actions probably saved this man's life. Wess told Carlos that his initial training as a First Responder and the Continuing Education programs he completed on the force made him feel much more comfortable in performing his job as a police officer. Carlos left the discussion with a new outlook on being a First Responder and a police officer.

First Responders are an integral component of the Emergency Medical Services System. This chapter marks the beginning of your educational process for becoming a First Responder. First Responders who initiate care until the ambulance arrives require a solid foundation of basic emergency procedures. This course will provide a road map for learning. This chapter outlines the job roles and responsibilities you will need to understand to help you to become a First Responder.

This chapter also describes the **Emergency Medical Services (EMS) system** and the role of First Responders within this system. The EMS system is the system of professionals who provide emergency medical care, beginning when someone initially realizes an injured or ill person requires emergency care, and continues through to the patient's admission to the hospital (Fig. 1-1).

THE EMERGENCY MEDICAL SERVICES SYSTEM

You are about to embark on a great journey that will affect not only your life, but also the lives of many others. You will learn to help patients who are strangers, partners, co-workers, neighbors, friends, and even loved ones. Clearly, being a First Responder is an important job.

Working or volunteering as a First Responder can be both a demanding and rewarding component of your life. Few other professions have such an impact on people's lives on a daily basis.

Everyone becomes involved in the EMS system for a different reason. Some students experience the loss of a friend or family member following a medical emergency and want to prevent others from experiencing the same loss. Others watch television dramas showing emergency

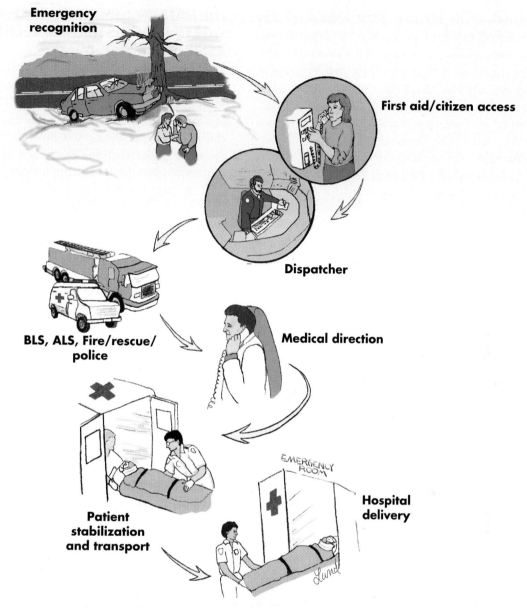

Fig. 1-1 The EMS system encompasses emergency recognition, system access, EMS personnel dispatch and response, care provided to the patient at the scene, medical direction when necessary, and patient stabilization, transportation, and delivery to the hospital.

medical care as an exciting, challenging, and fulfilling profession, and want to become involved. Still others are taking this course to fulfill a job requirement. Some people may be taking this course to springboard into another health care position. Regardless of your reason, welcome to the ranks of one of the most rewarding professions in the world.

Every day, people's lives are touched by EMS. From an elderly patient who must reach the doctor's office for an appointment, to a child with a life-threatening airway emergency, all of the patients you will encounter have one thing in common—they need help. They require the assistance of a competent, qualified, caring individual. The Emergency Medical Services system is a network of resources to provide emergency care and transport to victims of sudden illness and injury.

The EMS system also has a role in injury and illness prevention. Just as firefighters and police officers spend much of their time on prevention, EMS workers are beginning to make efforts directed at reducing preventable injury and illness. First Responders can impact lives by teaching people how to lead a healthy lifestyle and prevent injury where possible.

Another component of the EMS system is responding to emergencies. Once an event occurs that requires the services of EMS personnel, the event must be detected by informed bystanders who will activate the EMS system. Training the public to recognize emergencies and the proper way to access emergency services is one of the roles of the First Responder. Bystanders may be given care instructions over the telephone about how to help the patient until the First Responders arrive.

First Responders may be part of a designated EMS response or they may work as police officers, firefighters or rescue teams, or members of a business or industry response team. First Responders are often sent to the scene of an emergency to initiate emergency medical care until the transporting unit and additional EMS help arrives. In this role, the First Responders have an important job: the initial assessment and treatment of the ill and injured.

Once additional help arrives, the First Responders continue to provide care by helping the EMS personnel as they arrive at the scene. In some cases, this may require First Responders to help other EMS professionals transport the patient to the hospital, where care for the patient will be transferred to the in-hospital system.

The following sections will help you better understand the role of the EMS system, beginning with the national agency that sets standards for the education of First Responders.

THE NATIONAL HIGHWAY TRAFFIC SAFETY ADMINISTRATION TECHNICAL ASSISTANCE PROGRAM

The goal of the Department of Transportation (DOT) and the National Highway Traffic Safety Administration (NHTSA) is to reduce the number of deaths and disabilities caused by motor vehicle collisions on the nation's highways. NHTSA has therefore undertaken the role of the development of national standard curricula for EMS providers. NHTSA has also developed Technical Assistance Programs for individual states to ensure the effectiveness of EMS systems everywhere.

NHTSA has developed standards in ten areas to guarantee high quality EMS systems (Fig. 1-2):

- Regulation and policy
- Resource management
- Human resources and training
- Transportation
- Facilities
- Communications
- Public information and education
- Medical direction
- Trauma systems
- Evaluation

These aspects of the system are described below to help you better understand the overall system in which you will be working as a First Responder.

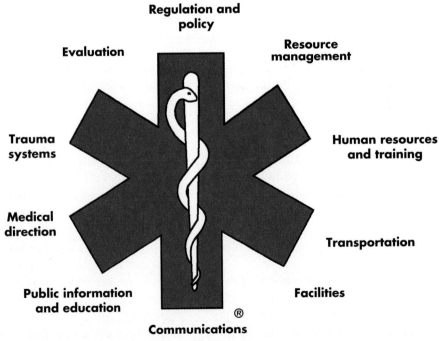

Fig. 1-2 The National Highway Traffic Safety Administration's 10 standards for EMS systems.

The **Regulation and Policy** standard ensures that all states have a lead EMS agency, funding, regulations, and operational policies and procedures. State legislatures must pass laws that promote quality EMS care and provide adequate funding. States finance their EMS systems in various ways, but all should have funds to provide high-quality, effective EMS care. As you train for your profession and begin working as a First Responder, you will become familiar with state and local rules and regulations, policies, and procedures.

The **Resource Management** standard coordinates resources throughout the state. This standard allows everyone access to basic emergency medical care, including treatment by personnel trained primarily at the First Responder level, and allows all patients to be transported in a well-equipped vehicle to a staffed, equipped, and prepared facility.

The **Human Resources and Training** standard requires all states to have good educational programs for First Responders and all EMS personnel, and identifies the minimum training for personnel who will be staffing transport vehicles.

The **Transportation** standard promotes safe and effective transportation for all patients. Ambulances and air medical units must meet minimum criteria and be inspected periodically. All aspects of the state EMS system must be in a constant mode of readiness.

The **Facilities** standard requires that providers transporting patients to a hospital are informed about the capabilities of each hospital in the area, including specialty facilities, such as trauma and burn centers, and children's hospitals. Prehospital care providers must understand the capabilities of different facilities and know which facility is the most appropriate for specific emergency situations.

The **Communications** standard ensures patients can call for emergency care and provides guidelines for emergency personnel to communicate effectively with the receiving hospital and other EMS personnel.

The **Public Information and Education** guideline promotes the public's involvement in the EMS system and injury prevention programs. First Responders often provide the public with information about system procedures and injury prevention. This education improves the system and helps patients receive quality care.

The **Medical Direction** standard involves physicians in the patient care system by developing protocols or patient care guidelines, by providing medical direction and consultation, and by evaluating patient care activities and quality improvement.

Trauma is a severe wound or injury. The **Trauma Systems** standard provides for the development of a statewide trauma plan. A trauma patient requires specialized medical trauma care, provided through the state's trauma system. Across the United States, there are many statewide trauma care systems, including designated trauma centers, trauma triage guidelines, data collection, trauma registry definitions, system management, and quality improvement.

The final standard involves **Evaluation** of the effectiveness of patient care, including the care provided by First Responders. In this way, the EMS system can continue to improve the quality of patient care delivered.

ACCESS TO THE EMERGENCY MEDICAL SERVICES SYSTEM

The manner in which the public contacts the EMS system is extremely important. In many areas of the United States, 9-1-1 is the universal access number to police, fire, and EMS (Fig. 1-3). There are also enhanced 9-1-1 systems that allow the person receiving the emergency call to know the location of the caller based on computer and phone records. However, some areas of the country do not have this capability and a seven-digit number is used to access the EMS system.

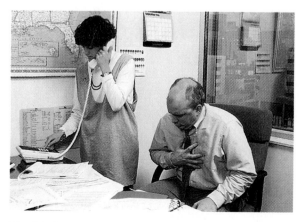

Fig. 1-3 In many areas of the United States, "9-1-1" is the universal number for access to police, fire, and EMS.

Regardless of the phone number used, First Responders should educate the public on proper access to the system. Public information campaigns, such as "Make the Right Call," teach the public the proper local access number and when to call for an ambulance. First Responders and other emergency providers at all levels should be active in these public service campaigns.

LEVELS OF EDUCATION

The **National EMS Education and Practice Blueprint** sets the standards for the education of prehospital emergency care providers. There are four established levels of prehospital care providers: the First Responder, EMT-Basic, EMT-Intermediate, and EMT-Paramedic.

The EMS system currently lists these four levels for certification or licensure, although not all states use every level. States can also augment the levels with additional care levels. Each recognized level has its own scope of practice.

The **First Responder** course is for those persons who, similar to law enforcement personnel or firefighters, are likely to encounter an ill or injured person but are not trained for ambulance service. The focus of this level is to provide initial stabilization until additional EMS resources arrive.

The **EMT-Basic** course prepares personnel to provide primary medical care before the patient reaches the hospital. Most states require the EMT-Basic course as the minimum accepted education level for ambulance staff. The **EMT-Intermediate** level is an advanced life support level that includes skills such as manual defibrillation and administration of intravenous fluids and some medications. The **EMT-Paramedic**, currently the highest skill level, includes more advanced techniques such as advanced airway management and administration of additional medications. The National Registry of EMTs prepares and conducts examinations designed to test the competency at all levels (Fig. 1-4). State regulations and local medical directors determine the specific procedures at all levels.

THE HEALTHCARE SYSTEM

The EMS system is an integral component of the overall healthcare system in the United States. This healthcare system has many components. Most important to First Responders are the prehospital setting and the hospital setting, although many other aspects are involved.

First Responders, EMT-Basics, EMT-Intermediates, and EMT-Paramedics are the primary emergency medical care providers outside of the hospital. The sequence of an EMS event begins when someone notices the patient's illness or injury and calls the EMS system through the local number. First Responders such as firefighters or lifeguards may already be at the scene and provide initial care until more advanced EMS personnel arrive. Also involved are professional dispatchers who not only forward the emergency call to the EMS unit, but may also give pre-arrival instructions to the EMS unit. In many systems, **emergency medical dispatchers** have received education for dispensing simple medical care instructions over the phone before the First Responders arrive.

The next step in the healthcare system is the hospital. This typically begins with the arrival to the emergency department, although some states permit EMS providers to transport a patient directly to a physician's office or clinic. Healthcare workers in the hospital include physicians, nurse practitioners, physician assistants, nurses, and nursing assistants. Other services are also provided, such as lab work, electrocardiograms, X-rays, and other services including clerical, communications, and housekeeping support.

Some patients may need the attention of a specialty care center. These patients may require transport to centers such as trauma facilities, burn centers, or children's hospitals. These specialty centers vary in different regions. Knowledge of the specialty centers in your area is important, including knowledge of the local

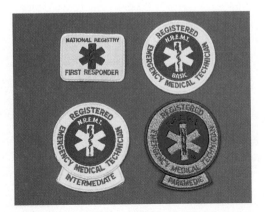

Fig. 1-4 National Registry of EMTs patches for the four EMS levels.

guidelines for transporting patients to one of these facilities. Your service area may have additional specialty centers, such as poison centers, to provide EMS personnel with information about special situations.

Your instructor or your local ambulance service can provide you with an overview of the EMS system in your community.

ROLES AND RESPONSIBILITIES OF THE FIRST RESPONDER

The roles and responsibilities of First Responders are continually evolving. Job descriptions established by each service define specific requirements. First Responders must understand these roles and responsibilities to be competent, professional members of the healthcare team (Box 1-1).

PERSONAL SAFETY

As a First Responder, you have a responsibility for your own safety. This role is discussed in depth in Chapter 2, "Well-Being of the First Responder." Ensuring personal safety includes maintaining a healthy body, remaining physically fit, and using body substance isolation precautions appropriately. Personal safety also includes surveying the emergency scene for hazards or potential hazards before entering. Chapter 7, "Patient Assessment," describes the appropriate measures to be taken in this important procedure.

SAFETY OF THE CREW, PATIENT, AND BYSTANDERS

First Responders are also responsible for the safety of fellow crew members, patients, and bystanders. Looking out for the well-being of your partners is extremely important. As you will learn in the next chapters, this also includes maintaining scene safety and coping with stress. You are responsible for providing the best possible care for patients, while carrying out safety precautions that will prevent further injury to patients from hazards at the scene. The safety of bystanders must also be considered. By securing a safe scene and communicating effectively with bystanders, you protect everyone's safety.

PATIENT ASSESSMENT AND CARE

Patient assessment is a primary responsibility (Fig. 1-5). In some cases, you may have to gain access to the patient before you can begin care. Special tools and equipment may be necessary to gain access, and additional education is required for these situations.

BOX 1-1 **Roles and Responsibilities of the First Responder**
• Personal safety
• Safety of the crew, patient, and bystanders
• Patient assessment and care
• Transport and transfer of care

REVIEW QUESTIONS

The Emergency Medical Services System

1. How many levels of prehospital care providers are established by the National EMS Education and Practice Blueprint?
   A. 3
   B. 4
   C. 5
   D. Not defined

2. Mark an "A" for advanced life support provider and a "B" for a basic life support provider for each of the following certification levels.
   ___ First Responder
   ___ EMT-Intermediate
   ___ EMT-Paramedic
   ___ EMT-Basic

3. The guidelines for the EMS curriculum are established by which agency?
   A. The National Registry of EMTs
   B. The National Association of EMTs
   C. The Department of Transportation/National Highway Traffic Safety Administration
   D. The National Association of EMS Physicians

4. In many communities, 9-1-1 is the phone number used to contact EMS, police, and firefighters. This number is considered:
   A. Community access
   B. National access
   C. Worldwide access
   D. Universal access

1. B; 2. First Responder: B, EMT-Intermediate: A, EMT-Paramedic: A, EMT-Basic: B; 3. C; 4. D

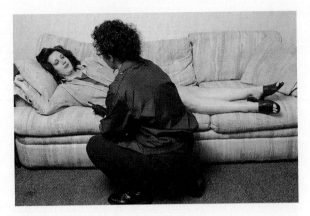

Fig. 1-5 First Responders assess patients to determine needs and provide appropriate care.

First Responders assess the patient's needs and provide basic medical care established by the assessment. Chapter 7 describes how to assess a patient. As a First Responder, you should practice and master these skills. The emergency care you provide is based on assessment findings. This approach allows for rapid management of life-threatening injuries and illnesses and helps to relieve the patient's discomfort quickly.

TRANSPORT AND TRANSFER OF CARE

First Responders are responsible for ensuring that EMS personnel with more training and the ability to transport the patient to the hospital are dispatched, and that care is continued for these patients. As additional EMS providers arrive, First Responders will assist them in their continued care.

When the patient has been evaluated and treated, EMS responders and First Responders prepare the patient for transport; therefore you must be able to assist in lifting and moving patients safely. You must be sure the environment is safe for lifting, for example, by moving debris off of a sidewalk before moving a patient over it. You also must use safe lifting and moving techniques as described in Chapter 5, "Lifting and Moving Patients."

First Responders may have to complete a prehospital care report that includes information about the scene, the patient's illness or injury, and care provided. This report will become part of the patient's record, and may be used in data collection for studies about EMS systems.

PROFESSIONAL ATTRIBUTES

In addition to these roles and responsibilities, First Responders must behave professionally. Professional attributes include physical appearance, a positive attitude, up-to-date knowledge and skills, making the patient's needs a top priority without endangering yourself or others, and expanding current knowledge of local, state, and national issues affecting EMS and healthcare.

First Responders are healthcare professionals and are an important component of the healthcare team. Therefore, you should strive to project a professional appearance. Overall grooming, hair, and clothing should be neat and clean at all times. Shoes or boots should be clean and polished. Many services have a uniform dress policy. Some services may have duty uniforms and dress uniforms to be worn at the appropriate times.

The patient's and family's first impression of healthcare personnel can come from their initial contact with you. An unkempt First Responder may imply sloppy patient care. Dressing in a crisp, clean uniform may reduce the patient's and family's anxiety. Maintaining calm and composure in emergency situations, and a caring, confident manner toward the patient and family while waiting for additional EMS personnel to arrive will also help relieve anxiety.

An additional role of the First Responder is liaison with other public safety workers. Some public safety agencies will require their employees to be First Responders. In other cases, the First Responder will interact with various providers of public safety, such as local, state, and federal law enforcement personnel, fire departments, and EMS providers. It is important that the First Responder develop a professional working relationship with the other public safety workers. This relationship will benefit the ultimate consumer of the First Responder's services—the ill or injured patient.

As you enter this facet of the world of healthcare, you are choosing a profession that demands lifelong continuing education and skills review. Medical care will continue to evolve, and technology will provide EMS with new options for patient care. Federal, state, and regional laws and regulations will also change the way in which care is provided. First Responders have an obligation to be knowledgeable and to provide technically proficient care.

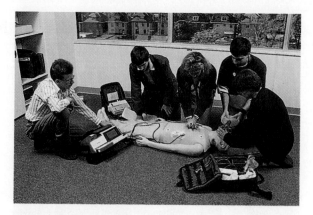

Fig. 1-6 Continuing education provides opportunities for First Responders to practice skills that are not often used.

As a First Responder you must keep abreast of changes and advances in medical care. You may elect to take a refresher course to update your skills and knowledge periodically.

Continuing education is an important aspect of your career. First Responders should attend continuing education courses whenever possible and should practice skills that are not often used (Fig. 1-6). Continuing education should not be postponed until you conclude your initial education program. You should begin to attend these programs immediately. Ask your instructor which programs can be taken before completing your initial education, and which can be taken afterward. Consider attending courses providing vehicle operation and rescue education programs. Many states require continuing education as a part of the recertification process or license renewal.

There are many journals that can help keep First Responders informed about trends in prehospital care. Several journals offer excellent information, such as *Journal of EMS (JEMS)*; *Emergency, Rescue, Prehospital and Disaster Medicine*; and *Emergency Medical Services*. Other journals targeted to specific professions that utilize First Responders also provide excellent information regarding trends in emergency medical services. Check with your instructor or service to see which journal is best suited to your needs.

Another way to stay informed regarding EMS issues is to join a professional organization. Several are of benefit to First Responders, including the National Association of EMTs (NAEMT) and the National Association of EMS Physicians (NAEMSP). Professional organizations keep their

members abreast of changes in EMS through newsletters, journals, and conferences. In addition to these national organizations, many states and local areas have professional associations for EMS providers. This is an ideal opportunity to learn more about issues that affect EMS and to participate in decisions affecting First Responders.

As described earlier, First Responders should be patient advocates. With the exception of their own safety and that of the crew, First Responders must put the needs of the patient first. Serving as a patient advocate requires good judgment, which will develop further with clinical experience.

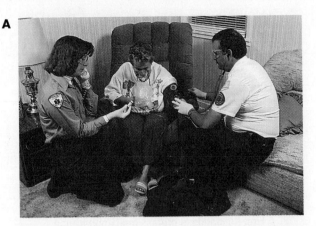
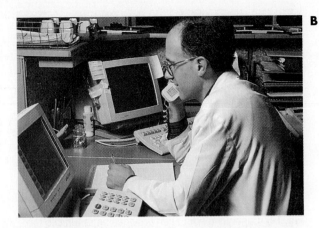

Fig. 1-7 Direct medical direction allows **A,** EMS providers to consult directly with **B,** emergency medical staff at the receiving hospital by radio or telephone to determine proper care for the patient.

MEDICAL DIRECTION

Medical direction is the process through which physicians monitor the care given to ill or injured patients by First Responders. In the past, some states required medical direction only at an advanced level and not for First Responders or EMT-Basics. The nationwide curriculum change for EMT-Basics in 1994 called for a physician medical director to authorize certain skills performed by EMT-Basics. The 1995 First Responder curriculum also includes medical direction for First Responders. Your local EMS service will be able to give you information about medical direction and First Responders. Every EMS system must have medical direction. The physician in charge of medical direction is often called the system medical director.

Care provided can be monitored through the two components of medical direction: direct medical direction and indirect medical direction.

DIRECT MEDICAL DIRECTION

Direct medical direction, also referred to as on-line medical direction, means direct communication between the physician and the provider in the field (Fig. 1-7, A and B). This communication may occur via a cellular telephone, radio, or telephone (land-line). In some cases, the physician may be present at the scene, allowing prehospital providers to speak directly with the physician. The role of a physician at the emergency scene may vary. Local protocol dictates the proper procedure for following the orders and advice of a physician at the emergency scene.

INDIRECT MEDICAL DIRECTION

Indirect medical direction, or off-line medical direction, consists of other ways physicians influence care. There are prospective aspects of indirect medical direction, including designing the EMS system, developing protocols and standing orders, and providing initial and continuing education, as well as retrospective aspects, including reviewing prehospital care reports and data collection. Medical directors should also participate in quality improvement, a system for evaluating and improving care provided within an EMS system. Indirect medical direction encompasses all components of physician involvement beyond direct medical direction (Fig. 1-8).

The relationship of First Responders and the medical director depends on the specific system. In many instances, the First Responder is a designated agent of the medical director. Often the care rendered by the First Responder is considered an extension of the medical director's authority. Check with your instructor regarding specific laws and regulations in your area.

Rural and frontier providers tend to use the indirect approach because of distance factors. Urban and suburban providers often interact with medical directors more frequently. Ideally, the relationship begins when the medical director becomes involved in the education of First Responders. This relationship continues as students complete courses and begin to provide patient care. The medical director participates in quality improvement of the service and aids in the development of protocols.

First Responders have a responsibility to interact with the medical director in a professional manner and to abide by the decisions of the medical director. The medical director is a resource for problem solving before, during, and after patient interactions. Try to become acquainted with the medical direction used in your EMS system. A strong working relationship with the medical director will enhance the quality and appropriateness of the medical care you provide.

CHAPTER SUMMARY

THE EMERGENCY MEDICAL SERVICES SYSTEM

The EMS system is one of many agencies and institutions involved in planning, providing, and monitoring emergency medical care. The National Highway Traffic Safety Administration helps states to develop EMS systems through established technical standards and assessments of EMS delivery in each state. These standards include: regulation and policy; resource management; human resources and training; transportation; facilities; communications; public information and education; medical direction; trauma systems; and evaluation. Each area addresses specific concerns for the delivery of quality EMS.

The four recognized levels of prehospital care providers as defined by the National EMS Education and Practice Blueprint are: First Responder, EMT-Basic, EMT-Intermediate, and EMT-Paramedic. All EMS personnel interact with other healthcare system professionals. First Responders should establish a strong working relationship with these other personnel.

ROLES AND RESPONSIBILITIES OF THE FIRST RESPONDER

The First Responder has many roles and responsibilities, including personal safety; the safety of crew, patient, and bystanders; patient assessment; patient care based on assessment findings; lifting and moving patients safely; transportation of patients and transfer of care; record keeping and data collection; and patient advocacy. The individual EMS system provides the First Responder with a job description outlining specific roles and responsibilities.

The First Responder is a healthcare professional with certain professional attributes, including attending continuing education programs; projecting a professional appearance; maintaining

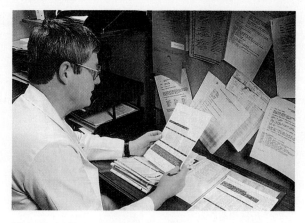

Fig. 1-8 Indirect medical direction, such as routine physician review of prehospital care reports, contributes to quality improvement and influences care to all patients.

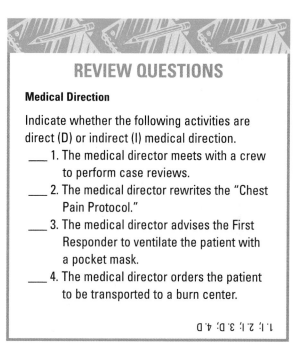

REVIEW QUESTIONS

Medical Direction

Indicate whether the following activities are direct (D) or indirect (I) medical direction.

___ 1. The medical director meets with a crew to perform case reviews.

___ 2. The medical director rewrites the "Chest Pain Protocol."

___ 3. The medical director advises the First Responder to ventilate the patient with a pocket mask.

___ 4. The medical director orders the patient to be transported to a burn center.

1. I; 2. I; 3. D; 4. D

knowledge and skills at a competent level; participating in issues that affect EMS on a local, state, and national level; and serving as a patient advocate.

MEDICAL DIRECTION

Quality care and medical direction go hand in hand. Medical direction establishes that all care given a patient is medically appropriate. Direct medical direction involves direct contact between the physician and providers in the field. Indirect medical direction includes other activities, such as system planning, protocol development, education, and quality improvement.

UNITED STATES DEPARTMENT OF TRANSPORTATION NATIONAL HIGHWAY TRAFFIC SAFETY ADMINISTRATION FIRST RESPONDER OBJECTIVES

Check your knowledge. The National Registry of EMTs and many state EMS agencies use the objectives below to develop First Responder certification examinations. Can you meet them?

COGNITIVE OBJECTIVES

1. Define the components of Emergency Medical Services (EMS) systems.
2. Differentiate the roles and responsibilities of the First Responder from other out-of-hospital care providers.
3. Define medical oversight and discuss the First Responder's role in the process.
4. Discuss the types of medical oversight that may affect the medical care of a First Responder.
5. State the specific statutes and regulations in your state regarding the EMS system.

AFFECTIVE OBJECTIVES

6. Accept and uphold the responsibilities of a First Responder in accordance with the standards of an EMS professional.
7. Explain the rationale for maintaining a professional appearance when on duty or when responding to calls.
8. Describe why it is inappropriate to judge a patient based on a cultural, gender, age, or socioeconomic model, and to vary the standard of care rendered as a result of that judgement.

Well-Being of the First Responder

TWO

I. Emotional Aspects of Emergency Care
   A. Death and Dying
   B. Stressful Situations
   C. Stress Management
   D. Critical Incident Stress Debriefing

E. Comprehensive Critical Incident Stress Management

II. Safety
   A. Scene Safety
   B. Personal Safety

KEY TERMS

Body substance isolation (BSI) precautions
Measures taken to prevent First Responders from coming in contact with a patient's body fluids.

Burnout A condition characterized by physical and emotional exhaustion resulting from chronic unrelieved job-related stress.

Critical incident Any situation that causes an emergency worker to experience unusually strong emotional reactions and that interferes with their ability to function, either immediately or at some time in the future.

Critical Incident Stress Debriefing (CISD) A debriefing process conducted by a team of peer counselors and mental health professionals to help emergency workers deal with their emotions and feelings after a critical incident.

Hazardous material Substance that poses a threat or unreasonable risk to life, health, or property if not properly controlled during manufacture, processing, packaging, handling, storage, transportation, use, and disposal.

Stress Bodily or mental tension caused by physical or emotional factors; can also involve a person's response to events that are threatening or challenging.

FIRST RESPONSE

A week after the fatal plane crash, John again woke from a nightmare of the crash scene. He still couldn't accept that a crash with no survivors happened in his town. He remembered the radio call to implement the airport disaster response and his hurried trip to the scene in the fire engine as a First Responder. Dozens of ambulances responded within minutes after John's arrival, but there were no survivors to receive medical care. The First Responders, EMTs, paramedics, nurses, and physicians felt helpless. John thought about the crash every day. He had lost his appetite and couldn't concentrate at work. Everyone involved in the response was supposed to talk to the Critical Incident Stress Debriefing (CISD) team, but John didn't feel that talking would help.

When John arrived at work that day, his supervisor, Mary, met him at the door. "I think we need to talk," Mary said. In the last few days, she had noticed his change in attitude and tried to approach him, but he didn't want to talk. She discussed the problem with John and asked him to see the CISD team.

After talking to the team and the other First Responders at the crash, John still thinks about the crash, but without the negative emotions and tension of several weeks ago. The team helped John work through his frustration at being unable to care for the victims of the crash, and to remember the value of the work he does every day.

EMS is a stressful profession. First Responders and other healthcare professionals are regularly called upon to help the sick, injured, and dying. First Responders must deal with physical illnesses and injuries, as well as with the emotions of the patient, the patient's family, and themselves (Fig. 2-1). First Responders must be prepared to deal with these stresses effectively.

First Responders also face personal risk in the form of scene hazards, exposure to disease, and stress. Knowing the warning signs of stress and how to protect yourself can help you to have a long and healthy career as a First Responder.

EMOTIONAL ASPECTS OF EMERGENCY CARE

DEATH AND DYING

Death is the natural end to all living things. At some time in our lives, we will all face death—the death of a friend or family member, a patient, or our own death. Different people have different ways of coping with death, but there are some similarities in general coping mechanisms. Familiarity with the normal grieving process provides insight to the reactions of patients, their family members, and yourself. People generally go through five stages:

DENIAL: "Not me." This is a defense mechanism that allows people to feel there must be a mistake when they learn they or someone they care about is dying—the medical tests were wrong, the results were misinterpreted, or something else went wrong. People often deny the facts even in the face of overwhelming evidence. This can make them very difficult to deal with. It is important to be straightforward and honest with both the patient and the family regarding questions you are asked about your knowledge of the patient's illness or condition.

ANGER: "Why me?" Once patients begin to accept the fact they are dying, a common response is anger. Patients may become angry at those nearby who are in good health, the doctor who informs them of their condition, their family, or First Responders who try to help. Remember that the patient is not actually angry with you and do not take any insults or anger personally. Be tolerant and patient, and do not become defensive. Listen empathetically to what the patient has to say, and answer all questions truthfully. Do not make false reassurance, such as saying, "Of course you will be all right," or "Don't worry, everything is fine."

BARGAINING: "OK, but first let me...." Once patients begin to accept their imminent death, they may try to postpone the inevitable event by bargaining. "OK, I know I'm going to die, but let me live awhile longer to see my first grandchild." Patients may try to bargain with doctors, themselves, or God.

DEPRESSION: "OK, but I haven't...." Once patients realize that bargaining won't work, sadness and despair may set in. They think of all of the happy things in their lives they will miss, and all of the things they will never get to do. These patients are often silent and retreat into their own world. They are preparing and grieving for their own death.

ACCEPTANCE: "OK, I'm not afraid." At this stage, people have made peace with themselves and are willing to accept that they are dying. Acceptance does not imply that the patient is happy about dying, only that they realize their fate. Some family members still may not accept death and may require more emotional support than the patient. Be supportive of family members and the patient's wishes.

BOX 2-1 Situations That Cause Stress

- Mass casualties
- Pediatric patients
- Death
- Infant and child trauma
- Amputations
- Violence
- Infant or child abuse, elder abuse, spouse abuse
- Death or injury of a co-worker or other public safety personnel

---

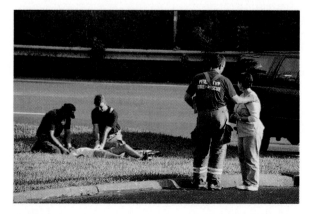

Fig. 2-1 First Responders must handle the emotions of patients and their family members, as well as their own emotions.

Not everyone moves through these stages in the same way or in the same time frame. Some patients may experience the stages in a different order or skip stages. Some people never make it through all of the stages, or they may return to a previous stage. The response to death is as varied as people are. The patient's progression through these stages is influenced by age, duration of illness, and family support.

Dealing with a dying patient and comforting the family members is not an easy task. Kindness, compassion, and understanding may help the patient or family members cope with their emotions. Listen empathetically and speak with a gentle tone of voice. Allow the patient and family members to express their emotions, including rage, anger, and despair.

Patients should always be treated with respect, and their privacy should be protected. Patients may feel the need to have some control over their treatment, and their wishes should be honored when possible. Always explain your actions to the patient and family members and treat the patient with dignity, even when they are unresponsive. Often a gentle touch is remembered more than the most expert care. Let the patient and family know that everything that can be done for the patient will be done, but do not falsely reassure them about the situation.

STRESSFUL SITUATIONS

Stress and working as a First Responder often go hand in hand. First Responders feel stress in many different situations. Although different people find different situations stressful, some situations cause almost all emergency workers to feel stress (Box 2-1).

First Responders not only have their own stress to deal with, but often also have to manage bystanders or patients who are experiencing stressful reactions.

Stressful situations may cause the First Responder to feel stress long after the incident. After caring for an injured child, for example, First Responders may be more protective of their own children in the days and weeks to follow. Stress can also be caused by a slow buildup of smaller stressful situations. You must know the warning signs of severe stress and be able to recognize them in yourself or co-workers to help manage stress.

STRESS MANAGEMENT

Stress is a bodily or mental tension caused by physical or emotional factors that involves the

---

BOX 2-2 Stress Warning Signs

- Irritability with co-workers, family, or friends
- Inability to concentrate
- Difficulty sleeping or nightmares
- Anxiety
- Indecisiveness
- Guilt
- Loss of appetite
- Loss of interest in sexual activities
- Isolation
- Loss of interest in work

---

person's response to events that are threatening or challenging. Not all stress is negative. If we didn't feel the stress of knowing there is an exam at the end of the course, we might not read the book for class. If not for the stress of being late for work, we might never get out of bed. Stress becomes a problem when it is felt so strongly that it begins to hinder our ability to function. Emergency workers are not immune to the stress of emergency situations. You must be aware of the signs of stress in yourself and in co-workers so you know when to take steps to manage stress.

There are warning signs of stress that need to be recognized in order to manage stress appropriately. The warning signs of stress are listed in Box 2-2.

The ways stress is handled are as different as people's reactions to stress. Too much stress can unquestionably affect your health and ability to perform your job. **Burnout** is a condition characterized by physical and emotional exhaustion resulting from chronic job-related stress. The following are some proven guidelines that help many people deal with their stress and avoid burnout (Fig. 2-2).

CHANGE YOUR DIET: A healthy diet keeps your body in good condition and prepared to respond to an emergency. Consume only small amounts of sugar, caffeine, and alcohol. Avoid fatty foods, but increase carbohydrates. Also avoid excessive salt, which may increase your blood pressure. It is easy to miss meals during a busy day; don't forget to take care of yourself and eat meals regularly.

STOP SMOKING: Cigarette smoking increases your blood pressure and heart rate, and doubles your chances of a fatal heart attack. Cigarettes contain hundreds of toxins that increase your chances of lung disease and cancer, and contribute to thousands of deaths every year. Although it is difficult

to quit smoking, most people can do it once they are committed to their decision. The benefits of quitting smoking are unquestionable. Cigarette smoking is the number one changeable risk factor for heart disease. Heart disease is the number one cause of death in the United States.

GET REGULAR EXERCISE: Regular exercise improves cardiovascular fitness, strength, and flexibility and lowers your chances of becoming ill or injured. Exercise contributes to psychological and physical well-being.

LEARN TO RELAX: Many people have learned to manage their stress by practicing relaxation techniques, meditation, visual imagery, and other methods. There are books and classes available to teach relaxation techniques.

BALANCE WORK, RECREATION, AND FAMILY: Plan time away from emergency work, and don't lose interest in your outside activities.

CHANGE YOUR WORK SCHEDULE: If you find that you are feeling severe effects of stress, request a change of duty assignment to a less busy area, or a change of shift that allows you to spend more time with friends and family. No one expects emergency workers to be immune to stress. It is not a weakness to need time to recover from stressful situations.

SEEK PROFESSIONAL HELP: You can benefit from professional help if the symptoms of stress are severe. Mental health workers, social workers, and clergy can all provide assistance with these sorts of issues.

First Responders and other emergency workers are not the only ones who experience stress on the job. Family and friends of emergency workers also experience stress. Spouses of First Responders often want to share the burden of stressful situations on the job, but may not understand the situations their spouse faces. At other times, family and friends may not want to hear about the emergency situations that their loved ones face. Families of emergency workers also deal with the fears of injury or death on the job, and separation from their loved ones. Rotating shifts, late calls, and on-call situations all add to the stress of emergency work. Talk with your family about these concerns and work out the best solution for you.

CRITICAL INCIDENT STRESS DEBRIEFING

Although First Responders deal with stressful situations regularly, some situations cause reactions more severe than usual. Stress is a normal response to an abnormal situation, but sometimes the level of stress can become overwhelming. The death or serious injury of a child may trigger greater stress for a First Responder with a child. For others, a patient who dies after a long rescue attempt may cause severe stress. Even though the types of incidents that cause severe stress vary, the result is often the same. A **critical incident** is a specific situation that causes an emergency worker to experience unusually strong emotional reactions and interferes with their ability to function, either immediately or in the future. First Responders may also place undue stress on themselves if they have unrealistic expectations about their abilities to help. It is important to realize that there are limitations in helping patients, and not every patient's situation will turn out for the best.

One way to deal with a critical incident is through a process called **critical incident stress debriefing (CISD)**. The debriefing process is conducted by a team of peer counselors and mental health professionals, and is designed to help emergency care workers accelerate the normal recovery process after dealing with a critical incident. Debriefings are held within 24 to 72 hours after a critical incident. During the discussion, emergency care workers are encouraged to discuss their fears, feelings, and reactions openly and honestly. The discussion is not an investigation into the causes of the stress, how the event was handled, or any other technical matters. It is a chance for emergency care workers to discuss the events and their feelings with people who will listen and provide understanding

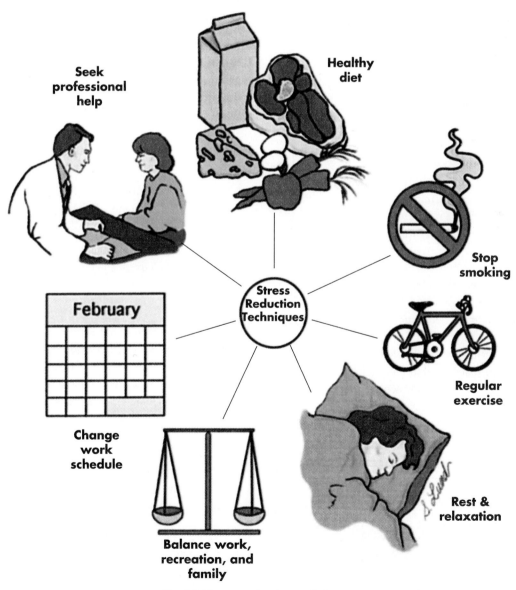

Fig. 2-2 Stress reduction techniques.

and support and who will not pass judgment or criticize. All personnel involved in the incident, including fire, police, dispatch and emergency medical service personnel should be involved in the debriefing. All information is kept confidential so that each person can feel free to discuss everything. The debriefing team then offers suggestion for dealing with and overcoming the stress.

Another technique used when dealing with critical incident stress is a defusing. A defusing is a much shorter, less formal, and less structured version of CISD. Defusings generally take place in 30 to 45 minutes, and occur a few hours after the event. Defusings allow for initial ventilation, which may eliminate the need for a formal debriefing. Defusings may also enhance the formal debriefing.

Find out how to access your local CISD team and remember that the service is there for you to use when you need it. Emergency workers should not feel embarrassed or uncomfortable when seeking help. We are all human and may need help dealing with our responses to emergency situations. Box 2-3 lists some common situations that may require CISD.

COMPREHENSIVE CRITICAL INCIDENT STRESS MANAGEMENT

In addition to dealing with stress after the occurrence of a critical incident, systems have been developed to help emergency workers, their families, and the community in general deal with stress in a more comprehensive manner. Preincident stress education helps emergency workers understand how to deal with stress they will face as part of their job. By knowing the signs of stress and how to find the help needed, emergency workers may be able to avoid burnout. In addition to preincident stress education, other health and wellness programs are in place to help emergency workers stay in good physical and psychological shape. On-scene

and one-on-one support provides a network of other emergency workers to rely upon during times of stress. This support is focused not only on disasters and critical incidents, but also on the daily stresses that emergency workers face. CISD is a part of the support provided. Families of emergency workers also learn how to deal with the stress their loved ones are facing, as well as the stress they face themselves.

In times of disaster, support services are provided to emergency workers, their families, and the community. The community as a whole may need to have a place to turn to discuss their feelings of loss and sorrow. An earthquake, for example, not

---

BOX 2-3 Situations That May Require CISD

- Line-of-duty death or serious injury
- Multiple casualty incident
- Suicide of an emergency worker
- Serious injury or death of children
- Events with excessive media interest
- Victims known to the emergency personnel
- Event that has unusual impact on the personnel
- Any disaster

REVIEW QUESTIONS

Emotional Aspects of Emergency Care

1. Number the stages of dealing with death and dying in order (O), and match (M) them with the phrase on the right that corresponds to the stage.

   O   M
   __ __ Anger   A. "Not me."
   __ __ Denial   B. "OK, I'm not afraid."
   __ __ Acceptance   C. "OK, but I haven't…"
   __ __ Bargaining   D. "Why me?"
   __ __ Depression   E. "OK, but first let me…"

2. Everyone moves through all of the stages of dealing with death and dying in the same order. True or False?

3. List at least three warning signs of stress.

   _____

   _____

   _____

4. Critical incident stress debriefing should:
   A. Take place at least two weeks after the incident
   B. Not include the person in charge of the call
   C. Be an open and honest discussion of feelings and emotions
   D. Involve criticism and judgment about actions taken on the call

1. Order—2, 1, 5, 3, 4; Matching—D, A, E, C; 2. False; 3. Irritability, inability to concentrate, difficulty sleeping/nightmares, anxiety, indecisiveness, guilt, loss of appetite, loss of interest in sexual activities, isolation, loss of interest in work; 4. C

only affects those working to help victims of the disaster, but everyone involved in the earthquake. Community outreach programs are designed to provide a way for the entire community to become involved in the healing process and aid in dealing with their feelings. Follow-up services are provided by the outreach programs to monitor how emergency workers are dealing with their own feelings after critical incidents, and to provide additional support if necessary. Some workers may not feel the effects of their stress for weeks or even months.

Comprehensive stress management programs are a way of dealing with the effects of stress before stressful events occur, during times of great stress, and after the events are over. Remember these situations do not have to be something as big as a natural disaster to cause stress, but any situation that involves a reaction to stress.

SAFETY

Safety should be your first priority every time you respond to a call for emergency help. As a First Responder, you are usually the source of scene safety for other emergency workers who arrive on the scene after you. In the excitement of an emergency, it is easy to rush to the aid of an injured person without taking the proper steps to ensure your own safety. The following sections on scene and personal safety will highlight the important steps that should be taken to protect yourself, co-workers, and the patient. Common sense and taking a moment to assess each situation play an important role in safety.

SCENE SAFETY

Every First Responder involved in an emergency call is responsible for the safety of that scene. As a First Responder, you are responsible for your own safety, the safety of your partner or other First Responders, the patient, and bystanders, in that order. It is in the caring nature of emergency workers to begin treating an ill or injured patient as soon as possible. However, to be able to help anyone, you must first take precautions so that you are not harmed. First Responders who are injured cannot provide care or help to anyone else, and must be cared for themselves by other emergency crews arriving on the scene, thus taking away from the care that can be provided to the patient.

You must work as a team and watch out for the safety of your partner, or any other First Responders or emergency personnel on scene. You must also take responsibility for the safety of patients and do your best to allow no further injuries. Traffic hazards, violent people, and environmental factors all pose a risk to patients. With the help of law enforcement personnel, you also protect bystanders by restricting them to areas out of the path of danger.

Scene safety begins when you receive a call. Scene safety includes an assessment of the surroundings that will provide valuable information to the First Responder and help ensure safety. As you arrive at every scene, ask yourself, "Is it safe to approach the patient?" In situations such as crash or rescue scenes, toxic substance scenes, crime scenes with the potential for violence, unstable surfaces that slope or are covered with ice or water, all need to be anticipated and planned for. First Responders must remember to evaluate the scene before entering and beginning care. If the scene is unsafe, make it safe. If you can't make the scene safe, do not enter. Instead, call for specialized resources that can make the scene safe.

Hazardous materials

A **hazardous material** is a substance that poses a threat or unreasonable risk to life, health, or property if not properly controlled during manufacture, processing, packaging, handling, storage, transportation, use, and disposal. Hazardous materials incidents should be handled by specialized hazardous materials teams. In general, specialty equipment and knowledge are needed, and crews not educated or equipped to handle the situation

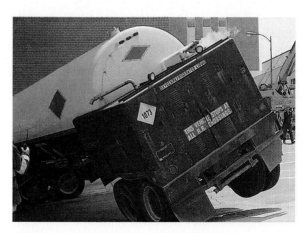

Fig. 2-3 A placard displayed on hazardous materials containers provides information about the materials inside.

should let the hazardous materials team handle the situation. Know how to call for the assistance of the specialty team as soon as a hazardous materials incident has been identified, and protect yourself and bystanders from harm.

Use binoculars to identify hazards at the scene. This allows you to identify any marking symbols without coming close to the hazardous material. For incidents involving motor vehicles carrying hazardous materials, a placard will be displayed on the vehicle. A placard is a diamond-shaped sign displayed on hazardous materials containers (Fig. 2-3). If the placard can be identified from a safe distance, information from that placard should be provided to the responding hazardous materials team so they are prepared for the type of incident. The *Hazardous Material Emergency Response Guidebook,* a publication of the United States Department of Transportation, contains concise reference information about hazardous materials and their identification numbers. This book allows you to identify the materials on the scene. For hazardous materials incidents at farms or industries, placards may not be displayed. In these situations, employees should know what chemicals are involved and can provide you with valuable information about them. Regardless of the type of hazardous material, do not attempt to enter the scene; wait for the hazardous materials team.

First Responders provide emergency care to patients only after the scene is safe. It is not safe to enter a scene to remove a contaminated patient until the hazardous materials specialists decontaminate the patient and inform you it is safe to do so. Premature entry could pose a risk to the patient, bystanders, and you.

If you are interested in receiving additional education for hazardous materials incidents, contact your local hazardous materials team or emergency management agency to find out about such education programs.

Motor vehicle crashes

Most motor vehicle crash scenes involve a variety of threats to life. First Responders called to motor vehicle crashes must be aware of the hazards common to these scenes. For example, along many highways there are electrical wires and poles that can become obstacles when struck by a vehicle. High voltage electricity could be conducted through those wires and they should never be touched until the utility company has turned off the power. Fires and explosions are also possible risks. You must carefully evaluate the situation before entering the

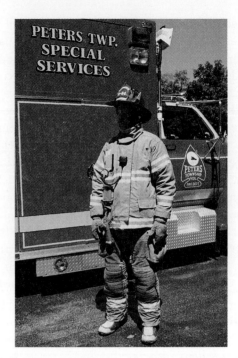

Fig. 2-4 Protective clothing is essential for all rescue situations. This equipment should include turnout gear, puncture-proof gloves, helmet with ear protection and a chin strap, eye protection (heavy goggles made specifically for working with power equipment), and boots.

scene. Broken glass, sharp jagged metal, and unstable surfaces are only a few of the concerns at most vehicle crashes. Traffic hazards and hazardous materials must also be dealt with, often requiring the help of other public safety workers.

Protective clothing is a must when working near vehicle crashes (Fig 2-4). The recommended protective clothing to be worn when working near vehicle crashes in listed in Box 2-4.

Besides basic motor vehicle crashes, there are other aspects of rescue and extrication. If you are interested in being a part of these operations, you must attend continuing education courses to prepare yourself for these incidents. These courses cover safety issues, equipment, and rescue techniques. In a variety of situations, the patient must be rescued from places that are difficult to access. Heavy rescue or specialty situations such as water rescue or entrapment in a heavily damaged car require special rescue teams.

Violence

Violent scenes should always be controlled by law enforcement personnel before you enter to provide patient care. Consider your own safety first. Allow law enforcement officials to determine that the scene is safe; then you can begin to provide care to the patient. At a crime scene, disturb as little evidence as possible. Evidence you protect at the scene may solve a crime case. Do not disturb anything unless you must to provide medical care. If you must disturb something, make note of what you see, where it was, how and where it was moved, by whom, and why. Dealing with the scene carefully will help maintain the chain of evidence.

Once you have taken the time to make sure the scene is safe, the next step to ensure your personal safety is to follow body substance isolation precautions.

PERSONAL SAFETY

Body substance isolation precautions

One of the first steps in personal protection is to prevent the spread of communicable diseases from patients to you. Although some patients clearly present a disease exposure risk, it is impossible to evaluate any patient as safe. Patients infected with diseases such as hepatitis or human immunodeficiency virus (HIV) do not have a certain appearance, dress, or particular socioeconomic class. Contact with the blood or other body fluid of any patient should be considered a risk, and you should follow steps to avoid such contamination. **Body substance isolation (BSI) precautions** are designed to prevent you from coming in contact with a patient's body fluids. Preventive measures to avoid exposure to communicable diseases are also a part of good patient care. First Responders could transfer a disease to other patients, healthcare workers, or family members if they are careless. To prevent the transmission of diseases between patients, equipment should be disinfected or cleaned according to service policy, and disposable items should be replaced after each patient contact.

The routine use of personal protective equipment will help reduce the risks of coming into contact with a communicable disease. Systems should have policies for the use of personal protective equipment that follow Occupational Safety and Health Administration (OSHA), state, and local regulations regarding body substance isolation. Body substance isolation equipment should be made available to you for use when there is a potential risk. To help prevent the spread of infection, take the measures described in the following sections.

Hand washing   Hand washing is the single most important procedure for preventing the spread of disease. Effective hand washing involves vigorously rubbing the hands together with lathered soap, and then rinsing under a stream of water (Fig. 2-5). Hand washing should last for at least 10 to 15 seconds. Dry hands thoroughly with a clean cloth or disposable towel. Be sure to wash hands thoroughly after every patient contact, even if you were wearing gloves. There are also waterless hand-washing substitutes available for use when you do not have access to a sink and water but need to wash your hands. These solutions are usually alcohol based. The rubbing

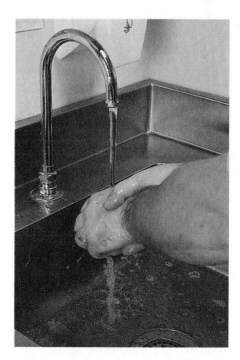

Fig. 2-5 Hand washing is the single most important procedure for preventing the spread of disease.

BOX 2-4 Recommended Protective Clothing for Working Near Vehicle Crashes

- Turnout gear, which is protective clothing that prevents or resists puncturing
- Puncture-proof gloves
- Helmet with ear protection and a chin strap to keep the helmet on your head (many helmets are equipped with face shields as well)
- Eye protection, such as heavy goggles made specifically for working with power equipment. Face shields and prescription glasses are not sufficient eye protection
- Boots with steel toes and insoles are recommended

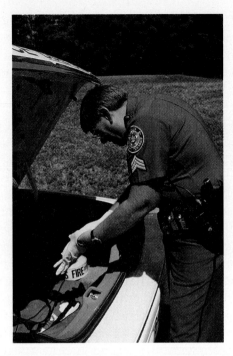

Fig. 2-6 First Responders should put on vinyl or latex gloves if it seems likely that the situation could include blood or other body fluids.

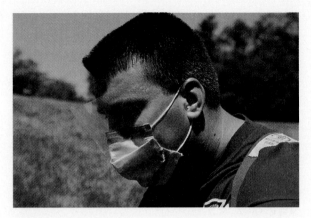

Fig. 2-7 First Responders should wear eye protection and a mask if body fluids could splash into the face.

action causes friction, and the alcohol kills most surface organisms. You must thoroughly wash your hands when you have access to a sink, even if you use waterless hand-washing substitutes.

Gloves   Wear disposable vinyl or latex gloves any time you are in contact with blood or other body fluids, when there is a high chance there will be blood or other body fluids present, or a chance you will come in contact with mucous membranes or broken skin. Gloves should also be worn if you will be dealing with equipment that has been in contact with blood or other body fluids or mucous membranes. If a patient complains of nausea but has not vomited, you face a high likelihood of contact with vomit during the call; it is too late to put on gloves once the patient begins to vomit. Prepare ahead and wear gloves if it seems possible that the situation could include contact with blood or other body fluids. Many First Responders find it convenient to put on gloves when they are approaching the scene, before patient contact (Fig. 2-6). Change gloves between contact with different patients to prevent cross-contamination. To remove gloves, turn them inside out using the cuff to pull them off so you do not touch the outside of the glove with your hands. When cleaning vehicles, utility gloves should be worn to protect your hands.

Eye protection   Eye protection is available in a variety of forms and should be worn when there is the possibility of blood or body fluids splashing into the face or eyes. Any type of eye protection that stops fluids from reaching the eyes is sufficient; high-quality, expensive goggles are not required. Remember, the splashing of body fluids can occur in many situations, not only in trauma situations. Assisting in childbirth, for example, will likely place you at risk for contact with splashing fluids. If you wear prescription glasses, you can apply removable side shields to them.

Masks   Masks can be worn by emergency workers to prevent body fluids from spattering into the nose and mouth. There are masks available that incorporate eye protection also. If it is likely that body fluids will come in contact with your nose and mouth, it is likely these fluids will also contact your eyes; therefore, eye protection should also be worn. There are masks available that have eye shields already attached (Fig. 2-7).

Masks can be worn by a patient who has an airborne disease. If the patient is unwilling to wear a mask, you should wear one. For a patient diagnosed with tuberculosis, specialty masks known as high-efficiency particulate air (HEPA) respirators are required. These masks are needed when working in enclosed spaces with a patient who has tuberculosis. This is an uncommon situation for a First Responder, but not an unprecedented one.

Gowns   Gowns are used for calls when large amounts of blood or other body fluids are expected, such as in assisting childbirth. Regular emergency services uniforms are also part of the protective barrier against body fluid contamination. Wearing a gown over your uniform keeps you from soiling your uniform. A change of uniform should always be readily available.

In addition to these body substance isolation precautions, First Responders should always use a barrier device when ventilating a patient. Barrier devices and techniques for ventilating patients are discussed in Chapter 6, "The Airway."

Advanced safety precautions

Before becoming First Responders or beginning patient contact, you should take steps to help ensure your physical well-being. Your immune status to commonly transmitted contagious diseases such as rubella, measles, mumps, and polio should be verified and you may also choose to be vaccinated against hepatitis B. In addition, you should receive a tetanus booster. Tuberculin-purified protein derivative (Mantoux) testing should be conducted in accordance with local or regional policies. Ask your instructor about the availability of immunizations in your community.

OSHA, states and regions require individual emergency services to have policies and regulations for BSI precautions. The requirements for notification and testing after an exposure incident depend on the region. It is vitally important that all healthcare workers understand their rights and responsibilities under these laws and fulfill

their obligations for reporting exposure. Each service will review its exposure control plan with the crew members.

Scene safety is discussed in more detail in Chapter 7, "Patient Assessment."

CHAPTER SUMMARY

EMOTIONAL ASPECTS OF EMERGENCY CARE

First Responders face many emotional situations, including patients and their family members who are dealing with death and dying. Patients respond differently to injury, illness, and death. People pass through a series of stages when faced with death: Denial ("Not me."); Anger ("Why me?"); Bargaining ("OK, but first let me…''); Depression ("OK, but I haven't…''); and Acceptance ("OK, I'm not afraid.").

Treat dying patients and their families with respect and dignity. Explain all your actions and honor the patient's wishes when possible. Patients may need to feel they have some control over the situation. Family members' responses to the impending death of a loved one may be stronger than the patient's, who may have already accepted their own death.

Almost all emergency workers experience severe stress when responding to situations such as mass casualty incidents, pediatric patients, death, infant and child trauma, amputations, violence, abuse, or death or injury of public safety personnel. First Responders may feel the effects of stress immediately after a call, or the reaction may be delayed or cumulative.

Stress can be detected by a variety of warning signs, including irritability to co-workers, family or friends, inability to concentrate, difficulty sleeping/nightmares, anxiety, indecisiveness, guilt, loss of appetite, loss of interest in sexual activities, isolation, and loss of interest in work.

Stress can be managed in many ways, not all of which work for all people. Some options for stress management include eating a balanced diet, not smoking, exercise, relaxation techniques, and balancing work, family, and recreation. Find professional help if stress is severe and you can't manage it alone. Families of emergency workers also feel the effects of stress. CISD allows emergency workers to discuss their emotions while counselors help them work through their problems.

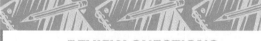

REVIEW QUESTIONS

Safety

1. First Responders must wear gloves only in trauma situations. True or False?

2. Hand washing is one of the best defenses against the spread of infectious diseases. True or False?

3. Hazardous materials placards identify the material inside the container bearing the placard. True or False?

4. First Responders should wait for law enforcement at all scenes of crime or violence, even if the patient states the violent individual has left the scene. True or False?

1. False; 2. True; 3. True; 4. True

SAFETY

As a First Responder, you are responsible for your own safety and the safety of your partners, the patient, and bystanders.

First Responders should not enter scenes that are unsafe or that require special knowledge and equipment. Specialty crews should be called to deal with hazardous materials and rescues. You may be able to identify hazardous materials by the placards on the container. Law enforcement personnel should be called upon to control scenes of crime or violence.

BSI precautions include hand washing, gloves, eye protection, masks, and gowns. These precautions should be followed any time there is a chance you will encounter body fluids. It is not always possible to determine at the beginning of a call if body fluids will be involved. It is often impossible to apply gloves once a patient begins to vomit or bleed, so evaluate the need for precautions early.

Healthcare workers who come in contact with patients should be vaccinated against common communicable diseases and tested for others on a regular basis.

UNITED STATES DEPARTMENT OF TRANSPORTATION NATIONAL HIGHWAY TRAFFIC SAFETY ADMINISTRATION FIRST RESPONDER OBJECTIVES

Check your knowledge. The National Registry of EMTs and many state EMS agencies use the objectives below to develop First Responder certification examinations. Can you meet them?

COGNITIVE OBJECTIVES

1. List possible emotional reactions that the First Responder may experience when faced with trauma, illness, and death and dying.
2. Discuss the possible reactions that a family member may exhibit when confronted with death and dying.
3. State the steps in the First Responder's approach to the family confronted with death and dying.
4. State the possible reactions that the family of the First Responder may exhibit due to their outside involvement in EMS.
5. Recognize the signs and symptoms of critical incident stress.
6. State possible steps that the First Responder may take to help reduce/alleviate stress.
7. Explain the need to determine scene safety.
8. Discuss the importance of body substance isolation.
9. Describe the steps the First Responder should take for personal protection from airborne and blood-borne pathogens.
10. List the personal protective equipment necessary for each of the following situations: hazardous materials; rescue operations; violent scenes; crime scenes; exposure to blood-borne pathogens; exposure to airborne pathogens.

AFFECTIVE OBJECTIVES

11. Explain the rationale for serving as an advocate for the use of appropriate protective equipment.

PSYCHOMOTOR OBJECTIVES

12. Given a scenario with potential infectious exposure, the First Responder will use appropriate personal protective equipment. At the completion of the scenario, the First Responder will properly remove and discard the protective garments.
13. Given the above scenario, the First Responder will complete disinfection/cleaning and all reporting documentation.

Legal and Ethical Issues

THREE

KEY TERMS

Abandonment   Termination of care without the patient's consent and without making any provisions for continuing care at the same or a higher level.

Advance directive   Order from a patient and their physician regarding what care should be provided or withheld in certain emergency situations.

Assault   Threatening or attempting to inflict offensive physical contact.

Battery   Offensive touching of a person without the person's consent.

Competence   The knowledge underlying an individual's ability to understand.

Confidentiality   The First Responder's responsibility to not share personal information about a patient except to another authorized person.

Consent   To give permission.

Duty to act   Legal obligation that certain personnel, either by statute or function, have a responsibility to provide patient care when the opportunity presents itself.

Expressed consent   Condition in which the patient agrees to the treatment plan and gives the First Responder permission to proceed, while understanding any risks associated with the treatment.

Implied consent   Condition in which First Responders have legal permission to provide treatment to a person who is mentally, physically, or emotionally unable to provide expressed consent or otherwise unable to agree to treatment when treatment is needed due to a serious or life-threatening injury or illness. Care is given on the assumption that the patient would ask for and agree to treatment if able to.

Negligence   Failure to act as a reasonable, prudent First Responder would under similar circumstances.

Refusal   The patient's ability to reject offer of care from the First Responder.

Scope of care   The range of duties and skills First Responders are allowed to and supposed to perform when necessary.

Standard of care   The minimum acceptable level of care readily provided within a general area.

FIRST RESPONSE

On a warm summer morning, 7-year-old Tory and her mother were at the playground where she was learning to ride her bicycle without training wheels for the first time. Suddenly, Tory lost her balance and crashed to the ground. Almost immediately she cried in an anguished voice, "Mommy, my arm! My arm!"

The child's crying drew a small crowd of onlookers. Tory's mother asked one of them to call 9-1-1 for an ambulance, while she tried to comfort her crying child. Tory was sitting on the ground supporting her right arm across her chest with her left hand. Her right forearm was obviously deformed, and it was already beginning to swell. The bystander returned and reported that the 9-1-1 operator said an ambulance would be sent right away, and police officers would arrive to help prior to the ambulance.

A few minutes later, police officers identifying themselves as First Responders arrived at the scene. They quickly reassured Tory's mother and calmed the child while assessing her for any additional injuries beyond the obvious one. Her mother answered their questions about Tory's allergies and past medical problems. Tory was wearing her bicycle helmet, and although there were no indications of head, neck, or back injuries, the police officers decided to have Tory stay in the position they found her upon their arrival at the scene. They informed Tory's mother the ambulance was en route and only 5 minutes from the scene, and that the EMTs on the ambulance would perform a more thorough assessment of Tory's arm before they splinted it.

Prior to the ambulance arriving at the scene, the police officers were able to obtain a great deal of information concerning Tory's past medical history, make her as comfortable as possible, move the crowd of onlookers away from the area, and place Tory's bicycle in the trunk of her mother's car.

The ambulance arrived and the First Responders were able to provide the EMTs with information concerning the patient and assist with the care provided. The police officers had served a vital role in the continuum of care.

Most of the time, when a call for help goes out, First Responders find a patient who is in some degree of distress from a medical or traumatic situation. These individuals want and expect to be helped on the scene and be transported to a hospital or other advanced-care facility. That is how things went in the opening scenario, but situations are not always that simple. As a First Responder you will play a vital role in this chain of events.

In addition to your essential medical knowledge and skills, you must also understand the legal issues involved in emergency medical care. For example, in the opening story, what would the legal consequences be if Tory had been alone and no parent or guardian could be found? What if her injury had occurred at home and Tory wouldn't say what happened but the story from her mother was inconsistent with her injury? How would the situation be different if the patient was a 260-pound person who, besides being obviously injured, was intoxicated, belligerent, and refusing treatment?

These are situations you can face on any call. How you medically, ethically, and legally handle such cases could mean the difference between a long and rewarding career in emergency services and a long and painful journey through the legal system.

SCOPE OF CARE

First Responders must function within both maximum and minimum performance guidelines called the scope of care. Scope of care (also referred to as scope of practice) identifies the range of duties and skills First Responders are allowed to and are supposed to perform when necessary.

For example, driving to the scene of a motor vehicle crash and evaluating the patient are within the scope of care for First Responders. Writing prescriptions and performing surgery are appropriate for physicians, but are beyond the First Responder's scope of care. Ignoring an accident victim's plea for help or failing to treat an obvious life-threatening injury would also be serious violations of the First Responder's scope of care because these actions are below the expected level of performance.

LEGAL RESPONSIBILITIES

First Responders have legal duties to their patients, the medical director, and the public in general. Most states have legislation that defines the scope of care for First Responders. These regulations are generally based on the United States Department of Transportation National Highway Traffic Safety Administration's National Standard Curriculum for the First Responder (Fig. 3-1). Consult with an attorney, the state Attorney General's office or its equivalent, the attorney for the ambulance service, or local, regional, or state EMS agencies with oversight authority if you have any questions about how state laws apply to your EMS activities.

First Responders have the duty to provide necessary care for the well-being of the patient as outlined by this scope of care. However, the scope of care does not automatically grant First Responders the authority to perform every identified skill.

As a First Responder, your legal right to provide certain care depends on the availability of medical direction. First Responders can perform certain procedures only after consulting with a medical direction physician, such as allowing a patient to refuse treatment or performing a skill such as automated external defibrillation. Whether permission is required depends on the nature of the skill, your own level of experience, the condition of the patient, and the physician's comfort level with your abilities.

The scope of care may be broadened through protocols, guidelines, or standing orders. These written policies allow First Responders in a particular area to carry out some treatments or procedures—in whole or in part—before consulting with the medical director. However, these are also at the discretion of the local, regional, or statewide medical director and must be approved by the agency with oversight authority.

The **standard of care** is the minimum acceptable level of care normally provided in the area. The care provided by a First Responder is judged against the standard of care, or against how another First Responder of similar training and experience would have provided care.

The way in which you obtain permission to give care also depends on various factors. You may be required to consult directly with a physician by radio or telephone, or face-to-face if there is a physician at the scene. In some cases, permission to carry out certain procedures is granted in advance by written protocols or standing orders. These enable you to carry out specified skills (e.g., AED) before speaking to a physician when the patient has specific signs and symptoms.

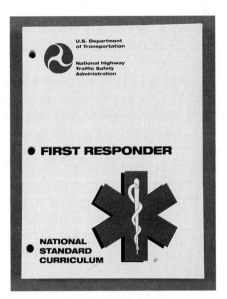

Fig. 3-1 In most states, legislation defines the scope of care for First Responders. Most states base their regulations on the United States Department of Transportation National Highway Traffic Safety Administration's National Standard Curriculum for the First Responder.

FIRST RESPONDER ALERT

Laws pertaining to patient care delivery vary from state to state. You should know how you are affected by your state's Medical Practice Act and other regulations. The information in this chapter is general and is not a complete guide to any state's legislative system, EMS laws, or regulations.

Standing orders may also be used in circumstances when direct consultation is not possible. This may occur with a patient who has a life-threatening problem requiring immediate attention or during multiple casualty incidents in which there is not time to speak to a physician about every patient. This may also occur if there is a failure of the communications system, such as when a severe storm knocks out telephone and power lines or in a disaster situation in which radio and telephone communications are already overburdened with other emergency transmissions.

Because First Responders function as an extension of the physician within the defined scope of care, the medical director has responsibility for any treatment rendered in the field. For this reason, the physician has the right to evaluate the performance of all First Responders he or she has responsibility for and to withhold medical direction privileges from anyone who fails to comply with the established standard of care.

ETHICAL RESPONSIBILITIES

As a First Responder you also have ethical responsibilities, including carrying out duties in a professional manner. A professional manner includes your attitude toward the care you give, regardless of whether you receive a salary for that service. In other words, there's more to being a First Responder than just responding to calls for help prior to more advanced personnel arriving at the scene. You must address your responsibilities to the patient, the medical director, and the general public on every call.

Think back to the case study at the opening of this chapter and try to view the events through Tory's eyes. It's not bad enough that you've wrecked your bicycle, but the pain in your arm won't stop. Your mother, who always knows what to do and makes you feel better when you get hurt, looks frightened and hasn't done anything to make the pain go away. There are several total strangers standing over you with frightened looks on their faces. And now, two policemen are trying to look at your injured arm, which only hurts worse because they're touching it.

For Tory, this is a terribly painful ordeal both physically and emotionally. For the First Responders, it is a routine call in which they have a medical responsibility to treat Tory's obvious injury as well as other potential injuries. They have a moral responsibility to try to make what may be the most frightening experience of her life a little less traumatic. That means they need to help her mother calm down so she can try to help Tory be less frightened. They must be courteous to the onlookers who, although they are not doing much, would like to help but do not know how. They have a responsibility to obtain and relay information about the patient and the situation to the EMS crew that arrives to continue care and transport Tory safely to the hospital. In other words, even the most routine call demands that you perform at nothing less than your very best, with all of your concerns relating back, either directly or indirectly, to the welfare of the patient.

Your responsibilities do not end when the call is over. You have a responsibility to practice and maintain all of your skills. Because one can never know when, where, or which skill will be needed next, you must practice all to the point of mastery. You also have a responsibility to maintain and upgrade your knowledge by participating in continuing education programs to remain up-to-date in patient care trends and treatments. All oral and written reports must be honest and accurate because of the associated medical/legal and educational issues. You must examine your own performance (driving ability, treatment, response times, communications skills, patient outcomes, etc.) in an effort to improve upon any areas of weakness and to advance to the currently available standard of care.

REVIEW QUESTIONS

Scope of Care

1. _____ identifies the range of duties and skills First Responders are allowed and are supposed to perform when necessary.

2. Laws pertaining to patient care vary from state to state. True or False?

3. You have no ethical or moral responsibility to maintain and upgrade your knowledge and skills by participating in continuing educational programs to remain current in patient care trends and treatments. True or False?

1. Scope of care; 2. True; 3. False

COMPETENCE AND CONSENT

UNDERSTANDING COMPETENCE

Competence is the ability of the patient to understand the reason a First Responder or other health professional may be at a scene to provide medical care. A patient is considered to be competent if they are willing and able to answer questions asked by the First Responder appropriately concerning the medical or trauma situation, and is able to understand the implications of decisions made concerning their care. First Responders will be called upon to make judgments concerning the patient's ability to make appropriate decisions concerning the care they will receive.

There are various reasons a patient may not be competent, including a patient who has ingested drugs or alcohol, a patient who has sustained serious injury, or one that is mentally incompetent. Therefore, a First Responder must first determine the competence of the patient before proceeding with evaluation of the patient or providing care.

CONSENT

Consent means that one gives approval for what another does or proposes to do. In general, consent means the patient must give you permission to carry out any treatments and procedures before those treatments and procedures can be carried out. Laws concerning the specifics of consent vary from state to state; therefore, you must be familiar with the statutes in your area and how they affect the scope of your practice.

It is important for you, as a First Responder, to understand that a competent adult patient has the right to refuse treatment. If the situation appears to be serious, then you should encourage the patient to allow you to provide care or suggest that they wait until more advanced personnel arrive at the scene.

Even in an emergency situation, a patient must consent to care before you can provide it. The patient may answer the question "May I help you?" in various ways. They may say "Yes" or "Please, look at my arm," or as in the opening story, Tory's mother directs the First Responders to provide care to her child. The patient must accept care based upon information provided by the First Responder about what will be done and the consequences of refusing or accepting care.

Expressed consent

Expressed consent means the patient directly agrees to accept your treatment and gives permission to proceed with it. In short, the patient expresses a desire for treatment.

Expressed consent depends on two criteria, and both must be met to obtain expressed consent:

1. The patient must be of legal age and able to make a rational decision. Legal age means an adult, which is defined differently in each state. You must know what is considered legal age in your own jurisdiction. Able to make a rational decision means that the patient is responsive and of sound mind, and has a full understanding of the consequences of his or her actions (or inactions).

2. You must explain to the patient all the steps of the procedure(s) and any associated risks. In other words, the patient has the right to know what to expect during a procedure, what can go wrong, and what the outcome could be if it does. This allows the patient to make an informed decision to let you perform the entire procedure, part of the procedure, or none of it at all.

You must obtain expressed consent from every responsive, mentally competent adult patient before you can legally begin to treat them. In order to obtain consent, the following steps should be performed. First, identify yourself by name and by level of training. This is accomplished by saying "Hello, my name is Jake Taylor, I'm a First Responder, may I help you?" Once the patient says "Yes" or nods, all procedures that will be performed should be explained to the patient, and the risks and benefits identified. The patient must understand and agree to each procedure before you begin.

Implied consent

Implied consent assumes that all responsive and rational patients suffering from an immediately life-threatening or disabling injury or illness would want to receive treatment and would provide expressed consent if they could. Therefore, implied consent applies in cases where the person requiring treatment is mentally, physically, or emotionally unable to provide expressed consent (Fig. 3-2). Life-saving measures should never be withheld because doing so would likely be considered negligence.

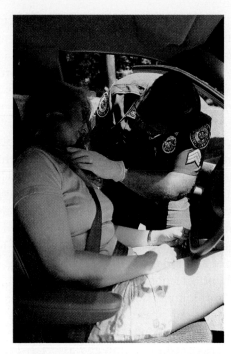

Fig. 3-2 Implied consent applies in cases where the person requiring treatment is unresponsive and therefore unable to provide expressed consent.

CHILDREN AND MENTALLY INCOMPETENT ADULTS

When a child requires medical care, consent for treatment must be obtained from a parent or legal guardian. Consent from an adult relative usually is enough if the parents are unavailable. If the parent gives consent, you have the legal right and obligation to treat the child, even if the child does not want to be treated.

Implied consent applies in situations involving children when no parent, guardian, or other adult relative is available to give expressed consent. The presumption is that they would want the child to be treated if they were present to give their consent.

The one exception occurs when a child is an emancipated minor. Emancipation, in this case, means the child is free from parental care and responsibility. Emancipated minors have control over their own lives and are free to make their own decisions. In short, they are legally considered adults. Emancipated minors have the right to consent to treatment or refuse care for themselves. In most states, minors are considered to be emancipated if they are married, pregnant, or out on their own and able to provide for themselves. The specific statutes pertaining to emancipation vary from state to state. Therefore, you must consult with

local authorities to determine the legal definition of emancipation in your area.

For a mentally incompetent adult, you must obtain consent the same way as for a child. Expressed consent from the patient's legal guardian is required before care can be given. Patients who cannot make or communicate decisions concerning themselves are considered to be incompetent. Persons who are mentally, emotionally, or developmentally unable to make rational decisions typically fit this definition. Also, as with children, if a life-threatening condition exists and no competent relative or guardian is available, life-saving measures should be carried out under implied consent.

Patients who are under the influence of drugs or alcohol and those who have a diminished level of consciousness because of their injury or illness may also be unable to make rational decisions. If no family member is available to give expressed consent on the patient's behalf, care should be given based on implied consent.

ADVANCE DIRECTIVES

An advance directive is a written document some patients use to state what care they want to receive, or refuse, should they become unable to express their wishes in the future. A living will is a type of advance directive that is becoming common. It is a written document that describes the kind of life-sustaining treatment that a patient wants (or does not want) if the patient later becomes unable to request, consent to, or refuse that treatment. The patient identifies how long and how extensive any resuscitative effort should be. The directive could indicate only compassionate care (accepting only nourishment, water, and possibly pain relief) or basic life support only be provided, or may indicate that every possible advanced procedure available be performed. The directive might also request several resuscitative attempts, one attempt only, or no attempts at all.

Life-sustaining treatment is an important phrase. It means that the living will applies only in life-threatening circumstances. In all other cases in which injuries or illnesses are less severe, appropriate care must be given when there is expressed or implied consent. For example, a patient's statement requesting no extraordinary life-saving efforts if diagnosed with terminal cancer doesn't mean a refusal of treatment for a broken arm.

Do Not Resuscitate (DNR) orders are another type of advance directive. They are written by the patient's physician, usually at the patient's request, stating that no (or very few) life-saving measures are to be taken if the patient experiences cardiac arrest (Fig. 3-3, A and B).

These orders are most commonly found in situations involving terminally ill patients being cared for at home or at long-term care facilities such as hospices or nursing homes. Because of issues concerning prolonged suffering, quality of life, and the cost of providing care for a loved one in a terminal and irreversible state, many patients are requesting that limited or no resuscitative efforts be performed.

An important consideration is that, although a written DNR order may exist, it may not be present at the scene. It may be kept on file at the patient's hospital or at the physician's office. Some patients and physicians provide copies of their orders to the local ambulance service so that responding crews can be given this information when they are dispatched. However, if you face a situation where you are informed of a DNR request but the physician's order cannot be produced, then there is little choice but to begin CPR or other life-saving measures. Consult with medical direction if you encounter a situation such as this.

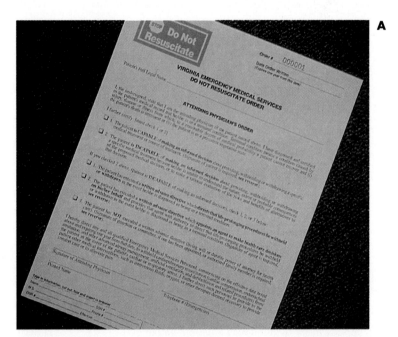

A

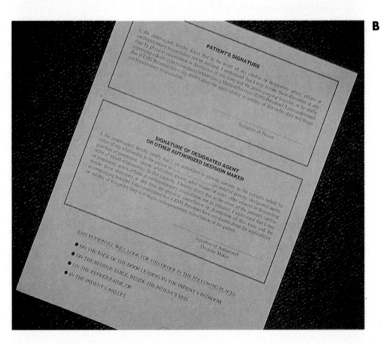

B

Fig. 3-3 Example of a Do Not Resuscitate (DNR) order. **A,** Front of form. **B,** Back of form.

Some states do not regulate emergency personnel in regard to DNR orders, living wills, or advance directives. In fact, in some states, DNR orders are considered beyond the First Responder's scope of care, leaving no choice but to start resuscitative efforts in these situations. You must therefore learn about any state and local laws or protocols that govern your actions regarding DNR orders, living wills, and advance directives.

REFUSALS

Competent adult patients have the right to refuse medical care. First Responders and other healthcare professionals have to be careful about refusals to avoid situations in which the First

---

REVIEW QUESTIONS

Competence and Consent

1. _____ is the ability for the patient to understand the reason why a First Responder or other health care professional may be at a scene and attempting to provide medical care.

2. It is not essential for the First Responder to determine if the responsive adult patient is competent prior to providing care. True or False?

3. List three reasons why a patient would be considered incompetent:

   _____

   _____

   _____

4. Competent adult patients have the right to refuse care. True or False?

5. The two most common forms of consent are _____ and _____.

6. Who must give consent to provide care for a child patient? _____ or _____.

7. When an advance directive is not present, what should you do for the patient?

   _____

1. Competence; 2. False; 3. Ingestion of drugs, intoxication, patient who has sustained serious injury, or patients who are mentally incompetent; 4. True; 5. Expressed and implied; 6. Parent or legal guardian; 7. Begin life saving measures

---

Responder abandons the patient by not providing or continuing care, or in which the patient accuses the First Responder of assault or battery.

RIGHT TO REFUSE

Adult patients who are of sound mind and who understand the consequences of their actions, even though injured or ill, have the legal right of refusal. Treating patients against their will may lead to charges of assault or battery being filed against you. Transporting patients against their will may even be interpreted as kidnapping.

The First Responder should never make an independent decision not to provide care to a patient. This is a very dangerous precedent for a First Responder to make. If you have responded to a scene and a patient is identified, you should determine the competence of the patient, begin to evaluate their medical condition, and provide appropriate care. Additional help should also be en route to the scene, or you should request additional medical help. You should never make an independent decision that the patient is not in need of medical care. Other health professionals in the system with significantly more knowledge and skills should assist in the decision not to provide care. It will be less likely for legal problems to occur from providing care to a patient, rather than from making an inappropriate decision and not providing care for a patient in need.

The patient also has the right to terminate treatment at any time after it has begun. For example, two First Responders find an adult male who has experienced a sudden and unexpected loss of consciousness at a fire scene. They begin to treat the patient under the conditions of implied consent. After a few moments, the patient regains consciousness and refuses further treatment and transportation to the hospital. He is an adult, and the only thing that has changed is that he is now responsive. As long as he is of sound mind (he understands what has happened and can make rational decisions about his current situation), he has the right to refuse any further care.

However, to avoid liability for negligence, the First Responders in this situation should not simply pack up and leave at the patient's first refusal of treatment. They should first try to persuade the patient to at least go to the hospital for further evaluation of the injury or illness, even if he doesn't want to be treated by them immediately.

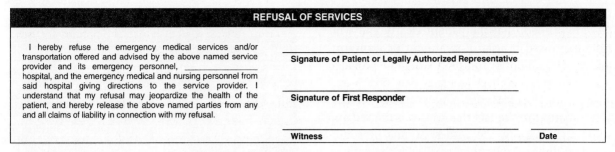

REFUSAL OF SERVICES

I hereby refuse the emergency medical services and/or transportation offered and advised by the above named service provider and its emergency personnel, _____ hospital, and the emergency medical and nursing personnel from said hospital giving directions to the service provider. I understand that my refusal may jeopardize the health of the patient, and hereby release the above named parties from any and all claims of liability in connection with my refusal.

Signature of Patient or Legally Authorized Representative

Signature of First Responder

Witness   Date

Fig. 3-4 A sample "release from liability" form.

The First Responders also must inform the patient of the potential risks and consequences of refusing further treatment or transport. In other words, a refusal of treatment must also be informed and expressed, just the same as a consent to treatment. In this situation, the First Responders must explain the potential seriousness of a sudden loss of consciousness and explain to the patient why medical evaluation is needed to find the underlying cause. Because the patient experienced unconsciousness without warning once, it could happen again, and the consequences could be life-threatening to the patient and to others.

The First Responders must be sure that the patient is not suffering from a mental impairment, either temporary (induced by drugs, alcohol, or the current injury or illness) or permanent (such as a mental illness), that prevents making a rational, informed decision. An impaired patient can be treated under implied consent, but unimpaired patients have the right to refuse treatment.

If the patient is mentally competent and still refuses treatment even though it is clearly needed, the First Responders should consult with a medical direction physician. This physician may be able to suggest alternatives or may talk directly with the patient to try to gain cooperation. It may also be appropriate to call for law enforcement personnel. However, police have little recourse unless the patient intends to do harm to self or another or unless the patient truly does have some type of mental impairment. In any case, the decision not to transport a patient is made in consultation with other EMS personnel. First Responders can also try to persuade the patient to allow the EMS personnel en route to perform an evaluation.

At this point, if the patient has sound judgment and still refuses treatment or transport, you must thoroughly document all assessment findings, any care that you gave, and the facts related to the

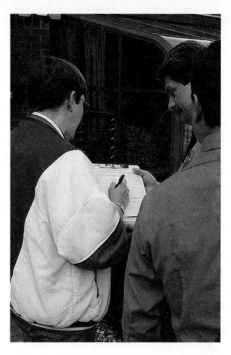

Fig. 3-5 Have a patient sign the "release from liability" form if the patient meets the criteria for sound judgement but still refuses care.

FIRST RESPONDER ALERT

Merely having a patient's signature on a refusal of treatment form does not relieve you from liability. Thorough supporting documentation is crucial. Your documentation in such cases may be the deciding factor as to whether you get into, or keep out of, court.

patient's refusal of treatment or transport. Then, the patient signs a "release from liability" form (Fig. 3-4). The form explains that, after being evaluated for a potential medical emergency, the patient refused the offered treatment against the better judgment of the First Responder. Also document that the potential consequences of refusal of care were explained, that the patient clearly and willfully expressed refusal of treatment or transport, and that treatment or transport would be provided if the patient called back at a later date (Fig. 3-5).

Try to have at least one witness sign the refusal form to attest to the fact that care was offered and refused. Preferably, the witness should be someone not affiliated with your service or the patient, such as a police officer, neighbor, or bystander. Documenting the witness's address, phone number, and reason for being there is important also in the event questions arise later.

Just as the patient has the right to refuse care, the patient also cannot be made to sign the refusal form. Having a witness sign the form attesting to that fact is even more important in this situation.

Finally, if the patient has a life-threatening condition and you have any doubt about the patient's ability to understand the risks of the refusal or about the soundness of the patient's judgment, you should provide care. It is worse to be sued for wrongful death resulting from gross negligence than for giving care without consent.

ASSAULT/BATTERY

Assault occurs when someone threatens or attempts offensive physical contact with another person, or makes another person fear such contact. Battery occurs when a person is touched offensively without consent. These definitions vary from state to state, so be sure to know your local laws.

Consent means all people have a legal right to determine what happens to their body. Assault and battery go against this right. That is why adults who are of sound mind and have a full understanding of the consequences of their actions, even though injured or ill, have the legal right to refuse treatment.

If you defy the patient's wishes in such circumstances and try to give treatment (even by simply laying a hand on the patient, as in taking a pulse), you may be found guilty of battery. You may be found guilty of assault even if you only cause the patient fear at the thought of being touched or treated after refusing care. For example, if you are a firefighter First Responder, saying something like, "If you don't let us splint your broken arm, we'll call the police and they'll come and hold you down so that we can," could certainly make a patient apprehensive about

> ### FIRST RESPONDER ALERT
>
> Once you accept responsibility for taking action (beginning care, stopping at a scene, or even taking the call from the dispatch center), an implied contract to provide service is established between you and the patient. Failure to provide or continue service could cause the patient harm and may potentially lead to a lawsuit for negligence against you.

being treated and could therefore be considered assault.

There may be situations when the patient is not able to make a rational decision about allowing someone to provide care to them, such as if the patient is intoxicated, has ingested drugs, or is mentally incompetent. It is assumed that the prudent individual would want care to be provided. Children may also refuse care; however, if the parent or legal guardian is present, they may direct you to provide care.

ABANDONMENT

Abandonment occurs when care is discontinued without the patient's consent and without ensuring that care is being continued at the same or a higher level. Once you begin care, you must not stop until a person of equal or greater training assumes responsibility for the patient. For example, you cannot turn patient care over to a bystander nor can you leave the scene of an accident once you start to provide patient care, except in the following situations:

- You relinquish care to someone with equal or greater qualifications
- Your personal safety is threatened by uncontrolled hazards at the scene
- The patient no longer needs or wants your services

NEGLIGENCE

In any of the previous examples, if a formal or implied contract existed and if the service or First Responder failed to follow through on it, then there was a failure to act. This could lead to charges of negligence.

Negligence occurs when a patient suffers damage or injury because a First Responder fails to perform at the accepted standard of care. The judgment of the First Responder's performance is based on what any other First Responder with similar education and experience would have done under similar circumstances.

Before negligence can be proven, four criteria must be met:

1. There was a duty to act. Duty to act means that, as a First Responder, you had the responsibility to provide services.
2. There was a breach of duty. You failed to act, or failed to provide the level of service that

another First Responder of equal education and experience would have provided in a similar situation.
3. Damage occurred. That is, the patient suffered some physical or psychological injury.
4. There was proximate cause. This means that the physical or psychological injury that the patient suffered was caused by your actions or inactions.

Again, all four of these criteria must be met. In other words: if you did not have a duty to act,

---

BOX 3-1 Criteria for Negligence

Duty to Act

In the simplest of terms, duty to act means that you, as a First Responder, have a legal responsibility to provide emergency medical care when called upon or presented with the opportunity to do so.

Duty to act is complex because it can involve either a legal or contractual obligation, which may be either formal or implied.

A formal obligation exists, for example, when a police or fire service has a written contract with a municipality to provide service. Specific clauses in the contract identify when and to what degree service will be provided, and when service can be refused.

An implied contract is not likely to be written, but is just as binding. For example, in the opening story of this chapter, an informal contract was established when the bystander called 9-1-1 on behalf of Tory's mother. The caller gave the 9-1-1 dispatcher the information about Tory's accident, and the dispatcher told the caller that an ambulance and First Responder police officers would be sent. In other words, a call for help was accepted and help was promised as soon as possible; a contract had been made, even if it was only implied.

In some states you will be "licensed," while in others you will be "certified." In either case, the implication is that you are educated and able to provide appropriate care and will do so when the need arises. In other words, all First Responders have met some minimum educational requirement. As a result of this education, First Responders may have an implied duty to act merely by being "licensed" or "certified." However, the laws pertaining to duty to act vary widely from state to state. Check with your ambulance service and local, regional, or state EMS agencies to determine when you have a duty to act.

In addition to the legal duty to act, First Responders must consider the moral or ethical obligation to help care for an ill or injured person when requested to.

Breach of Duty

Breach of duty occurs when you fail to act or fail to act appropriately. If you are on duty in a voluntary or career system, you are obligated to respond to requests for help. You should be careful how you respond to a call for help, remember the goal is to arrive at the scene safely without injuring yourself or others. Once at the scene, you are obligated to act in a safe and appropriate manner. Do not assume that others at the scene are providing care for the patient or are capable of providing care for the patient. If you are identified as the First Responder, you must perform to that level of training.

Injury or Damages

Injury or damage can be physical or psychological. In order for negligence to be proven, there must be some form of damage that occurred to the patient. A physical injury may occur if a patient is treated inappropriately; psychological damage if the patient's needs and wishes are not respected.

Proximate Cause

Finally, your actions or lack of actions caused the patient injury or damage. If it can be proven that your actions or lack of actions caused the injury or damage, the four components needed to prove negligence are met. Therefore, be careful in how you care for a patient.

there was no negligence; if you did act and you acted appropriately, there was no negligence; if the patient did not suffer an injury (either physical or psychological), there was no negligence; and finally, even if the patient did suffer a physical or psychological injury, if it was not as a result of your actions or inactions, there was no negligence. Box 3-1 reviews each of the four components of negligence.

PATIENT CONFIDENTIALITY

Confidentiality comes from the word confide. To confide in someone means to entrust that person with something. When receiving treatment, patients entrust First Responders with their lives, possessions, personal information, and privacy.

CONFIDENTIAL INFORMATION

You will learn a significant amount of personal information from patients in the course of assessing them and providing care. The patient's age, past and recent medical history, and personal information obtained during the physical examination are confidential. Treatments given also become confidential information.

Like everyone else, the patient has a right to privacy. All of the information stated above is considered the property of the patient. No one but the patient has the right to share this information with others.

The patient usually must sign a written release form before any personal information can be given out. You must not speak to friends, family, the media, or anyone else about the details of a call, including the patient's name, the injury or illness, what the patient said or did, what care was provided or refused, or where the patient was transported.

RELEASING CONFIDENTIAL INFORMATION

In certain situations, a signed release form is not required for you to share patient information with others. Some examples are:

1. When patients are delivered to other healthcare providers, you must relay information about them and their conditions and treatments to provide a complete transfer of care (such as reporting to an EMT or paramedic when a patient is transferred to the ambulance).

REVIEW QUESTIONS

Refusals

1. A First Responder should never make an independent decision not to provide care to a patient. True or False?

2. A patient has the right to _____ treatment at any time after it has begun.

3. If the patient has a life-threatening condition and you have any doubt about the patient's ability to understand the risks of the refusal or about the soundness of the patient's judgement, you should _____ _____.

4. In general, assault occurs when someone threatens or attempts offensive physical contact with another person, or makes another person fear such contact. True or False?

5. If you defy the patient's wishes in such circumstances and try to give treatment (even by simply laying a hand on the patient, as in taking a pulse), you may be found guilty of _____.

6. Abandonment occurs when care is discontinued without the patient's consent and without ensuring that care is being continued at the same or a higher level. True or False?

7. List the four criteria that must be present for a First Responder to be guilty of negligence:

   _____
   _____
   _____
   _____

8. _____ _____ _____ means that you, as a First Responder, have a legal responsibility to provide emergency medical care when called upon or presented with the opportunity to do so.

9. Negligence occurs when a patient suffers damage or injury because a First Responder fails to perform at the accepted standard of care. True or False?

1. True; 2. Terminate (stop); 3. Provide care; 4. True; 5. Battery; 6. True; 7. Duty to act, breach of duty, damage and proximate cause; 8. Duty to act; 9. True

2. Certain incidents require notifying law enforcement, and you must provide appropriate information in those situations. A police report may be required for industrial accidents, animal bites, rape, suspected child abuse, assault, or gunshot wounds. Because reporting regulations vary from state to state, check with your local law enforcement agency to find out what incidents must be reported.

3. First Responders can be subpoenaed for information. A subpoena is a legal document from a court requiring information or an action. In such a case you must honor the subpoena or face the consequences for refusing to follow a court order.

In any other situation, the patient must sign a release before confidential information can be released. If anyone requests confidential information, they must have the request authorized in writing before a First Responder can honor such a request.

SPECIAL SITUATIONS

MEDICAL IDENTIFICATION INSIGNIA

When assessing a patient or giving care, you may come across a medical condition identification insignia on a necklace, bracelet, or even ankle bracelet. Its purpose is to inform healthcare providers of the wearer's medical condition in case the person is unresponsive or cannot communicate directly (Fig. 3-6). Patients wear such devices because they have a potentially serious medical condition such as diabetes, severe allergies, epilepsy, or asthma that requires rapid intervention. A caduceus is sometimes engraved on one side and the patient's medical problem on the other. There may also be an identification number or telephone number for obtaining more information about the patient's medical condition.

Some patients carry a wallet card identifying their medical condition(s). Most patients carrying a wallet card also wear an insignia necklace or bracelet. If the insignia device suggests checking the wearer's wallet for additional information, then you should do so if you can retrieve the wallet without causing unnecessary movement or worsening of the patient's medical condition.

POTENTIAL CRIME SCENES

You may know that you are going to a crime scene when you are dispatched. In this case, police are probably already on the scene or being dispatched. Your first concern should be your own safety. Stand by at a safe location near the scene and wait for the police to arrive. After the police secure the scene, you can enter and begin to treat the patient.

If the police are already on the scene, check with them first to see if the scene has been secured. Enter the scene and treat the patient only after the scene is safe.

In some cases, you may not be aware that a violent crime has taken place until after you are already on the scene. If violence is still occurring or seems possible, call for police assistance immediately and take measures to ensure your own

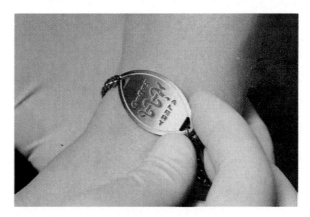

Fig. 3-6 The Medic-Alert® tag informs healthcare providers of the wearer's medical condition if the person is unresponsive or cannot communicate directly.

REVIEW QUESTIONS

Patient Confidentiality

1. Like everyone else, the patient has a right to
   _____.

2. The patient usually must sign a written release form before any personal information can be given out. True or False?

3. Name two or more of the situations when confidential information is allowed to be provided:

   _____

   _____

   _____

1. Privacy; 2. True; 3. Transfer of care, incidents requiring reporting, subpoena

safety, even if that means leaving without providing care. If you find it necessary to leave the scene without the patient, go to a safe location from which you can quickly return to the scene. Remain at this location of safety until police arrive to secure the scene, and then return to provide patient care when needed or called upon.

In any event, your primary concern, once the scene is safe and personal safety is assured, is to provide emergency medical care to the patient. Any time care is delayed in any of these situations, such as while awaiting police arrival or leaving the scene for safety reasons, be sure to document the reason for the delay and the event(s) that caused it.

If possible, try not to disturb anything at the scene unless absolutely necessary to provide patient care. Blood trails, the position of furniture, small items on the floor, and the location and position of the victim are all evidence and may provide clues about the crime. If something must be moved, try to remember its exact location, and tell the police.

If the victim has been shot or stabbed, try to avoid cutting, tearing, or otherwise damaging or destroying knife or bullet holes in the clothing. The clothing is an important piece of evidence, and the police can learn much about the crime and the perpetrator from the size, shape, and location of holes that are still intact.

Finally, pay close attention to what you see and hear in a possible crime scene, especially anything out of the ordinary. Include any observations in the prehospital care report. If you observe things that you do not include in the prehospital care report form because they do not involve patient care (for example, the patient's state of dress or the presence of money strewn about the scene), make additional documentation listing this other information. Most services have generic, special, or supplemental report forms for documentation of non-patient care issues and events. All this information is extremely important, particularly if the patient must be transported before the police arrive on scene. Your observations may be crucial pieces of information.

DOCUMENTATION

Fundamental medical documentation is essential to the First Responder. You are responsible for becoming familiar with state, local, and system

REVIEW QUESTIONS

Special Situations

1. When assessing a patient or giving care, you may come across a medical condition indentification insignia on a _____, _____, or _____ _____.

2. The purpose is to inform healthcare providers of the wearer's medical condition in case the person is unresponsive or cannot communicate directly. True or False?

3. Some patients carry a wallet card identifying their medical condition(s). Most patients carrying a wallet card also wear an insignia necklace or bracelet. True or False?

4. What should your first concern be for as you approach a potential crime scene?

   _____

5. What should you do if you arrive at a scene that has evidence of a crime scene?

   _____

6. If the victim has been shot or stabbed, try to avoid cutting, tearing, or otherwise damaging or destroying knife or bullet holes in the clothing. True or False?

1. Necklace, bracelet, or ankle bracelet; 2. True; 3. True; 4. Your own safety; 5. Contact the police; 6. True

requirements for appropriate documentation. Some systems have an established form for the First Responder to complete following every response. If so, you should obtain the necessary training to assure that you are able to complete the form in accordance to set standards.

You may encounter other unusual situations that require additional reports or notifications. Suspected child, elder, or spouse abuse commonly requires additional reporting. Crimes of violence such as a shooting, suicide, stabbing, or rape may also require additional reporting. These reports may be required by service policy or local or state law. In some states, First Responders can be found negligent for failing to notify law enforcement when there is suspicion of abuse.

Exposure to an infectious disease also requires a special report. This type of reporting enables tracking of both the patient and you for follow-up evaluations or treatments to ensure the health and welfare of both as well as that of the general public.

Because the requirements vary from service to service and state to state, you must check with your service and local law enforcement agency to determine exactly what situations require special reporting measures. Box 3-2 lists situations that commonly require special reporting.

CHAPTER SUMMARY

SCOPE OF CARE

First Responders have legal responsibilities to patients, the medical director, and the public at large. These responsibilities are identified by the First Responder's scope of care and the standard of care in the area.

First Responders provide care measures as outlined by the state's EMS legislation. That legislation identifies the scope of practice (i.e., the maximum and minimum performance guidelines for functioning). Any legal questions about a First Responder's actions are based on how those specific activities compare with the actions of any other First Responder with the same education and experience under similar conditions.

COMPETENCE AND CONSENT

There are three components that you should keep in mind when considering competence of a patient. The first component is understanding what competence means: the ability for a patient to understand. Second, you must be able to determine if the patient is competent. Remember, there are a variety of reasons that a person may not be competent. Finally, you need to realize the differences between those patients who are competent and not competent and make appropriate decisions as to how you will provide care. Consent can be either expressed or implied, depending on the patient's age and mental state.

Living wills and Do Not Resuscitate orders state what care a patient would like or would like to be withheld in the event they cannot make decisions for themselves.

REFUSALS

Adult patients who are of sound mind and understand the consequences of their actions have the legal right to refuse treatment or transport to a care facility, even when obviously ill or injured. First Responders who treat the patient without consent may be found guilty of battery for touching the patient against his or her will. Even if the First Responder only suggests that treatment will be provided and thereby instills some fear in the patient, assault could be charged.

You will be held accountable for the act of abandonment if you discontinue care without the patient's consent. You will also be held accountable for the act of abandonment if care is not continued for the patient by an individual of equal or higher medical certification.

REVIEW QUESTIONS

Documentation

1. Fundamental medical documentation is essential for higher levels of EMS personnel, such as EMT-Intermediates or paramedics, but not for First Responders. True or False?

2. You may encounter unusual situations that require additional reports or notifications. List three:

   _____

   _____

   _____

3. Exposure to an infectious disease does not need to be reported. True or False?

1. False; 2. Suspected child, elderly, spouse abuse; violence such as a shooting, suicide, stabbing or rape; animal bites; certain communicable diseases; 3. False

---

BOX 3-2 Cases Reportable Under Law in Most States

- Neglect or abuse of children
- Neglect or abuse of older adults
- Rape
- Gunshot wounds
- Stab wounds
- Animal bites
- Certain communicable diseases

Failure to provide care, or providing care incorrectly or inappropriately, may make First Responders liable for negligence. Starting but failing to follow through with care or to transfer care to another provider with equal or greater education may make a First Responder liable for abandonment.

CONFIDENTIALITY

There are a few instances when First Responders either may or must release confidential patient information; these are all related to line of duty events (transferral of the patient's care to another, for third-party billing purposes, or when subpoenaed). Other unusual situations may require First Responders to release confidential patient information. These situations depend on the nature or circumstances of the incident (child, elderly, spouse abuse; rape; shootings or stabbings; treating or transporting a patient without consent; exposure to infectious disease; etc.).

SPECIAL SITUATIONS

Medical condition identification insignia are designed to alert healthcare providers that the patient has a serious medical condition. They are usually readily visible and easily seen during the physical examination. Other patients may carry a wallet card with medical information listed on it in place of a necklace or bracelet, but usually this is carried in addition to a necklace or bracelet.

When dispatched to treat a patient who was injured as a result of a crime, a First Responder's first concern is for personal safety. If the scene is not secure and there are indications of personal danger, First Responders should take whatever measures are necessary to ensure their safety.

DOCUMENTATION

Documentation is essential to transfer information to the receiving facility. You must become familiar with state, local, and system requirements for appropriate documentation.

UNITED STATES DEPARTMENT OF TRANSPORTATION NATIONAL HIGHWAY TRAFFIC SAFETY ADMINISTRATION FIRST RESPONDER OBJECTIVES

Check your knowledge. The National Registry of EMTs and many state EMS agencies use the objectives below to develop First Responder certification examinations. Can you meet them?

COGNITIVE OBJECTIVES

1. Define the First Responder scope of care.
2. Discuss the importance of Do Not Resuscitate (DNR) [advance directives] and local or state provisions regarding EMS application.
3. Define consent and discuss the methods of obtaining consent.
4. Differentiate between expressed and implied consent.
5. Explain the role of consent of minors in providing care.
6. Discuss the implications for the First Responder in patient refusal of transport.
7. Discuss the issues of abandonment, negligence, and battery, and their implications to the First Responder.
8. State the conditions necessary for the First Responder to have a duty to act.
9. Explain the importance, necessity, and legality of patient confidentiality.
10. List the actions that a First Responder should take to assist in the preservation of a crime scene.
11. State the conditions that require a First Responder to notify local law enforcement officials.
12. Discuss issues concerning the fundamental components of documentation.

AFFECTIVE OBJECTIVES

13. Explain the rationale for the needs, benefits, and usage of advance directives.
14. Explain the rationale for the concept of varying degrees of DNR.

The Human Body

FOUR

KEY TERMS

Atria   The two upper chambers of the heart which function to receive blood and pump it to the ventricles.

Diaphragm   The large, dome-shaped muscle separating the thoracic and abdominal cavities; used in breathing.

Epiglottis   A leaflike flap that prevents food and liquid from entering the windpipe during swallowing.

Hormones   Chemicals that regulate body activities and functions.

Nasopharynx   The part of the pharynx that lies directly behind the nose.

Oropharynx   The part of the pharynx that is just behind the mouth and extends to the level of the epiglottis.

Perfusion   The process of circulating blood to the organs, delivering oxygen, and removing wastes.

Pharynx   A muscular tube commonly referred to as the throat.

Pulse points   A location where an artery passes close to the skin and over a bone, where the pressure wave of the heart contraction can be felt.

Ventricles   The two lower chambers of the heart that pump blood out of the heart.

FIRST RESPONSE

It was a quiet, North Carolina summer evening. Just as the sun was going down, Unit 44 approached the scene. A drunk driver struck a 14-year-old boy while he was riding his bike. Trooper Benfield saw that the boy was bleeding profusely from the wrist. With each beat of his heart, blood spurted from the wound. He feared that the young man had cut his radial artery and knew he had to stop the bleeding quickly. He put pressure on the injury and remembered that the brachial artery was the major artery supplying the arm. He put pressure on the inside of the upper arm and the bleeding slowed. The responding EMS crew said that his quick thinking probably saved the boy's life.

The driver was shaken up, but uninjured. He barely remembered the accident after he sobered up and was convicted of driving under the influence. The young man was riding his bike again three days later.

The human body is the envy of modern engineering. An engineer has yet to come close to creating anything as well designed and constructed. Although no body system functions independently, the complexity of the human body can be better understood by considering its separate parts. A body system is a group of organs that work together to perform a function. Although each body system is described in the following sections as an independent component, they are all interconnected.

THE RESPIRATORY SYSTEM

The respiratory system plays a crucial role in the delicate balance of life. The body is composed of trillions of cells that need oxygen to convert food into energy. This process gives off carbon dioxide as a waste product. The respiratory system takes oxygen from the air and makes it available for the blood to transport to every cell and rids the body of excess carbon dioxide.

THE AIRWAY

Air enters and exits the respiratory system through the mouth and the nose. These two structures play an important role in warming, cleaning, and humidifying inhaled air. The **pharynx** is a muscular tube commonly referred to as the throat.

The pharynx is divided into two areas: the **nasopharynx** and the **oropharynx**. The nasopharynx lies directly behind the nose. The oropharynx is just behind the mouth and extends to the level of the epiglottis. The **epiglottis** is a leaflike flap that prevents food and liquid from entering the windpipe (trachea) during swallowing. The pharynx is a common pathway for both food and air. Because air and food pass through the pharynx, it is often the location of airway obstructions by foreign bodies. Figure 4-1 shows the upper airway.

Just below the epiglottis is the opening to the windpipe. The voice box (larynx) is just below this opening. The vocal cords are bands of cartilage that vibrate when we speak.

THE LUNGS

The windpipe extends from the voicebox and is the common pathway for the air that enters the lungs. The trachea splits into two branches, each leading to one lung. These branches subdivide into smaller and smaller air passages until they end at the microscopic air sacs of the lungs. These air sacs are only one cell thick and are surrounded by capillaries. This is where gas exchange actually occurs (Fig. 4-2).

The process of ventilating the lungs with a constant supply of fresh air uses two sets of muscles: the **diaphragm** and the muscles between the ribs (intercostal muscles). The diaphragm is the large, dome-shaped muscle separating the thoracic and abdominal cavities. When the diaphragm contracts, the dome of the diaphragm flattens and lowers.

Contraction of the intercostal muscles (the muscles between the ribs) causes them to move upward and outward. Inhalation begins with the contraction of the diaphragm and the intercostal

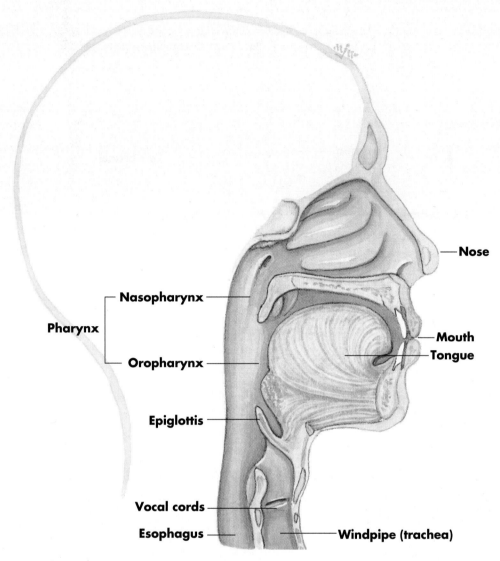

Nose

Nasopharynx

Pharynx

Mouth

Tongue

Oropharynx

Epiglottis

Vocal cords

Esophagus

Windpipe (trachea)

Fig. 4-1 The upper airway.

muscles. This increases the size of the chest, and air is pulled into the lungs through the mouth and nose, much like pulling the plunger back on a syringe. Inhalation is an active process resulting from muscle contraction, and therefore the muscles must act for inhalation to occur (Fig. 4-3A). The exchange of oxygen for carbon dioxide occurs, and then you exhale.

Exhalation begins with the relaxation of the intercostal muscles and the diaphragm. As these muscles relax and return to their resting position, the size of the chest decreases and air rushes out through the mouth and nose. Normally, exhalation is a passive process, and therefore, muscle action is not needed for exhalation to occur (Fig. 4-3B). In some cases of disease or obstructions, exhalation becomes an active process. A cough is also an example of a forced exhalation.

Gas exchange

There are two sites for the exchange of oxygen and carbon dioxide: the lungs and the tissues. During inhalation, air is drawn into the lungs. Normally, air contains 21% oxygen and almost no carbon dioxide. As this oxygen-rich air enters the lungs, blood with low levels of oxygen and high levels of carbon dioxide flows through the capillaries in the lungs. Oxygen enters the blood and carbon dioxide is removed (Fig. 4-4).

The oxygenated blood is then pumped by the heart to the rest of the body. As this oxygen-rich blood approaches its destination, the blood vessels decrease in size until they branch into thin-walled capillaries. The blood in the capillaries is highly oxygenated and low in carbon dioxide. However, the tissue is low in oxygen and high in carbon dioxide. The capillaries give up oxygen to the cells, and the

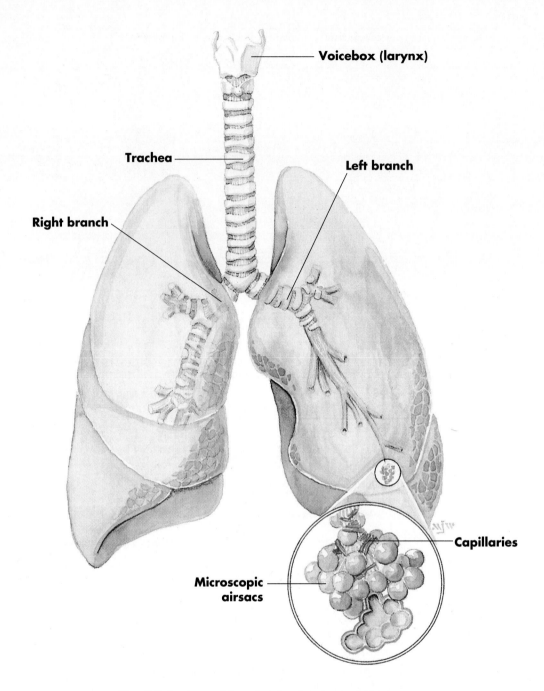

Voicebox (larynx)

Trachea

Left branch

Right branch

Capillaries

Microscopic airsacs

Fig. 4-2 Anatomy of the windpipe (trachea) and lungs.

cells give carbon dioxide to the blood in the capillaries (Fig. 4-5). The blood is then collected in the veins and returned to the lungs for re-oxygenation.

THE RESPIRATORY SYSTEM OF INFANTS AND CHILDREN

Infants and children are not just small adults. There are considerable differences between pediatric and adult patients. The most obvious difference in the respiratory system is the smaller size of the airway structures. The smaller diameter of the airway makes obstructions much more common in young patients. Airway obstructions can occur when foreign bodies are lodged in the trachea or with even a small amount of swelling of the airway.

Two factors combine to make infant's and children's airways more easily obstructed. First, the tongue is much larger in proportion to the size of

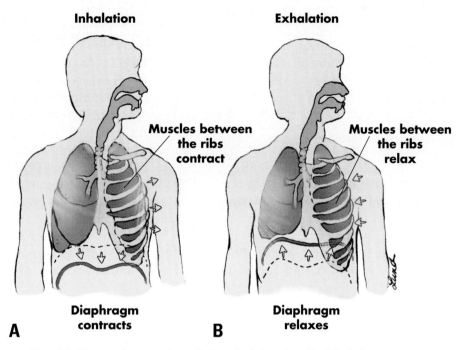

Fig. 4-3 The mechanics of ventilation. **A.** Inhalation. **B.** Exhalation

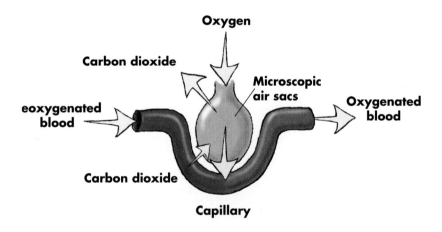

Fig. 4-4 Gas exchange in the lungs.

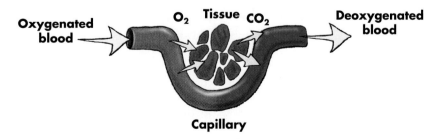

Fig. 4-5 Gas exchange in a cell.

the mouth in infants and children. Second, the younger the patient, the softer the trachea. Because of these factors, the airway can be more easily obstructed. The most common cause of cardiac arrest in infants and children is uncorrected respiratory problems.

THE CIRCULATORY SYSTEM

In the growing fetus, the heart begins to pump in the 4th week of development and, on average, will keep beating continuously for the next 75 years. Contracting over 100,000 times a day, the heart is a marvel of endurance and reliability. The heart pumps blood containing oxygen and nutrients to the body's organs through the circulatory system. The exchange of oxygen and nutrients for waste products occurs in the smallest vessels of the circulatory system. This process is so vital to life that any interruption for more than a few minutes can mean death to the individual.

THE HEART

The heart is a pump consisting of four chambers. The two upper chambers are called the **atria**, which function to receive blood and pump it to the lower chambers of the heart. The two lower chambers are the **ventricles**, which pump blood out of the heart. Because of one-way valves between the chambers, heart contractions move blood in only one direction.

The left ventricle pumps blood rich in oxygen to the body to be used by the cells. After the oxygen is used, blood is returned from the veins of the body into the right atrium, which pumps it to the right ventricle. The right ventricle pumps this oxygen-poor blood to the lungs for oxygenation. The oxygen-rich blood is returned into the left atrium. The left atrium pumps blood to the left ventricle, and the circuit starts all over again (Fig. 4-6).

The heart has specialized cells that generate electrical impulses and serve as the heart's pacemaker. Electrical signals are carried through the

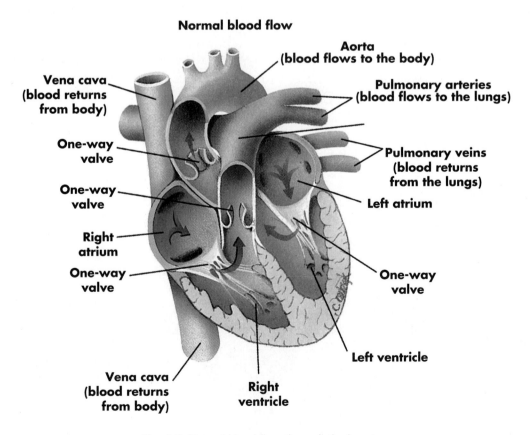

Normal blood flow

Vena cava
(blood returns
from body)

One-way
valve

One-way
valve

Right
atrium

One-way
valve

Vena cava
(blood returns
from body)

Right
ventricle

Aorta
(blood flows to the body)

Pulmonary arteries
(blood flows to the lungs)

Pulmonary veins
(blood returns
from the lungs)

Left atrium

One-way
valve

Left ventricle

Fig. 4-6 Normal blood flow through the heart.

heart by conductive tissue. These signals give the heart the amazing ability to beat on its own. The number of times the heart beats per minute is the heart rate, which varies with age, physical condition, situation, and a number of other factors.

BLOOD VESSELS

Blood vessels are the "pipes" of the body. These vessels carry blood to every organ. Arteries carry blood away from the heart. The major artery of the body is the aorta, which is a vessel

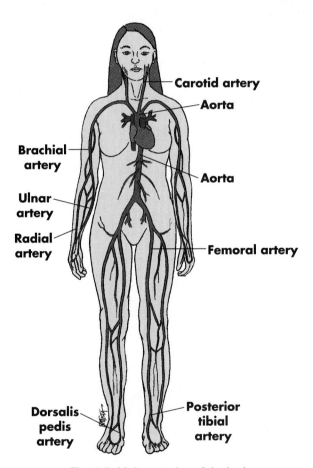

Fig. 4-7 Major arteries of the body.

approximately the diameter of your thumb. It originates from the base of the heart and arches in front of the spine, then descends through the chest and abdomen. The carotid artery is the major artery of the neck, and pulsations can be palpated on either side of the neck. The femoral artery is the major artery of the thigh, and pulsations can be palpated in the groin. The radial artery is the artery of the lower arm, and pulsations can be palpated on the thumb side of the wrist. The brachial artery is the artery of the upper arm, and can be palpated on the inside of the arm between the elbow and the shoulder. Figure 4-7 shows the location of the major arteries in the body.

Arteries branch as they get further away from the heart and eventually lead to capillaries, which are the smallest blood vessels in the body. Capillaries are tiny blood vessels that connect arteries to veins. The exchange of oxygen and nutrients for carbon dioxide and other wastes occurs in the thin-walled capillaries (Fig. 4-8). The capillaries are microscopic structures, only about one twenty-fifth of an inch in length and just one cell thick, but they are present in astronomical numbers everywhere in the body. If all of the capillaries in your body were placed end to end, they would extend for 62,000 miles!

Many capillaries join together to form veins, which return the oxygen-poor blood back to the heart. Figure 4-9 shows the location of the major veins of the body.

THE BLOOD

An average-sized adult man has about 5 to 6 liters of blood circulating in the body. This complex fluid serves many functions and contains many components. One of the main functions of the blood is to deliver oxygen and remove

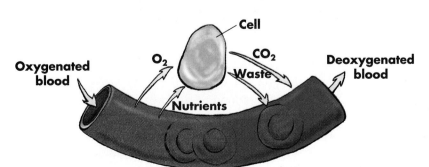

Fig. 4-8 The exchange of gases, nutrients, and wastes between tissue cells and capillary blood.

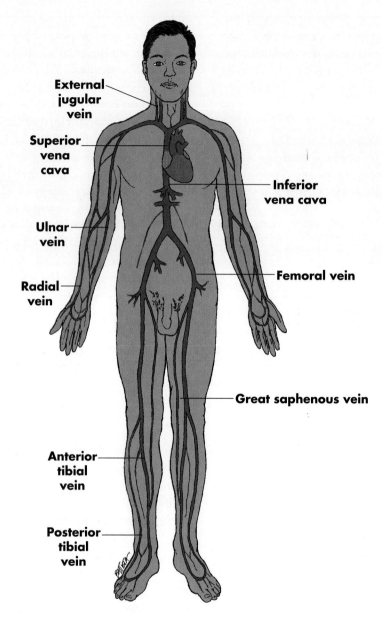

External
jugular
vein

Superior
vena
cava

Inferior
vena cava

Ulnar
vein

Femoral vein

Radial
vein

Great saphenous vein

Anterior
tibial
vein

Posterior
tibial
vein

Fig. 4-9 Major veins of the body.

carbon dioxide. Blood also plays an important role in clotting and in the body's defense against infection.

THE CIRCULATION OF BLOOD

As the left ventricle contracts, pumping blood to the body, a wave of pressure is sent through the arteries. This pressure wave can be felt anywhere an artery passes close to the skin and over a bone. These locations are called pulse points and occur both in the extremities and near the trunk. The most common pulse points of the

body are the carotid, femoral, radial, and the brachial (Fig. 4-10).

For the cells of the body to function properly, they must have a continuous supply of oxygenated blood. This supply requires adequate pressure in the heart and vessels to circulate the blood to all parts of the body. The process of circulating blood to the organs, delivering oxygen, and removing wastes is called perfusion. When perfusion is inadequate, a state known as shock develops. Shock is a widespread decrease of perfusion and is also known as hypoperfusion.

REVIEW QUESTIONS

The Respiratory and Circulatory Systems

1. What are the two main muscles of respiration?

   _____

   _____

2. Inhalation is an (active or inactive) process, while exhalation is an (active or inactive) process.

3. Where is blood re-oxygenated and carbon dioxide removed?

   _____

4. Which of the following is NOT a characteristic of the respiratory system of infants and children:
   A. Proportionally larger tongue
   B. Slower respiratory rates
   C. Smaller airway structures
   D. Softer trachea

5. Place the following in order of blood flow from the right atrium:
   A. left ventricle _____
   B. lungs _____
   C. left atrium _____
   D. body _____
   E. right ventricle _____

6. Blood carries oxygen to the _____ and carbon dioxide to the _____ for removal.

   6. Tissues, lungs
   2. Active, inactive; 3. The lungs; 4. B; 5. E, B, C, A, D;
   1. The diaphragm and the muscles between the ribs;

THE MUSCULOSKELETAL SYSTEM

THE SKELETAL SYSTEM

The skeletal system is the scaffolding of the body. Not only do bones give the body shape and rigidity, but they also protect the vital internal organs. For example, the skull completely surrounds the delicate brain and protects it from everyday bumps and bruises. The ribs, breastbone (sternum), and spinal column play important roles in protecting the heart and other important organs from damage.

Along with muscles, bones also serve as attachment points to enable the body to move. The

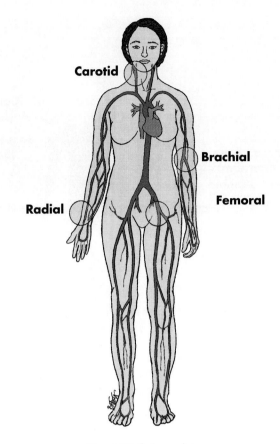

Fig. 4-10 Pulse points.

skeleton creates levers and fulcrums throughout the body. The contracting of muscles moves these levers with incredible precision. Figure 4-11 shows the major bones of the body.

The head, spinal column, and thorax

The skull houses the brain and forms the face. The brain is the most important organ in the human body and is protected by the rigid bones of the skull. The spinal column extends from the base of the skull to the pelvis and consists of 33 small bones (Fig. 4-12). The bones in the neck and back each have a vertical hole in them and stack on top of each other. The holes line up to create a tube for the spinal cord. If one of these bones becomes misaligned or damaged, it can cause permanent damage to the spinal cord.

The bones of the spinal column in the upper back serve as a point of attachment for the 12 pairs of ribs. The first ten pairs of ribs are attached in front to the breastbone (sternum). The 11th and 12th ribs are the floating ribs, so called because they simply extend from the spinal column. The floating ribs

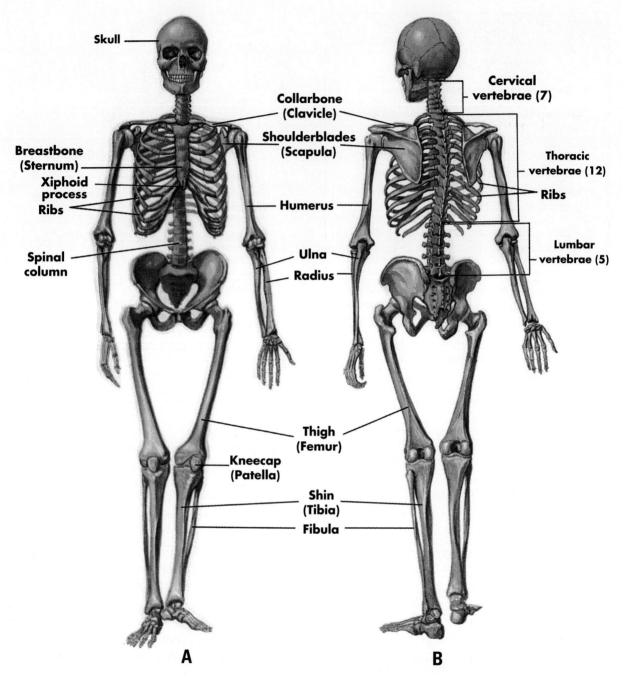

Fig. 4-11 A and B The skeletal system.

help protect the kidneys. The attached ribs provide protection to all of the organs in the chest and assist in breathing.

The thorax consists of the ribs and the breastbone (sternum). At the very end of the sternum is the xiphoid process. The xiphoid process is an important landmark when performing chest compressions during CPR. The xiphoid process is sharp and delicate and can cause damage to internal organs (such as the liver) if your hand placement is incorrect.

The pelvis and lower extremities

The spinal column forms the back of the pelvis. Fused bones create the remainder of the pelvis, which serves as an attachment point for the legs at the socket for the hip joint.

The femur is the long bone of the thigh. One end of the femur fits into the hip joint and allows the leg to move easily. The other end meets the bones of the lower leg at the knee. The kneecap (patella) protects you from injury if you fall directly onto your knee.

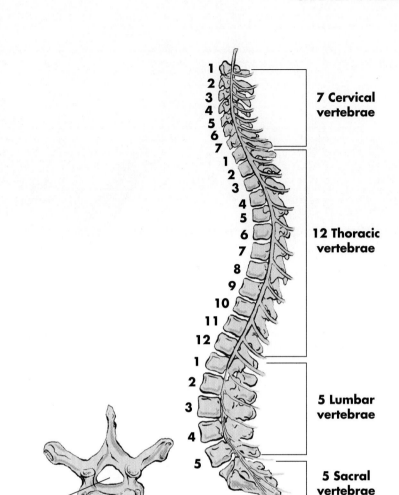

1
2
3
4
5
6
7

7 Cervical vertebrae

1
2
3
4
5
6
7
8
9
10
11
12

12 Thoracic vertebrae

1
2
3
4
5

5 Lumbar vertebrae

5 Sacral vertebrae

Fused coccyx

Hole for spinal cord

A

B

Fig. 4-12 The spinal column is comprised of 33 vertebrae. **A** single vertebrae. **B** The spinal column.

The lower leg has two bones. The shin (tibia) is the main weight-bearing bone of the lower leg. The fibula does not bear weight but assists in the movement of the ankle. Small bones provide structure to the heel, feet, and toes (Fig. 4-13).

The upper extremities

The arms join the trunk at the shoulder, which consists of the collar bone (clavicle) and the shoulder blade (scapula). The humerus is the bone of the upper arm. The forearm is made up of the radius and the ulna. Small bones make up the wrist, hand, and fingers. These small bones enable the hand and wrist to move in many intricate positions (Fig. 4-14).

Joints

A joint is a place where bones come together. Joints serve many functions, but most importantly, they provide a system of fulcrums and levers that make movement of the body possible.

THE MUSCULAR SYSTEM

No movement in the body could occur without muscles. Every physical activity, from riding a bike to turning the pages of this book, occurs with the contraction of muscles. Additionally, muscles protect vital organs and help give the body shape.

There are three types of muscles found in the human body: skeletal, smooth, and cardiac. All three types of muscle have the unique ability to contract (shorten) (Fig. 4-15).

Skeletal muscles

As the name implies, these muscles are attached to bones. When these muscles shorten, they provide the force to move the levers of the skeletal system, allowing the body to move (Fig. 4-16). Skeletal muscles make up the major muscle mass of the body. Weight lifters and athletes exercise to strengthen and develop skeletal muscles.

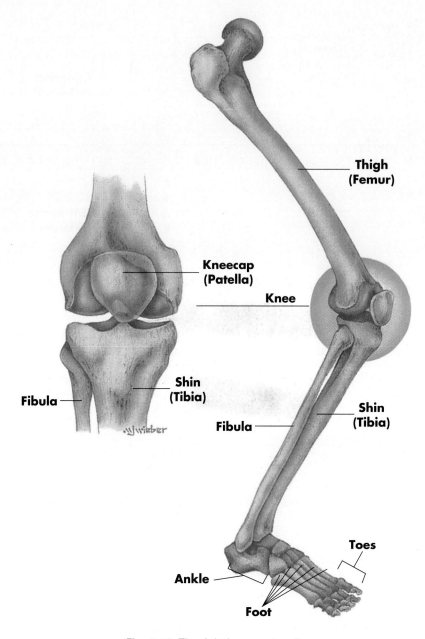

Fig. 4-13 The right lower extremity.

Tap your right foot three times. To accomplish this task, your brain sent a signal to the muscles in your calf to shorten, and your foot extended. Then your brain told your calf to relax and the muscles in the front of your lower leg to contract; this process was repeated twice more. Although you did not have to consciously think about each step, it was voluntary because you chose to do it. Therefore, skeletal muscles are called voluntary muscles.

Smooth muscles

These muscles are found in the walls of tubular structures in the gastrointestinal tract and the urinary system. Smooth muscles are also found in the blood vessels and the bronchi. Because they are circular, contraction changes the inside diameter of the tube (Fig. 4-17). This contraction is very important for controlling flow through the tubes of the body.

For instance, when you are cold, the body decreases blood flow to the arms and legs because significant body heat can be lost through the skin in these areas. The blood flow to the extremities is reduced by contracting the smooth muscles in the arteries that lead to the arms and legs.

You have no control over this process. Smooth muscles carry out many of the automatic muscular functions such as digestion, blood vessel control, and modifying the diameter of your airway.

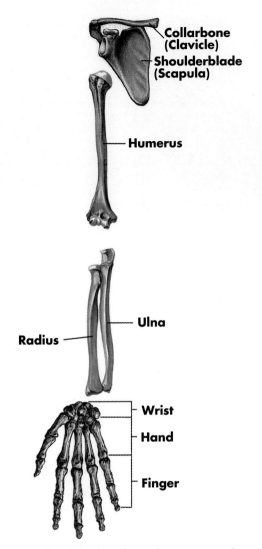

Fig. 4-14 The right shoulder and upper extremity.

Because no conscious thought is required for these activities, the smooth muscles are called involuntary muscles.

Cardiac muscle

The heart is the most important muscle in the body. The heart muscle has tremendous stamina. Imagine squeezing a tennis ball 60 times per minute. How long do you think that you could keep up with that pace? Certainly not 60 times per minute, 24 hours a day, just as the heart does.

To accomplish this amazing feat of stamina, the heart must have a continuous supply of blood. The heart has its own special arteries to deliver oxygen and nutrients to the heart muscle. Cholesterol in the bloodstream is deposited on the inside walls of these arteries. Eventually, these deposits can decrease blood flow to the heart. If the flow of blood is interrupted for more than a few minutes, part of the heart will be damaged. The damaged muscle causes the most common sign of a heart attack — chest pain.

Cardiac muscle is the only type of muscle that has the ability to contract on its own, and is found only in the heart. Because your heartbeat is not under conscious control, cardiac muscle is also involuntary muscle.

THE NERVOUS SYSTEM

The human nervous system is incredibly well developed and complex. It is the root of all

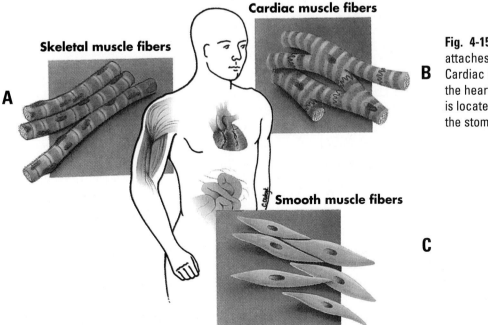

Fig. 4-15 **A,** Skeletal muscle attaches to the bone. **B,** Cardiac muscle is located in the heart. **C,** Smooth muscle is located in organs such as the stomach and intestine.

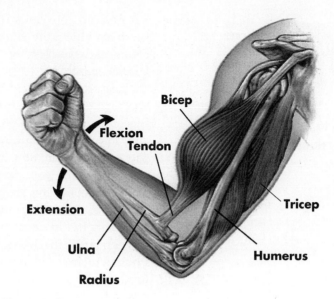

Fig. 4-16 Skeletal muscles provide the force to move the body.

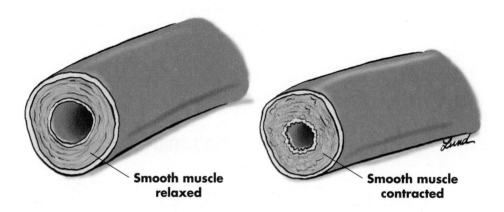

Fig. 4-17 Smooth muscles are found in the walls of some tubular structures and can contract or relax to change the diameter of the tube and thus affect flow through it.

thought, memory, and emotion. It also controls the voluntary and involuntary activities of the body. Anatomically, the nervous system has two components: the central nervous system and the peripheral nervous system (Fig. 4-18).

The central nervous system consists of the brain, which is located within the skull, and the spinal cord, which is located within the spinal column from the base of the skull to the lower back. The central nervous system is responsible for all higher mental functions, such as thought, decision making, and communication, and also has an important role in the regulation of body functions.

The peripheral nervous system consists of sensory and motor nerves that lie outside the skull or spinal cord. These nerves serve as wires, carrying information between the central nervous system and every organ and muscle in the body.

Sensory nerves carry information from the body to the central nervous system. They provide information about the environment, pain, pressure, and body position to the brain for decision making. Motor nerves carry information from the central nervous system to the body. Signals from the motor nerves cause contraction of skeletal muscles, which are responsible for all body movement (Fig. 4-19).

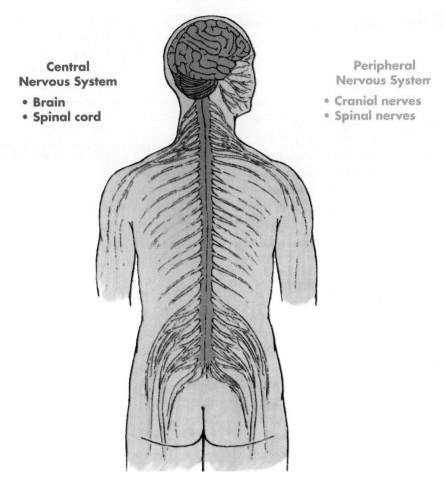

**Central
Nervous System**

• Brain
• Spinal cord

**Peripheral
Nervous System**

• Cranial nerves
• Spinal nerves

Fig. 4-18 The central nervous system consists of the brain and spinal cord. The peripheral nervous system consists of nerves that lie outside the skull and spinal cord.

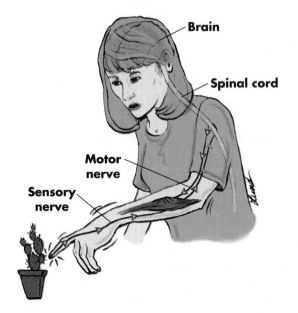

Brain

Spinal cord

Motor
nerve

Sensory
nerve

Fig. 4-19 Pain, such as pricking your finger, stimulates the sensory nerves, which carry the information to the brain. The brain then signals the motor nerves to withdraw your finger.

THE SKIN

Most people think of the skin as just a covering for the body. In reality it is a very important organ that performs many functions. The skin protects the body from the environment. Not only does it keep us from drying out, it also serves as a barrier to prevent invasion of the body by bacteria and other organisms.

The skin also plays a crucial role in temperature regulation. When you are too hot, the blood vessels dilate and the skin secretes sweat, which evaporates and cools the body. When you are cold, the blood vessels to the skin contract to decrease the heat loss to the environment.

Skin is also an important sensory organ. Special receptors in the skin can detect heat, cold, touch, pressure, and pain. Information from these receptors is transmitted to the central nervous system by sensory nerves.

THE DIGESTIVE SYSTEM

Food provides our bodies with substances that cells need to produce energy and build new tissue. The digestive system breaks down food so that it can be absorbed into the blood and delivered to the cells as nutrients, vitamins, and minerals (Fig. 4-20).

Food passes through the hollow organs of the digestive system from the mouth to the anus. The breakdown of food begins in the mouth as the food is chewed and mixes with saliva. This breakdown continues in the stomach, where the food is churned and combined with stomach acids. Chemicals from the liver and pancreas further break down food into its component parts.

Once food has been broken down, nutrients are absorbed into the blood as the food passes through the small intestine. Liquid is removed from the food as it passes through the large intestine, which is also called the colon. Undigestible material is eliminated from the body as feces.

THE ENDOCRINE SYSTEM

The endocrine system is a very complicated system, consisting of a number of glands inside the body that produce chemicals called hormones. These chemicals, when secreted into the bloodstream, regulate body activities and functions in many body systems. Two examples of such hormones are

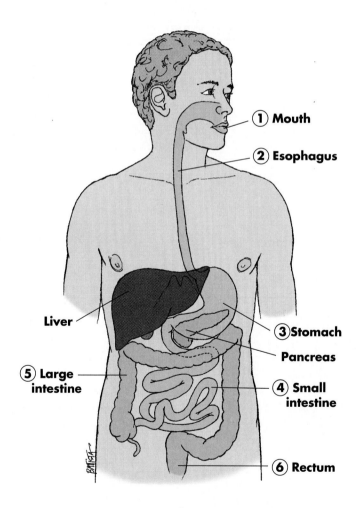

Fig. 4-20 The pathway food follows through the digestive system. The liver and pancreas add chemicals to aid in the breakdown of food.

adrenaline, which helps prepare the body for emergencies, and insulin, which is crucial for the body's use of sugars.

REVIEW QUESTIONS

The Musculoskeletal, Nervous, Skin, Digestive, and Endocrine Systems

1. List the two main functions of the skeletal system.

   _____

   _____

2. What is name of the tip of the breastbone?
   A. xiphoid process
   B. patella
   C. sternum
   D. tibia

3. The bone of the upper thigh is the:
   A. humerus
   B. patella
   C. fibula
   D. femur

4. Name one of the bones of the forearm.
   A. tibia
   B. humerus
   C. ulna
   D. femur

5. The peripheral nervous system consists of _____ nerves, which carry information to the central nervous system, and _____ nerves, which carry information to the body.

6. The chemicals released by the endocrine system are called _____.

1. Give the body shape, protect internal organs; 2. A; 3. D; 4. C; 5. Sensory, motor; 6. Hormones

CHAPTER SUMMARY

THE RESPIRATORY SYSTEM
The respiratory system makes oxygen available to the blood and rids the body of carbon dioxide. The respiratory system can be divided into the airways, which are the passageway through which air flows, and the lungs, where gas exchange actually occurs.

THE CIRCULATORY SYSTEM
The circulatory system delivers oxygen and nutrients to and removes waste products from the organs and tissues of the body. This is accomplished by pumping blood through the lungs and to the body tissues through a network of blood vessels.

THE MUSCULOSKELETAL SYSTEM
The skeleton gives the body shape, protects vital organs, and provides for body movement. The skeleton can be divided into the head, spinal column and thorax, the pelvis and lower extremities, and the upper extremities. The muscles provide movement by contracting. There are three types of muscles: skeletal muscles, which are attached to bones and move the skeleton; smooth muscles, which affect the flow of fluid or gas through the tubes of the body; and cardiac muscle, which enables the heart to beat.

THE SKIN, NERVOUS SYSTEM, DIGESTIVE SYSTEM, AND ENDOCRINE SYSTEM
The skin provides a barrier for protection and interaction with the environment. The nervous system controls all voluntary and involuntary actions of the body. The digestive system breaks down food so that it can be absorbed into the blood and delivered to the cells as nutrients, vitamins, and minerals. The endocrine system regulates body function through the release of chemicals called hormones into the bloodstream.

UNITED STATES DEPARTMENT OF TRANSPORTATION NATIONAL HIGHWAY TRAFFIC SAFETY ADMINISTRATION FIRST RESPONDER OBJECTIVES

Check your knowledge. The National Registry of EMTs and many state EMS agencies use the objectives below to develop First Responder certification examinations. Can you meet them?

COGNITIVE OBJECTIVES

1. Describe the anatomy and function of the respiratory system.
2. Describe the anatomy and function of the circulatory system.
3. Describe the anatomy and function of the musculoskeletal system.
4. Describe the components and function of the nervous system.

Lifting and Moving Patients

KEY TERMS

Body mechanics   The principles of effective use of the muscles and joints of your body when lifting and moving patients.

Emergency move   A patient move used when there is an immediate danger to the patient or crew members if the patient is not moved, or when life-saving care cannot be given because of the patient's location or position.

Non-urgent move   A patient move used when there is no present or anticipated threats to the patient's life and care can be adequately and safely administered.

Recovery position   The patient positioned on his/her left side, used to help maintain an open airway by preventing the tongue from occluding the posterior aspect of the mouth and allowing gravity to assist in draining secretions.

FIVE

FIRST RESPONSE

Fire fighters Joe and Jake responded to an emergency call for an 82-year-old woman, complaining of being very ill. Dispatch has reported that the patient believes carbon monoxide is in her home, but is feeling too weak to get out of her bed. The patient is reported to be in the upstairs bedroom. When Joe and Jake arrive at the scene, they use their self-contained breathing apparatus to protect themselves from carbon monoxide. They open doors and windows as they search for the patient. Joe finds the patient in a second floor bedroom, and he and Jake prepare to immediately remove her from the house. The ambulance crew is en route to the scene and will arrive within five minutes. Joe and Jake take a blanket and place it on the floor next to the bed. They lift the elderly woman from the bed and gently place her on top of the blanket. They use the blanket to move her gently down the steps and out to the front of the home to the EMS crew that has just arrived on the scene. Joe and Jake then assist the EMS crew with moving the patient onto the stretcher and into the ambulance.

Lifting and moving patients is a common practice for anyone involved in EMS. As a First Responder, the amount of lifting and moving that you do will be determined by the system in which you work. For the most part, the role of the First Responder is to assist other EMS personnel with lifting and moving patients. However, for emergency situations, it may be necessary to rapidly move the patient to a safe location prior to the arrival of more advanced EMS personnel.

First Responders may be called upon to move patients before the arrival of other EMS personnel, or may assist other EMS personnel with moving. Therefore, it is important that you understand the techniques for lifting and moving, including how to position patients and how to best assist other EMS personnel with lifting and moving patients.

EMS personnel frequently sustain disabling injuries while performing their duties. Most of these injuries can be prevented by using the proper lifting and moving techniques discussed in this chapter.

ROLE OF THE FIRST RESPONDER

There are three situations when First Responders commonly move patients: 1) when there is immediate danger to the patient or crew, 2) when it is necessary to prevent further injury to the patient, and 3) when assisting other EMS personnel. In most situations, First Responders will not move the patient until other EMS personnel are on the scene.

If there is a threat to the patient's life, such as a fire, explosion, or hazardous substance, the First Responder may move patients to an area of safety. Remember, never enter a scene until it is safe. If you determine that personnel with additional training or equipment are necessary to move the patient, wait until they are available before moving the patient.

The patient's condition determines how they should be positioned. Patient positioning will be discussed later in this chapter.

Once additional EMS personnel arrive at the scene, you should assist them with lifting and moving the patient. Because you will most likely be assisting other EMS personnel when lifting and moving, you should become familiar with the equipment used by your local EMS services.

BODY MECHANICS AND LIFTING TECHNIQUES

One of the most common ways to injure yourself as a First Responder is through use of poor body mechanics when lifting or moving patients. Body mechanics are the principles of effective use of the muscles and joints of your body when lifting and moving patients. Use of proper body mechanics is essential in performing your duties and greatly reduces your chances of being injured.

GUIDELINES FOR LIFTING

When lifting a patient, keep your back straight and use your legs, not your back, to lift. The closer you hold the patient's weight to your body, the less strain is placed on the muscles of your back. When lifting, do not twist your torso. This increases the strain on your lower spine. Figure 5-1, A and B, demonstrate improper lifting techniques with the back bent and the torso twisted. Figure 5-1C demonstrates proper lifting techniques. Notice the position of the First Responder's back and torso in each picture.

Lifting patients poses a great risk for injury for health care providers. The risk of lower-back injury is high. First Responders can damage their backs over long periods of time by using poor body mechanics when lifting patients and EMS equipment. Chronic back pain may not be disabling, but can limit lifestyle and work capabilities. A sudden traumatic back injury, such as a ruptured disk, can also occur. This injury causes immediate and crippling pain that could end your career.

When preparing to lift a patient, consider the patient's weight and determine if the patient can be safely lifted with the available crew members. Every First Responder has different lifting capabilities, and it is your responsibility not to surpass your own limit.

Position your feet approximately shoulder width apart, making sure you have good traction under your feet and that you are positioned close to the patient. Always communicate with your crew. Don't be afraid to let others know if you need help carrying a patient. Don't try to be a hero; you may injure yourself and place the patient and others who are lifting at risk.

Proper lifting depends on understanding several key principles. These include, but are not limited to, the weight of the patient and number and size of crew members. Again, be sure you can handle the lift. At the very minimum, two people are required for a successful lift. Call for more help if necessary. The more help available, the easier and safer the lift will be. Use an even number of people to maintain the balance of the patient and the lifting and moving device. Don't try to lift more than you can handle. Always request additional personnel.

You must also know the weight limitations of any equipment being used. Most lifting and moving equipment has a warning label similar to that shown in Figure 5-2. Check the manufacturer's guidelines for equipment weight limits. You may have to improvise if the patient's weight exceeds the capacity of the equipment. There is no set rule other than to use skillful common sense in moving the patient. If the situation appears unsafe to you, do not move the patient until you are comfortable with the method to be used.

When lifting from the ground, use the power lift position. This position keeps your back locked

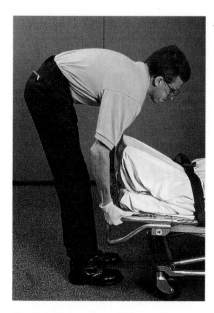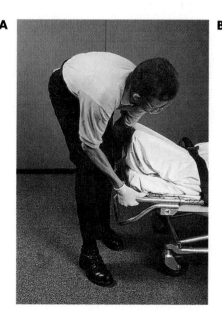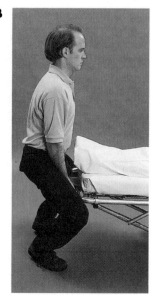

Fig. 5-1 A, Improper lifting technique with the back bent. **B,** Improper lifting technique with the torso twisted. **C,** Proper lifting technique with knees bent.

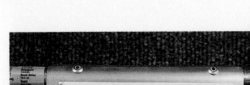

Fig. 5-2 Warning labels on lifting equipment specify weight limits

TECHNIQUE 5-1 Power lift

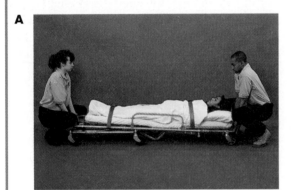

A

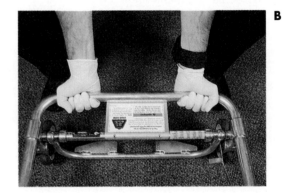

B

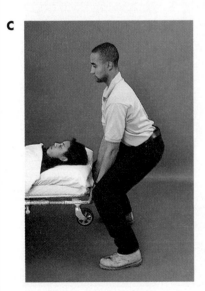

C

Fig. 5-3 A, Stand facing the stretcher with your feet shoulder width apart. This can be done at either the ends or the side of the stretcher. Squat down to the stretcher, bending at the knees. Keep your back tight, with the abdominal muscles locking your back in a normal slight inward curve. **B,** To get the maximum force from your hands, the palm and fingers should come into complete contact with the object and all fingers should bend at the same angles. Your hands should be at least 25 cm (10 in.) apart. **C,** Keep your feet flat and distribute your weight to the balls of your feet, or just behind them. Stand up, making sure that your back is locked and your upper body comes up before your hips.

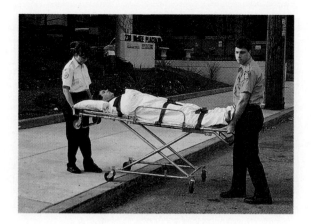

Fig. 5-4 When carrying the stretcher with only two crew members, face each other in opposing positions-from either the sides or ends of the stretcher.

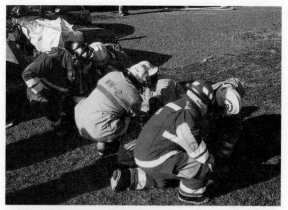

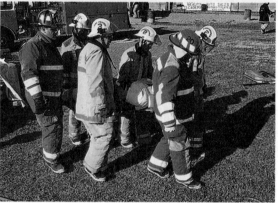

Fig. 5-5 A, Multiple rescuers preparing to lift a backboard using the one-handed technique. **B,** Multiple rescuers carrying a patient.

during the lift. The power lift (see Technique 5-1, Fig. 5-3) is the ideal method for lifting from the ground, particularly for crew members with weak knees or thighs. If only two crew members are present, maintain balance by standing opposite each other at the sides or ends of the stretcher when lifting the patient.

GUIDELINES FOR CARRYING

Sometimes First Responders will assist other EMS personnel in carrying patients from the scene to the ambulance. Be sure to take your direction for this from the more advanced personnel at the scene. As a general rule, always try to wheel patients to the ambulance rather than carry them. Let the stretcher wheels do the work for you. However, in some situations, such as uneven ground or areas with multiple obstacles, the crew has to physically carry a patient and device to the ambulance. In this case, the safety precautions and guidelines are the same as for lifting a patient.

Ideally, First Responders should work with partners of similar height and strength to maintain better balance when lifting and carrying. This is usually impossible, so you will have to adapt to height and strength differences. Be careful not to hyperextend your back or lean to either side to compensate for any imbalance when carrying a patient. When carrying a stretcher or backboard with only two crew members, face each other in opposing positions from the sides or ends (Fig. 5-4). The more people available to help, the easier it is to carry the patient. The stretcher or backboard can be carried using the one-handed technique

with multiple rescuers (Fig. 5-5, A and B). This is much safer than a two-person carry, because the stretcher or backboard is balanced, the weight is evenly distributed, and there is less weight for each person to carry.

When you assist in carrying a patient down stairs, a stair chair should be used (Fig. 5-6). Stair chairs allow the crew more flexibility for handling and transporting the patient. The patient is seated in the stair chair, and straps are applied to secure them to the chair. The smaller size of the stair chair makes it easier to maneuver in tight, steep areas. Although a stair chair is the best method for steep stairs, it should not be used for a patient with a possible spinal injury. In this case, the patient can be transported down stairs immobilized on the long spine board.

GUIDELINES FOR REACHING

Reaching for patients can also lead to injury. Reaching may simply be reaching across the stretcher to fasten a buckle or straining to pull the patient onto a backboard. Try to keep your

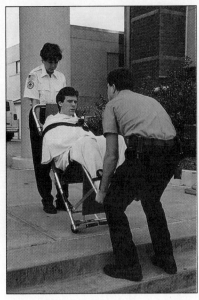

Fig. 5-6 A stair chair provides more flexibility for handling and transporting the patient in narrow or steep areas.

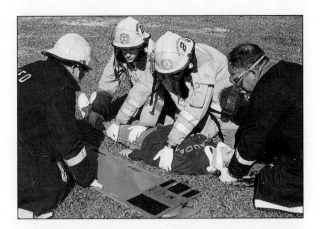

Fig. 5-7 When reaching across a patient on the ground, keep your back straight while leaning over the patient, lean from the hips and use your shoulder muscles.

REVIEW QUESTIONS

Body Mechanics and Lifting Techniques

1. Bending the back during lifting may cause serious back injury. True or False?

2. Feet should be about _____ width apart when lifting a patient.

3. It is better to _____ rather than _____ a patient.

1. True; 2. Shoulder; 3. Push; pull

---

back in a locked position, avoid leaning back over your hips, and avoid twisting your back. All of these actions place strain on the spine and increase the chance of injury. Generally, try not to reach more than 0.5 m (20 in.) in front of you, and avoid situations where you must reach for longer than 1 minute to perform a task. Reaching for longer than 1 minute may fatigue body muscles, increasing the chance of injury. When assisting in rolling a patient onto a long backboard, keep your back straight when leaning over the patient, lean from the hips, and use your shoulder muscles to help with the roll (Fig. 5-7).

GUIDELINES FOR PUSHING AND PULLING

Whenever possible, it is preferable to push rather than pull a patient into position, although in some situations, pulling may be the only option. Again, keep your back locked in position. The back is simply not strong enough to bear the weight of your body along with the added stress of the patient's weight. Keep the weight of the patient close to your body. When pulling the patient, keep the line of pull through the center of your body by bending your knees. The line of pull is the path from the patient directly to you. Push the patient with your arms between your waist and shoulder.

Be careful whenever the weight load is below your waist level, or above the level of your shoulders. If the weight is below waist level, kneel down to prevent back injury. Keep your elbows bent with arms close to the sides when you push or pull.

You should have training sessions with the ambulance service in your area to practice lifting and moving techniques with them. This is an excellent continuing education program that should be conducted annually and with new recruits. During this period of instruction, ask questions about the equipment, the advantages and disadvantages of different each different type, and methods for use.

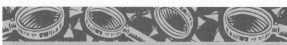

PRINCIPLE 5-1 Considerations for an Emergency Patient Move

There is an immediate danger to the patient or First Responders if the patient is not moved in these situations:

1. Fire or danger of fire.
2. Explosives or other hazardous materials.
3. Inability to protect the patient from other hazards at the scene.
4. Inability to gain access to other patients in a vehicle who need life-saving care.
5. Any other situation that has the potential for causing immediate injury.
6. Life-saving care cannot be given because of patient location or position, for example, a cardiac arrest patient sitting in a chair.

PRINCIPLES OF MOVING PATIENTS

GENERAL CONSIDERATIONS

Deciding to move any patient depends on two major considerations: the seriousness of the patient's condition and the presence of any life-threatening conditions at the scene. The three basic types of patient moves are emergency moves, non-urgent moves, and patient positioning.

An emergency move is required when there is immediate danger to the patient or you if the patient is not moved, or when life-saving care cannot be given because of the patient's location or position. This includes situations where there is a fire or a danger of fire; explosives or the danger of an explosion; inability to protect the patient from other hazards at the scene (traffic hazards or environmental factors such as extreme cold or lightning); and inability to gain access to other patients who need life-saving care. It may also be necessary to move a patient to a different location or position to provide care. For example, if a patient is in cardiac arrest and found sitting in a chair, they must be moved to the floor to begin CPR.

A non-urgent move is appropriate when there is no threat to life, and care can be adequately and safely administered. If there is no threat to the patient's life, then the patient should not be moved until more advanced EMS personnel are at

FIRST RESPONDER ALERT

Always suspect a spinal injury when moving a trauma patient, especially if the mechanism of injury involved forces that might cause spinal damage. Every precaution should be taken to protect the patient's spine from additional risk.

the scene. Remember, your role is primarily to assist with the lifting and moving of the patient.

Patients may require positioning to prevent further harm. Patients can be positioned for airway control or allowed to remain in a position of comfort.

EMERGENCY MOVES

Once you have determined an emergency move is necessary (see Principle 5-1), take caution not to aggravate a possible spinal injury. There is no time to properly immobilize the spine in an emergency move, but you should attempt to protect the spine by pulling the patient in the direction of the long axis of the body while keeping the patient's body in a straight line.

A patient who is lying on the floor or ground can be moved in several ways. The general principle is to maintain as much in-line spine control as possible. The clothes drag uses the patient's clothing as the point for balance (Fig. 5-8). Your arms cradle the patient's head as you pull on the clothing around the shoulders. The blanket drag has the same principle, except the patient is placed onto a blanket (Fig. 5-9). If a patient is difficult to handle because of size or lack of cooperation, securing your arms under the patient's arms will help to maintain balance and control (Fig. 5-10).

Always suspect a spinal injury when moving a trauma patient, especially if the mechanism of injury involved forces that might cause spinal damage. Every precaution should be taken to protect the patient's spine from additional risk. Never pull the patient's head away from the neck and shoulders.

NON-URGENT MOVES

For a non-urgent move, the role of the First Responder is to assist other EMS personnel. Remember to ask for directions and listen carefully to those individuals directing the movement of the patient.

For a non-urgent move, there are two major techniques to move the patient from the ground to a stretcher: the direct ground lift (Technique 5-2, Fig. 5-11) and the extremity lift (Technique 5-3, Fig. 5-12). For a non-urgent move, transferring a supine patient from a bed to a stretcher may be accomplished by the direct carry (Technique 5-4, Fig. 5-13) or the draw sheet method (Technique 5-5, Fig. 5-14).

PATIENT POSITIONING

The patient's condition determines how they should be positioned. An unresponsive patient without a suspected spine injury should be placed in the recovery position to allow secretions to drain from the patient's airway. To place the patient in the recovery position, roll the patient onto the left side, place the left arm under the head, and bend the left knee to balance the patient (Fig. 5-15).

A patient who has suspected trauma should not be moved until additional EMS resources can evaluate and stabilize the patient, unless there is immediate danger to you or the patient. Once additional EMS personnel have arrived at the scene, assist them as directed.

A patient without injuries, but with complaints of chest pain, discomfort, or difficulty in

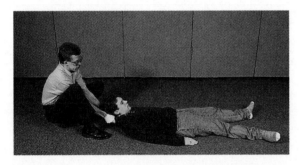

Fig. 5-8 The clothes drag technique for moving a patient.

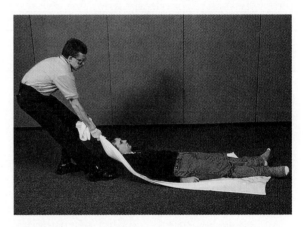

Fig. 5-9 The blanket drag technique for moving a patient.

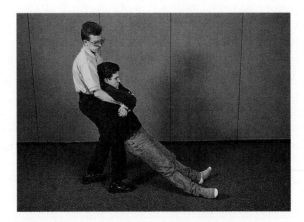

Fig. 5-10 Pulling the patient under the arms is also a technique for moving or lifting a patient.

TECHNIQUE 5-2 Direct Ground Lift (No Suspected Spine Injury)

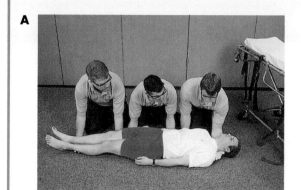

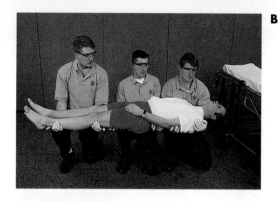

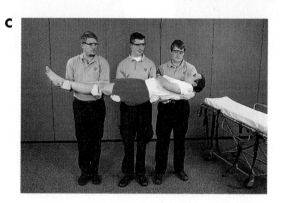

Fig. 5-11 A, Two or three rescuers line up on one side of the patient and kneel (preferably the same knee for all EMS personnel) for lifting power. The patient's arms are placed on the chest if possible. Rescuer 1 at the patient's head places one arm under the patient's neck and shoulder, cradles the patient's head, and places the other arm under the patient's lower back. Rescuer 2 places one arm under the patient's knees and one arm above the patient's buttocks. Rescuer 3 (if available) places both arms under the patient's waist and Rescuers 1 and 2 should slide their arms either up to the midback or down to the buttocks, depending on the weight distribution. **B,** On signal from the Rescuer at the head, all three Rescuers lift the patient onto their knees and roll the patient in toward their chests. **C,** Again on signal, the Rescuers stand and move the patient to the stretcher. To lower the patient, the steps are reversed.

TECHNIQUE 5-3 Extremity Lift (No Suspected Spine Injury)

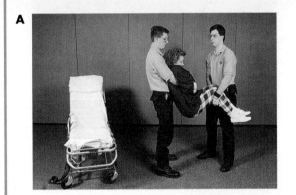 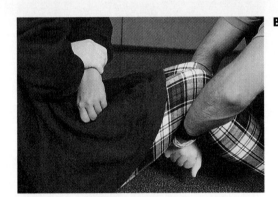

Fig. 5-12 A, Rescuer 1 kneels at the patient's head and Rescuer 2 kneels at the patient's side by the knees. Rescuer 1 places one hand under each of the patient's arms and grasps the wrists. Rescuer 2 reaches under and grasps the patient's knees, reaching as closely under the patient's hips as possible to redistribute the weight. (Otherwise, Rescuer 1 lifting the patient's head and chest will have to bear the major portion of the patient's weight.) Both Rescuers then move up to a crouching position. **B,** Both Rescuers stand up simultaneously and move with the patient to a stretcher.

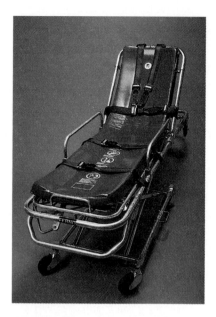

Fig. 5-16 The wheeled stretcher.

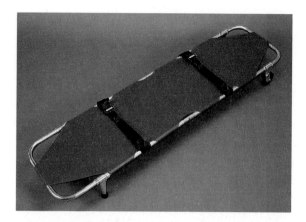

Fig. 5-17 A portable stretcher.

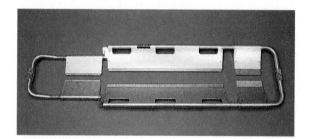

Fig. 5-18 A scoop stretcher.

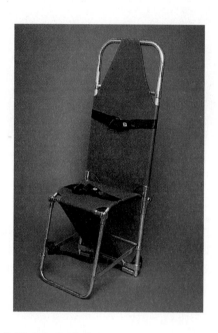

Fig. 5-19 A stair chair.

rolling them on a wheeled stretcher. This saves the crew from injury or exhaustion caused by carrying a patient. However, a wheeled stretcher can be used only on smooth terrain. Direct the stretcher by guiding the foot end, while another crew member at the head of the patient pushes the stretcher. This prevents the patient from becoming dizzy or disoriented.

Lifting the stretcher is preferred over rolling in narrow, steep spaces, but this technique requires more crew strength. The stretcher must be carried over steps, because it is difficult to roll wheels over steep steps. With two rescuers, one stands at the patient's head and the other at the feet. This allows for greatest control and balance. A four-

person carry is better because it provides more stability and places less strain on the rescuers. Each crew member carries a corner. The four-person carry is considered much safer over rough terrain.

When assisting in loading the patient into a ambulance, the primary concern is safety. Follow the equipment manufacturer's directions, and ensure all stretchers and patients are secured before the ambulance moves. Be careful of traffic around the ambulance.

PORTABLE STRETCHER

A portable stretcher (Fig. 5-17) is used to transport a second patient, or for extrication from areas

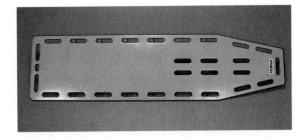

Fig. 5-20 The long backboard.

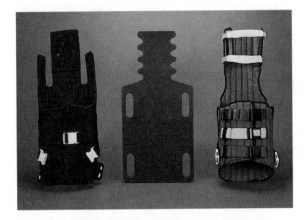

Fig. 5-21 The XP1 (left), short wooden backboard (center), and KED (right).

REVIEW QUESTIONS

Equipment

1. The _____ is used to fully immobilize the spine of a patient.

2. When using multiple rescuers to lift or carry a stretcher, the carry will be much safer than when only two rescuers carry the stretcher. True or False?

3. An unresponsive patient without a suspected spine injury is placed in the _____ position.

1. Long backboard; 2. True; 3. Recovery

where a wheeled stretcher does not fit. The portable stretcher is commonly folded in half to allow for easy storage. The principles are the same for securing the patient as for the wheeled stretcher.

SCOOP STRETCHER

A scoop stretcher (Fig. 5-18) is used to lift a patient who is lying down onto the stretcher for transport. The scoop stretcher is hinged and opens at the head and feet to "scoop" around and under the patient. Once the scoop stretcher is fastened, the patient can be lifted onto the wheeled stretcher. Because there is controversy regarding the use of a scoop stretcher for patients with a suspected spine injury, follow local protocol. If you do use a scoop stretcher for patients with possible spine injury, use it to transfer a patient to a long backboard.

STAIR CHAIR

The stair chair (Fig. 5-19) is the preferred method for transporting the patient down stairs or through narrow hallways to a stretcher. After securing the patient to this device, two EMS providers can safely carry the chair. Most stair chairs have wheels at the rear, which are used to roll the patient to the stretcher. Stair chairs cannot be used to move patients with a suspected spine injury or unresponsive patients.

BACKBOARDS

Backboards come in both long and short forms. The long backboard (Fig. 5-20) is used to immobilize the entire patient. Straps must be secured across the patient's torso, waist, and legs along with a cervical immobilization device for the patient to be properly immobilized. There are several varieties of long boards available.

Short boards are available in two types: the traditional wooden device and vest-type extrication devices (Fig. 5-21). These are used to immobilize the patient's spine during extrication and must be used in conjunction with the long backboard after extrication to provide full spinal immobilization.

For each device, follow the manufacturer's directions for use and maintenance.

CHAPTER SUMMARY

ROLE OF THE FIRST RESPONDER

The role of the First Responder in lifting and moving a patient is limited. First Responders should generally move patients with other EMS personnel. First Responders should be able to move patients who are in immediate danger, position patients to prevent further injury, and assist other EMS personnel in lifting and moving patients.

BODY MECHANICS AND LIFTING TECHNIQUES

Use your legs, not your back, to lift a patient. The power-lift method is used to minimize strain on the back when lifting. Do not attempt to lift a weight beyond your physical limitations. Carrying the patient requires excellent balance and more work by the crew than rolling the patient on a wheeled stretcher. Reaching for the patient puts stress on the back. Never try to reach overhead or hyperextend the back, as these lead to possible injury. It is preferable to push, rather than pull, a patient or stretcher into position.

PRINCIPLES OF MOVING PATIENTS

The three types of moves are emergency moves, non-urgent moves, and patient positioning. An emergency move is for patients who are in immediate danger or when life-saving care cannot be given because of the patient's location or condition. The role of the First Responder with non-urgent moves is to assist other EMS personnel. Remember to ask for directions and listen carefully to those individuals directing the movement of the patient. A patient who has no life-threatening conditions may be moved when the patient is ready for transportation. Responsive patients with no suspected spinal trauma can remain in a position of comfort. Unresponsive patients with no suspected spinal trauma should be placed in the recovery position.

EQUIPMENT

You should meet regularly with your local EMS personnel and practice working with the following devices: wheeled stretchers, portable stretchers, scoop stretchers, stair chairs, and backboards. These are all tools used to move the patient from the scene to the ambulance for transport.

UNITED STATES DEPARTMENT OF TRANSPORTATION NATIONAL HIGHWAY TRAFFIC SAFETY ADMINISTRATION FIRST RESPONDER OBJECTIVES

Check your knowledge. The National Registry of EMTs and many state EMS agencies use the objectives below to develop First Responder certification examinations. Can you meet them?

COGNITIVE OBJECTIVES

1. Define body mechanics.
2. Discuss the guidelines and safety precautions that need to be followed when lifting a patient.
3. Describe the indications for an emergency move.
4. Describe the indications for assisting in non-emergency moves.
5. Discuss the various devices associated with moving a patient in the out-of-hospital arena.

AFFECTIVE OBJECTIVES

6. Explain the rationale for properly lifting and moving patients.
7. Explain the rationale for an emergency move.

PSYCHOMOTOR OBJECTIVES

8. Demonstrate an emergency move.
9. Demonstrate the use of equipment to move patients in the out-of-hospital arena.

The Airway

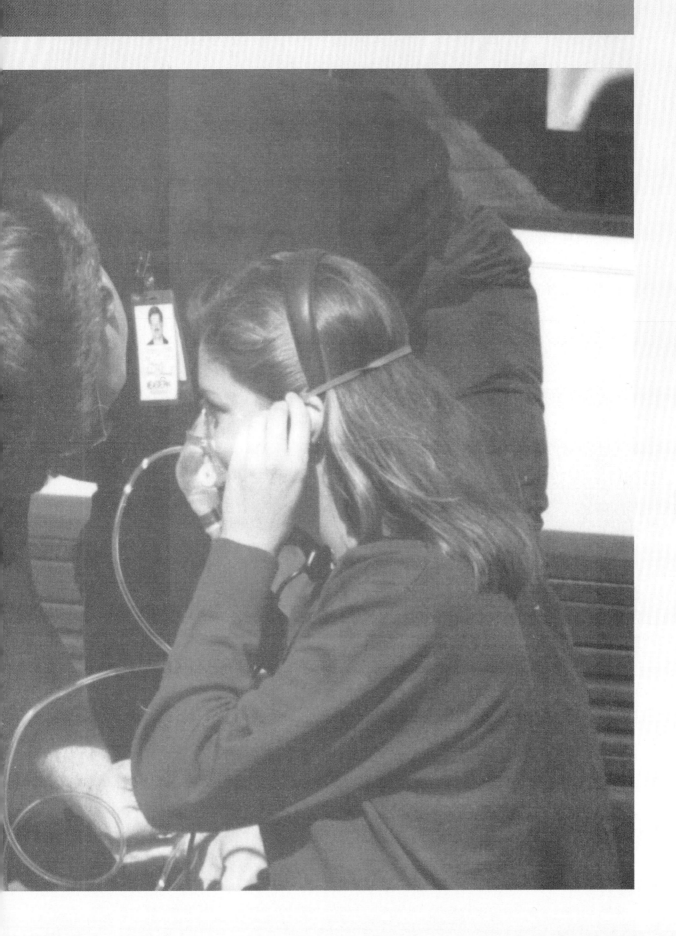

The Airway

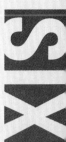

I. The Respiratory System
   A. Components and Function of the Respiratory System
   B. Considerations for Infants and Children
II. Opening the Airway
   A. Manual Positioning
   B. Inspecting the Airway
   C. Airway Adjuncts
III. Clearing the Compromised Airway and Maintaining an Open Airway
   A. The Recovery Position
   B. Finger Sweeps
   C. Suctioning
IV. Assessing Breathing
   A. Determine the Presence of Breathing
   B. Determine the Adequacy of Breathing
V. Artificial Ventilation
   A. Mouth-To-Mask Ventilation Technique

B. Mouth-To-Barrier Device Ventilation Technique
C. Mouth-To-Mouth Ventilation Technique
D. Special Considerations for Trauma Patients
E. Assessing the Effectiveness of Artificial Ventilations
VI. Special Situations in Airway Management
   A. Patients with Laryngectomies
   B. Ventilating Infants and Children
   C. Facial Trauma
   D. Dental Appliances
VII. Foreign Body Airway Obstruction (FBAO)
   A. FBAO in the Responsive Patient
   B. FBAO in the Adult Patient
   C. FBAO in Infants and Children

KEY TERMS

Accessory muscles   Muscles in the neck, chest, and abdomen used to assist breathing. The use of accessory muscles indicates difficulty in breathing.

Agonal respirations   Weak and ineffective chest wall movements immediately after cardiac arrest.

Airway   The respiratory system structures through which air passes.

Barrier devices   Typically a piece of plastic that is designed to create a barrier between the patient's and rescuer's mouth during ventilation.

Bulb syringe   A device that is used to suction the mouth and nose of infants.

Diaphragm   The large, dome-shaped muscle that separates the thoracic and abdominal cavities; the main muscle used in breathing.

Epiglottis   The flap-like structure that prevents food and liquid from entering the windpipe during swallowing.

Finger sweep   Placing a gloved finger deep into the patient's mouth to remove solids or semi-solid obstructions.

Gag reflex   A reflex that causes the patient to retch when the back of the throat is stimulated; this reflex helps the unresponsive patient protect their airway.

Heimlich maneuver   Abdominal thrusts used to relieve a foreign body airway obstruction.

Laryngectomy   A surgical procedure in which the larynx is removed.

Larynx   The voice box; contains the vocal cords that vibrate during speech.

Nasopharyngeal airway   A flexible tube of rubber or plastic that is inserted into the patient's nostril to provide an air passage.

Nasopharynx   The region of the pharynx that lies just behind the nose.

CONTINUED

Oropharyngeal airway   A curved piece of plastic that goes into the patient's mouth and lifts the tongue away from the back of the throat.

Oropharynx   The region of the pharynx that lies just below the nasopharynx; the back of the throat.

Pharynx   Part of the airway behind the mouth and nose, divided into two regions, the nasopharynx and the oropharynx.

Resuscitation masks   Small, lightweight masks that can be used when ventilating a patient.

Stridor   A harsh sound heard during breathing, usually during inhalation, that indicates an upper airway obstruction.

Suction   Using negative pressure to remove liquids or semi-liquids from the airway.

Suction catheter   A flexible or rigid tip placed on the end of suction tubing. The suction catheter goes into the patient's mouth.

Trachea   The windpipe.

Tracheal stoma   A permanent artificial opening into the trachea.

Universal distress signal   Both hands clutching at the neck; a sign of upper airway obstruction.

Wheeze   A high-pitched whistling sound caused by narrowed air passages that can indicate an airway obstruction.

FIRST RESPONSE

Sergeant Mike Benfield is a proud father; he is constantly showing pictures of Cathy, his wife, and two children, Julie and Jeffrey, to everybody at the station. He had just come home from a midnight shift and was eating breakfast with Cathy when Julie came running downstairs screaming for her parents to come quickly. They burst through the door to find the limp little body of their eight month old son Jeffrey. He was playing with his sister's stuffed animals when he'd suddenly stopped breathing.

Mike looked at his son who was blue around the lips and unresponsive and he knew that he had to do something quickly. Cathy said, "I'll call 9-1-1, you help Jeff!" and Mike took hold of his son. He remembered what he learned from his First Responder class as he opened the little boy's airway and checked for breathing. He sealed his lips around his son's mouth and nose. When he attempted to ventilate, no breath went in. He repositioned his son's head and tried again, to no avail. He began performing back blows and chest thrusts. On the third chest thrust a button popped out of Jeffrey's mouth. He still was not breathing, so Mike performed mouth-to-mouth ventilations. Within a minute, Jeffery started to breathe on his own. By the time EMS arrived, he was crying and fully responsive. Mike had him checked out at the emergency department, and they were all home before lunch.

Nothing is more immediately life threatening than something that compromises the airway or prevents a patient from breathing. One of the popular memory aids to remember the priorities in managing emergencies is "A, B, C—Airway, Breathing, and Circulation." You will hear this many times as a First Responder and it emphasizes the importance of proper airway management and ventilation. As a First Responder, the patient care skills you learn in this chapter will be the most important skills you will learn.

THE RESPIRATORY SYSTEM

The respiratory system includes the parts of the body through which air passes. These tubes and passageways make up what is known as the **airway.** Because the body requires a continual supply of fresh air, anything that blocks or obstructs the airway is a serious life threat. As a First Responder, you must ensure that the patient's airway remains clear and open.

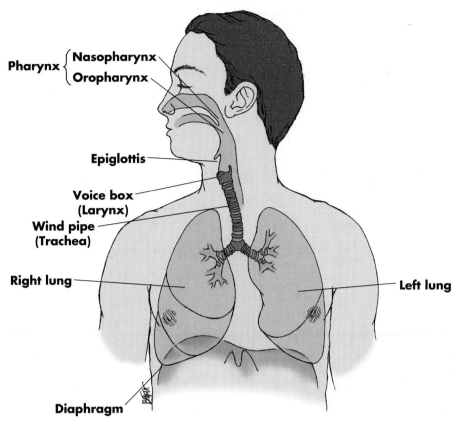

Fig. 6-1 Respiratory system anatomy.

COMPONENTS AND FUNCTION OF THE RESPIRATORY SYSTEM

The main purpose of the respiratory system is to deliver oxygen to the body and remove carbon dioxide. This process is so essential for life that any interruption of respiration can be fatal within minutes.

Familiarity with the anatomy of the airway helps you understand airway management (Fig. 6-1). The airway begins with the mouth and nose and continues into the pharynx. The pharynx is divided into two regions: the nasopharynx and the oropharynx. The area just behind the nose is the nasopharynx; the oropharynx lies just below the nasopharynx and is the back of the throat.

Covering the passageway into the windpipe, or trachea, is the leaf-shaped epiglottis. The epiglottis is a flap-like structure that prevents food and liquid from entering the trachea during swallowing.

The voice box, or larynx, is the first part of the windpipe. The voice box forms the prominence commonly called the Adam's apple. The windpipe descends from the voice box and divides into two main branches that lead to each lung. Within the lungs, the passageway continues to divide into smaller and smaller branches, ending at tiny air sacs where the exchange of oxygen and carbon dioxide takes place (Fig. 6-2).

The diaphragm is the main muscle that makes breathing possible. The diaphragm is a large, dome-shaped muscle that separates the chest from the abdomen. When the diaphragm contracts, it flattens. Contraction of the diaphragm increases the size of the chest, and air is pulled into the lungs through the mouth and nose. The exchange of oxygen and carbon dioxide takes place in the lungs. During exhalation, the diaphragm relaxes and moves upward. This movement decreases the size of the chest, moving air out through the mouth and nose.

CONSIDERATIONS FOR INFANTS AND CHILDREN

Because the airway structures in infants and children are smaller than those in adults, the airway is more easily blocked. The tongue is larger in relation to the size of infant's or child's mouth (Fig. 6-3). The large tongue can easily fall against the back of the throat and block the airway if the patient is on his back.

Because the windpipe in infants and children is very narrow, it can become easily obstructed by even a small amount of fluid or swelling. The windpipe of an infant is so soft and flexible that it can be kinked by positioning the head incorrectly, especially by tilting the head back too far. Excessive head tilt can also cause damage to the spine. It is very important to carefully maintain the airway in infants and children because uncorrected respiratory problems are the primary cause of cardiac arrest in pediatric patients.

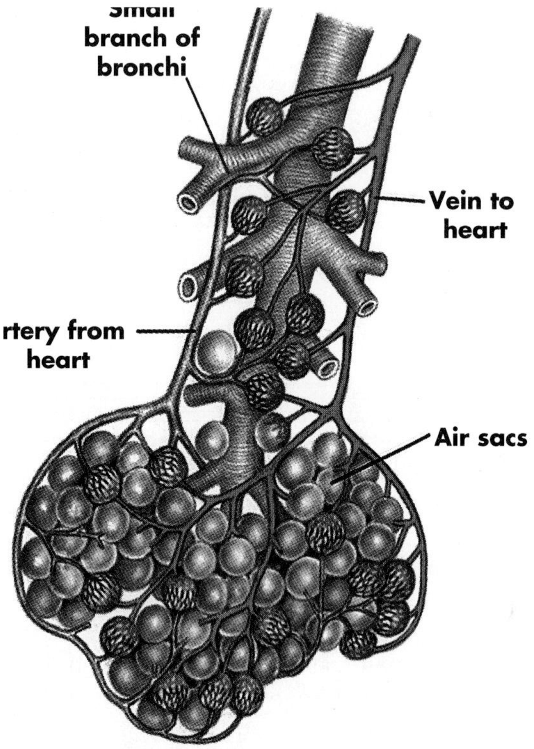

OPENING THE AIRWAY

Anything that interferes with the continuous flow of air in and out of the lungs is an immediate life threat. Ensuring that the patient's airway is open and clear is your most important patient care responsibility as a First Responder.

MANUAL POSITIONING

Unresponsive patients lose muscular control of the jaw. If the patient is lying on his back, the jaw falls backwards and the base of the tongue touches the back of the throat (Fig. 6-4). These actions close the airway and make it impossible to move air from the mouth and nose into the lungs. The tongue is the most common cause of airway obstruction in the unresponsive patient.

Head-tilt, chin-lift

Research has indicated that the head-tilt, chin-lift consistently provides the optimal airway. The head-tilt, chin-lift is the most common method of opening the airway in the uninjured, unresponsive patient. Since the tongue is attached to the lower jaw, tilting the head back and forwardly displacing the jaw will lift the base of the tongue away from the back wall of the

Small branch of bronchi

Vein to heart

rtery from heart

Air sacs

Fig. 6-2 In the lungs, capillaries surround the air sacs.

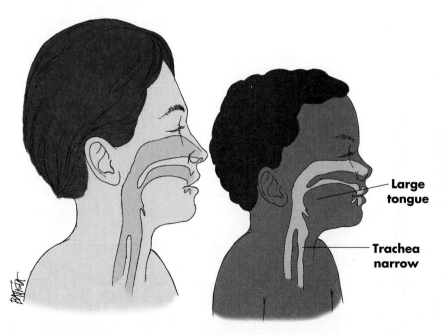

Fig. 6-3 In infants and children, the airway is more easily obstructed, and the tongue takes up proportionally more space in the mouth.

Large tongue

Trachea narrow

throat. This simple technique requires no equipment and should be performed immediately whenever you are treating an unresponsive, uninjured patient.

The first step in performing the head-tilt, chin-lift is to place the hand closest to the head on the patient's forehead and apply firm backward pressure to tilt the head back. Next, place the fingers of your other hand on the bony part of the patient's chin. Lift the chin forward and support the jaw while tilting the head back (Fig. 6-5).

When performing the head-tilt, chin-lift be sure that you do not press on the soft tissues of the chin. This can push the tongue against the roof of the mouth and cause an airway obstruction, especially in children. The thumb is not used to lift the chin, but rather to keep the patient's mouth open.

When using this technique with infants and children, avoid tilting the head past the point where the nose is perpendicular to the surface upon which the patient is lying. Tilting the head too far can kink the windpipe and cause spine damage. If an elderly patient has a curvature of the upper back that places the head in a hyperextended position, you should use padding under the head to maintain the correct position.

Jaw thrust without head-tilt

If the patient is injured, moving the neck can damage the patient's spinal cord. However, in

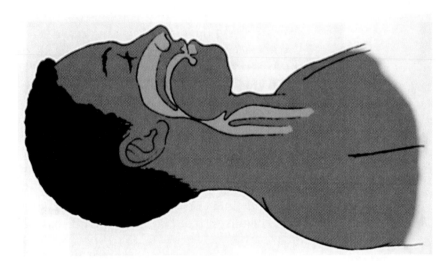

Fig. 6-4 Unresponsive patients lose muscular control of the jaw. This may cause the tongue to contact the back of the throat, obstructing the airway.

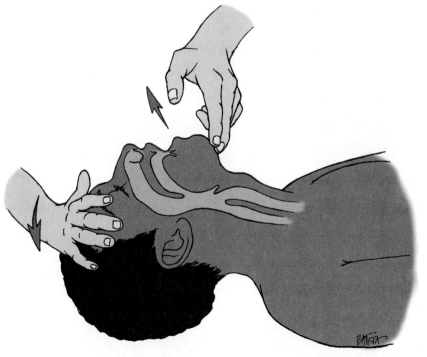

Fig. 6-5 When you tilt the head back and lift the chin, the base of the tongue and the epiglottis are lifted out of the airway.

many situations, you will not know if the patient has injured their spinal cord. If the mechanism of injury suggests that there may be injury, the jaw thrust without head-tilt should be performed when opening the airway. Mechanism of injury is discussed in Chapter 7, "Patient Assessment."

The jaw thrust without head-tilt is used to open the airway of unresponsive, injured

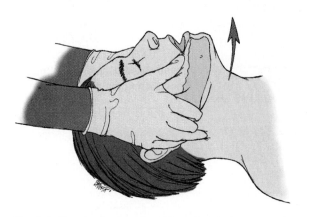

Fig. 6-6 Use the jaw thrust without head-tilt to open the airway in an injured patient.

patients. Although this technique is effective, it is technically difficult and fatiguing to perform. You should practice this skill often to maintain your proficiency.

To perform the jaw thrust without head-tilt, place the tips of your index fingers between the jaw and the earlobe, and the meaty parts of your thumbs on the cheekbones. Lift the jaw forward with both hands and use your thumb tips to keep the mouth open (Fig. 6-6).

INSPECTING THE AIRWAY

If there is fluid or solid material in the mouth, manual positioning techniques will effectively open the airway. Foreign material can block the passage of air from the mouth and nose and can prevent air from passing through the airway structures into the lungs. This can occur even if you have performed the head-tilt, chin-lift or the jaw thrust without head-tilt correctly. For this reason, you should visually inspect the airway in any unresponsive patient and any responsive patient who is not able to protect their own airway. To inspect the airway, open the patient's mouth with a gloved hand and look inside the mouth. You may find the airway to be clear (patent), or, as you inspect the airway, you may find fluids or solids (i.e., candy or food, teeth, dentures) that may block the free passage of air.

AIRWAY ADJUNCTS

Oropharyngeal airways and nasopharyngeal airways are devices that help open and maintain the airway. One of these two devices should be used

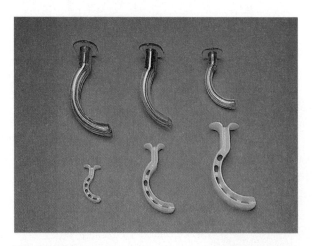

Fig. 6-7 Oropharyngeal airways are available in several sizes and types.

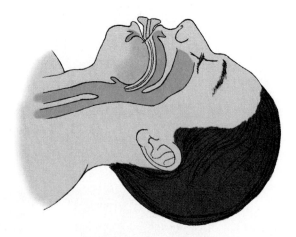

Fig. 6-8 The oropharyngeal airway displaces the tongue from the back of the patient's throat.

when unresponsive patients are unable to control their airway.

Oropharyngeal airways

The oropharyngeal airway (Fig. 6-7) is a curved piece of plastic that goes into the patient's mouth and lifts the tongue away from the back of the throat (Fig. 6-8). It is also called an oral airway or an OP airway.

The gag reflex causes the patient to retch when the back of the throat is stimulated. This reflex helps unresponsive patients protect their airway.

Unresponsive patients who lose the gag reflex are at very high risk for airway obstruction and inhalation of material into the lungs. The oral airway should be used only if the patient is unresponsive and has no gag reflex. If it is used in a patient who has a gag reflex, the patient may gag or vomit. This can seriously threaten the airway. Technique 6-1 illustrates the steps for inserting an oral airway in an adult and Technique 6-2 illustrates the steps for inserting an oral airway in an infant or child.

TECHNIQUE 6-1   Method for Inserting the Oral Airway (Adults Only)

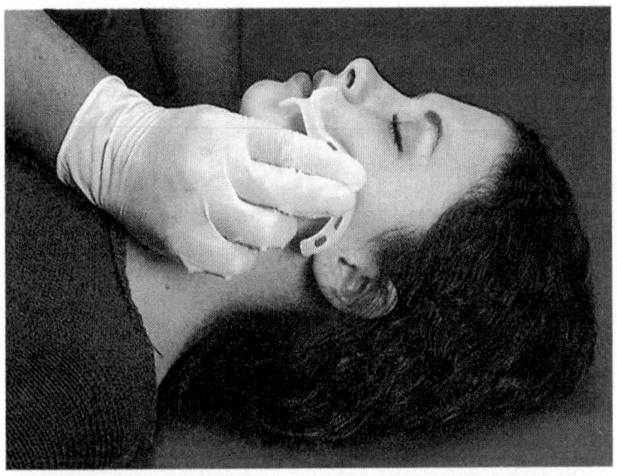

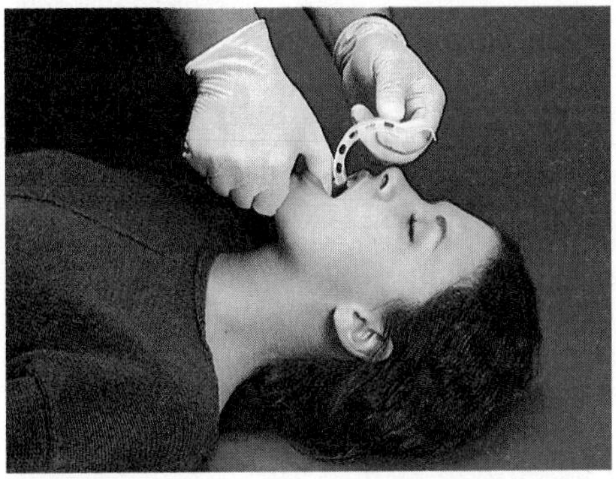

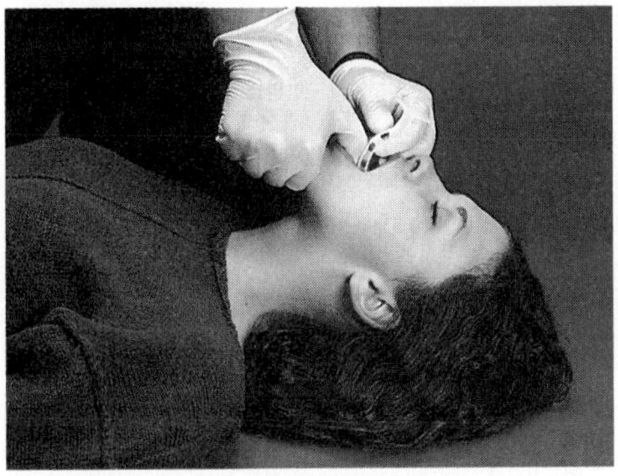

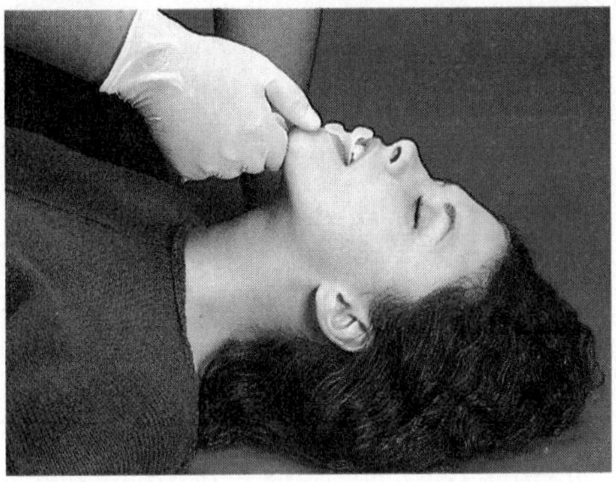

Fig. 6-9 Take body substance isolation precautions. **A,** Select the properly sized airway, which should measure from the corner of the patient's mouth to the earlobe or the angle of the jaw. Position yourself at the patient's side. **B,** Open the patient's mouth by lifting the jaw and tongue. Insert the airway upside down (with the tip facing toward the roof of the patient's mouth). **C,** Advance the airway gently until you feel resistance. **D,** Turn the airway 180 degrees so that it **E,** comes to rest with the flange on the patient's teeth. Ventilate the patient as needed.

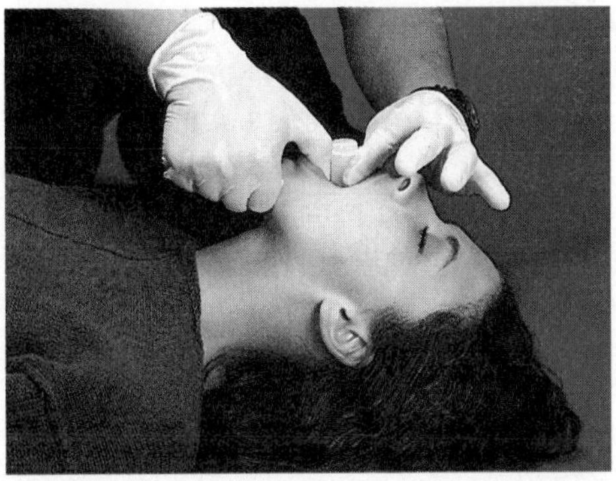

TECHNIQUE 6-2 Method for Inserting the Oral Airway (Preferred Method for Infants and Children)

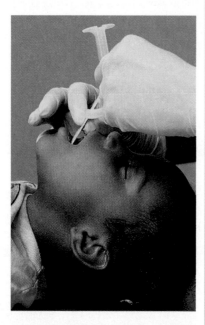

Fig. 6-10 Take body substance isolation precautions. Select the properly sized airway, which should measure from the corner of the patient's mouth to the earlobe or angle of the jaw. Position yourself at the top of the patient's head. Open the patient's mouth and use a tongue depressor to press the tongue forward and out of the airway. Insert the airway right side up (with the tip facing toward the floor of the patient's mouth). Advance the airway gently until the flange comes to rest on the patient's lips or teeth. Ventilate the patient as needed.

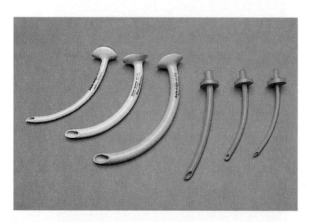

Fig. 6-11 Different types and sizes of nasopharyngeal airways.

Nasopharyngeal airways

The **nasopharyngeal airway** is a flexible tube of rubber or plastic (Fig. 6-11). It is inserted into the patient's nostril to provide an air passage (Fig. 6-12). The nasopharyngeal airway is commonly called a nasal airway or NP airway. The nasopharyngeal airway is less likely to stimulate vomiting and is a

REVIEW QUESTIONS

The Respiratory System and Opening the Airway

1. What is the main muscle used in respiration?
   _____

2. Normal inhalation is a process initiated by _____ of the diaphragm, whereas exhalation is a process that occurs during _____ of the diaphragm.

3. Why is airway obstruction more common in infants and children?
   _____
   _____

4. What is the proper way to size an oral airway?
   _____
   _____

5. What is the proper way to size a nasal airway?
   _____
   _____

6. Place the following steps in order for inserting an oral airway in an adult:
   A. Advance the airway gently until you feel resistance.
   B. Select the properly sized airway.
   C. Ventilate the patient as needed.
   D. Take body substance isolation precautions.
   E. Insert the airway upside down.
   F. Position yourself at the patient's side.
   G. Turn the airway 180 degrees so that it comes to rest with the flange on the patient's teeth.
   H. Open the patient's mouth by lifting the jaw and tongue.

1. The diaphragm; 2. contraction, relaxation; 3. Because of the larger tongue and smaller airway structures; 4. The oropharyngeal airway is sized by measuring from the corner of the patient's mouth to the earlobe or angle of the jaw; 5. The nasopharyngeal airway is sized by measuring from the tip of the patient's nose to the earlobe. Also consider the diameter of the patient's nostril when choosing a nasal airway; 6. B, F, H, E, A, G, C.

valuable adjunct in patients who are responsive but who need assistance in keeping the tongue from obstructing the airway. This type of airway is well tolerated in patients of all ages and are the easiest airway adjunct to use if the patient is actively seizing. Technique 6-3 describes the steps for inserting a nasopharyngeal airway in patients of any age.

It is important to select the correct airway size. The proper nasal airway size measures from the tip of the patient's nose to the earlobe. You should also consider the diameter of the nostril. The airway should not be so large that it causes blanching of the skin around the nostril. If you meet resistance, do not force the airway. Remove it from that nostril, relubricate it, and try the other side. Even a well-lubricated nasopharyngeal airway may be uncomfortable for the patient.

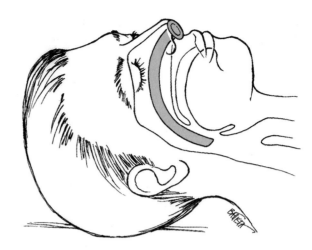

Fig. 6-12 Nasopharyngeal airways can be used in responsive and semiresponsive patients to maintain an open airway.

TECHNIQUE 6-3 Inserting a Nasopharyngeal Airway

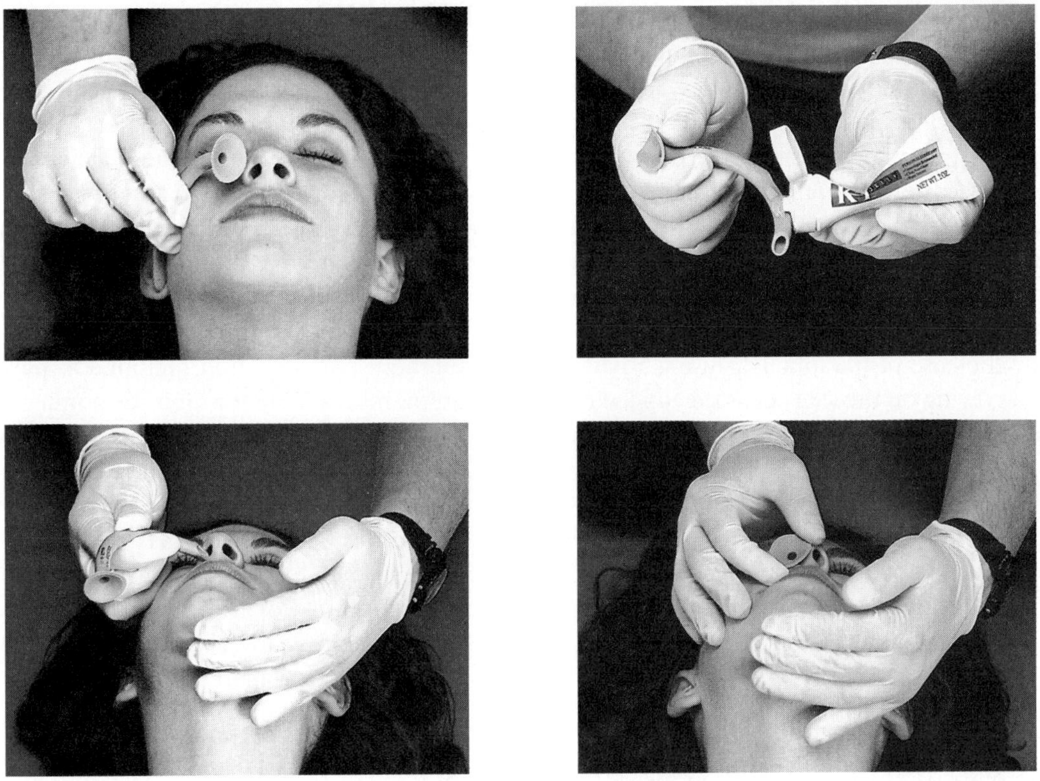

Fig. 6-13 Take body substance isolation precautions. **A,** Select the properly sized airway by measuring from the tip of the patient's nose to the earlobe. Also consider the diameter of the patient's nostril when choosing a nasal airway. **B,** Lubricate the airway with a water-soluble lubricant. **C,** Insert the airway into the patient's nostril with the bevel toward the base of the nostril or the nasal septum. Most nasal airways are designed to be inserted into the right nostril. **D,** Advance the airway gently until the flange comes to rest at the patient's nostril. Ventilate the patient as needed.

CLEARING THE COMPROMISED AIRWAY AND MAINTAINING AN OPEN AIRWAY

Threats to the airway are quickly fatal and require immediate action. There are three techniques that are used to clear and maintain the airway. The specifics of each situation dictate which of these techniques is most appropriate. These three techniques are not sequential; you will have to decide which is most appropriate and effective depending on the nature of the problem.

THE RECOVERY POSITION

The recovery position is an important technique for maintaining an open airway in the unresponsive, uninjured patient who is breathing adequately. It uses patient positioning and gravity to prevent the tongue and foreign material from obstructing the airway. Placing the patient on his side allows fluids to drain from the mouth and prevents gravity from causing the base of the tongue to contact the back of the patient's throat. By placing the patient in the recovery position, obstructions are less likely to occur and the airway is more likely to remain open. The recovery position makes it easier to monitor the patient until additional EMS resources arrive and assume care.

A simple illustration of the effectiveness of the recovery position is the fact that most people will stop snoring if they lay on their side. Snoring is caused by the base of the tongue causing a partial obstruction. Lying on the side keeps the tongue out of the airway. Technique 6-4 demonstrates the steps of placing the patient in the recovery position.

FINGER SWEEPS

Occasionally, solid or semi-solid objects (i.e., broken teeth, dentures, candy, and vomit) become lodged in the airway. If you see any of these objects when you visually inspect the airway, quickly remove them with a hooked finger placed deeply into the mouth. **Finger sweeps** are generally more effective if the patient is on his side. If the patient is uninjured, he can quickly be placed on his side before you perform the finger sweep. If the patient is injured, you should perform the finger sweep while the patient remains in the position in which they were found.

Liquid or semi-liquids should be wiped out with the index and middle fingers covered with a cloth.

You should observe proper body substance isolation precautions since your hands will be exposed to the patient's body fluids. You should also make sure the patient is completely unresponsive so they do not bite your fingers. Assessing responsiveness is discussed in Chapter 7, "Patient Assessment."

Placing the fingers into the mouth of children can push the obstruction further into the airway or stimulate swelling. Never perform a finger sweep on infants or children unless you can see an obstruction. Technique 6-5 illustrates the steps of performing a finger sweep.

SUCTIONING

Fluid such as blood, vomit, mucous, or saliva in the airway can obstruct the passage of air into the lungs. This fluid can also be inhaled into the lungs, causing damage to lung tissue. **Suction** should be used if the recovery position and finger sweeps are ineffective in draining fluid from the airway, or if the patient is injured and cannot be placed in the recovery position.

Suction devices are important emergency equipment and are often included as part of the equipment available for First Responders. If possible, have a portable suction device within reach whenever you are treating a patient. Some portable suction devices are electric and have rechargeable battery systems (Fig. 6-16). Some hand-operated suction units have become very popular because of their lightweight compact design, reliability, and low cost (Fig. 6-17). Most suction units are capable of clearing small solid objects but are inadequate for removing larger solid objects such as teeth, foreign bodies, or food.

Portable electric suction units generate negative pressure using a vacuum pump. The suctioned material empties into a collection canister. With most devices you attach a **suction catheter** to the end of tubing before you place it into the patient's mouth. A suction catheter is a flexible or rigid tip placed on the end of suction tubing that

TECHNIQUE 6-4 Placing the Patient in the Recovery Position

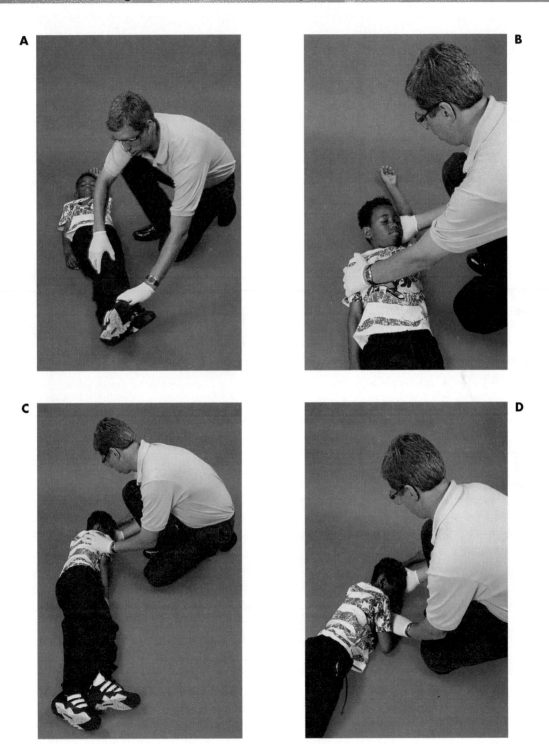

Fig. 6-14 Take body substance isolation precautions. **A,** Lift the patient's left arm over his head and cross his left leg over the right. **B,** Support the face and grab the patient's right shoulder. **C,** Roll the patient onto his left side. The head, torso, and shoulders should move simultaneously without twisting. **D,** Place the patient's right hand under the side of his face. The head should be as close to midline as possible.

TECHNIQUE 6-5 Finger Sweeps

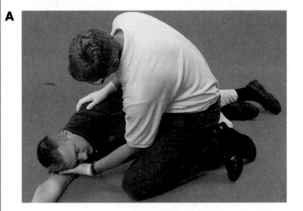

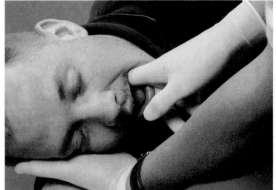

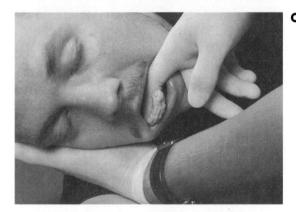

Fig. 6-15 Take body substance isolation precautions. **A,** If the patient is uninjured, turn him on his side and kneel in front of him. **B,** Insert your index finger along the cheek, deeply into the mouth. **C,** Sweep your finger across the back of the throat and attempt to hook any foreign bodies.

FIRST RESPONDER ALERT

Gurgling is the most common sign of liquid in the airway! Any time you hear gurgling:
1. Open the airway immediately.
2. If the patient is uninjured, place him in the recovery position.
3. If the patient is injured, suction the airway immediately.

goes into the patient's mouth. Most suction catheters have a hole that you must cover with your finger during suctioning. If the material that you are suctioning is so thick that it clogs the suction catheter, use the tubing without a catheter attached. If there is a large volume of material that needs to be cleared from the airway and the patient is uninjured, roll him onto his side and continue to suction.

There are a variety of suction catheters available, but the most appropriate for First Responders are rigid catheters, also called "hard," "tonsil tip," and "tonsil sucker" catheters (Fig. 6-18). These hard plastic catheters are easy to control while suctioning. They are used to suction the mouth and oropharynx of unresponsive patients. The tip of the catheter should always remain visible when you insert it into the mouth. Never insert the catheter so far that you lose sight of the tip, or past the base of the tongue.

You are not able to suction and ventilate a patient at the same time. In order to avoid depriving the patient of oxygen, be sure to limit the time of suctioning to 15 seconds for adults, 10 seconds for children, and 5 seconds for infants. Ventilate the patient between suctioning attempts.

The rigid catheter is used for infants and children. In younger patients, however, stimulation of the back of the throat can cause changes in the

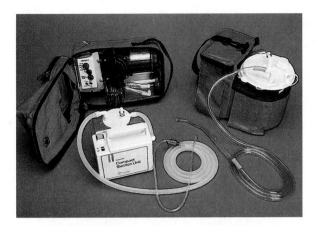

Fig. 6-16 Examples of portable suction units.

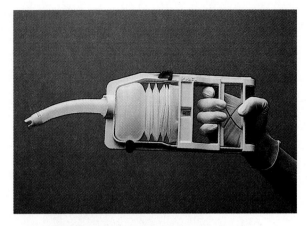

Fig. 6-17 A hand-operated portable suction unit.

heart rate. If you use a rigid suction catheter, avoid touching the back of the airway to decrease the chances of slowing the heart rhythm. If you see a change in heart rate, stop suctioning and provide ventilation.

Principle 6-1 lists the key principles for using suction. Technique 6-6 describes one technique for suctioning an adult with a portable electric suction unit.

A **bulb syringe** is used to suction infants (Fig. 6-20). This simple device is effective for suctioning the nose and mouth of a newborn and can be used to suction an infant up to 3 to 4 months of age. This device is useful to clear obstructions from the nasal passages because newborns and infants are not able to voluntarily breathe through their mouths. Technique 6-7 describes the use of the bulb syringe.

ASSESSING BREATHING

DETERMINE THE PRESENCE OF BREATHING

Once you open the airway, the next priority is to assure that the patient is breathing. This is fairly simple in the responsive patient, because you can ask, "Can you breathe?" In order to talk, the patient must move air past the vocal cords. If the patient speaks to answer you, they must be able to move some air past their vocal cords. If the responsive patient is unable to speak, it is probably due to an airway obstruction. Later in this chapter you will learn how to manage the foreign body airway obstruction.

Determining if an unresponsive patient is breathing is more of a challenge. Immediately after you

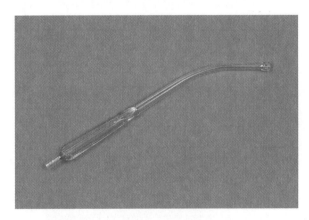

Fig. 6-18 The rigid suction catheter is the most versatile for use by First Responders.

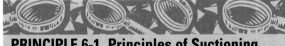

PRINCIPLE 6-1 Principles of Suctioning

1. Make sure the suction unit is working before you use it.
2. Follow body substance isolation precautions.
3. Use a rigid catheter.
4. Do not insert the catheter further than the base of the tongue.
5. Ensure that the patient does not become deprived of oxygen, by limiting the time of suctioning to 15 seconds for adults, 10 seconds for children, and 5 seconds for infants.
6. Keep the catheter and the tubing clean.

open the airway, place your ear next to the patient's mouth and look at the chest (Fig. 6-22). Check to see if you can feel or hear any exhaled breath and watch the chest for rise and fall. Look, listen, and feel for breathing for three to five seconds.

TECHNIQUE 6-6 Suctioning

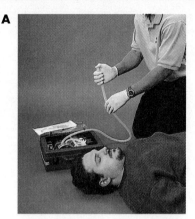

A

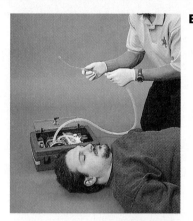

B

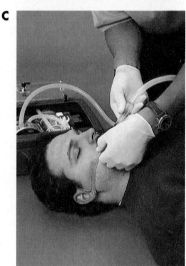

C

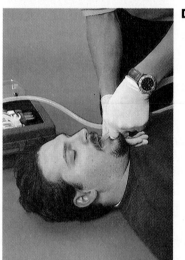

D

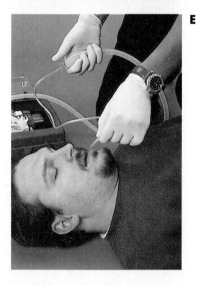

E

Fig. 6-19 Inspect the portable suction unit before use to ensure it is working and cleaned properly. Take body substance isolation precautions. Turn on the power. **A,** You will hear the motor start. You should check to be sure that the suction is working by placing your thumb over the end of the suction tubing. **B,** Attach a rigid catheter to the end of the suction tubing. **C,** Measure the distance from the corner of the patient's mouth to the earlobe and place your fingers at this mark on the catheter. Insert the catheter into the mouth without suction. This makes it easier to control the tip of the catheter during insertion. You can either keep your finger off of the hole in the catheter or turn the unit off until after you place the catheter into the patient's mouth. If there are copious amounts of fluid in the mouth, suction immediately upon placing the catheter into the patient's mouth. **D,** Insert the catheter until your fingertips reach the patient's lips. This prevents inserting the catheter too far. **E,** Once you have placed the catheter into the patient's mouth, apply suction by turning the unit on or occluding the hole in the catheter. To prevent the patient from becoming deprived of oxygen, never suction the adult for more than 15 seconds, a child for more than 10 seconds, or an infant for more than 5 seconds. To prevent the suction catheter or tubing from becoming clogged, you can intermittently suction water to clear the lines.

In some cases, you may see the chest rise and fall and yet feel no air moving through the mouth and nose. This is usually caused by an airway obstruction and must be managed promptly. In the first few minutes after a cardiac arrest, some patients have reflex gasping for air, called agonal respirations. This should not be confused for breathing.

DETERMINE THE ADEQUACY OF BREATHING

Once it is determined that the patient is breathing, whether responsive or unresponsive, evaluate the effectiveness of the breathing. To breathe effectively, the patient must breathe at an adequate rate and depth. Normal breathing should be effortless and cause the chest wall to rise and fall. Under normal circumstances, the diaphragm is the major muscle of breathing. When breathing becomes labored, the muscles of the neck and abdomen are also used. Any use of these muscles, called accessory muscles, is an indication of difficulty breathing.

The number of breaths in one minute is called the respiratory rate. Box 6-1 lists the average respiratory rates for patients of different ages. Normal breathing should cause the chest to move. If the chest is not moving, or is moving very little, the

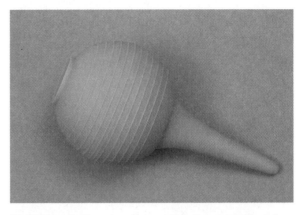

Fig. 6-20 A bulb syringe is an effective piece of equipment to clear the airway of newborns and infants.

TECHNIQUE 6-7 Bulb Syringe

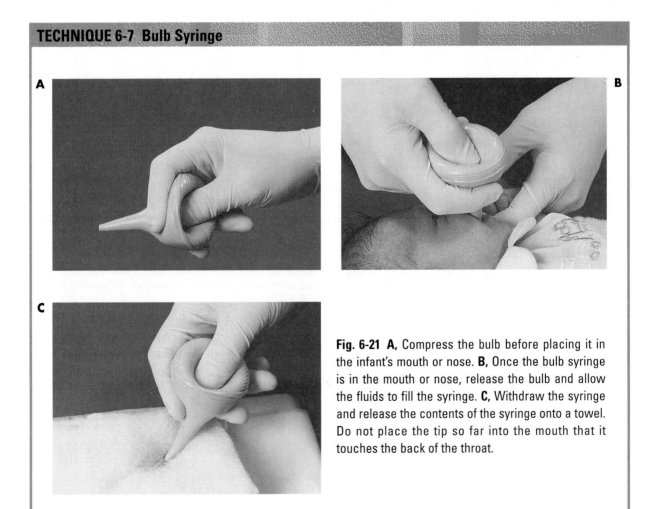

Fig. 6-21 A, Compress the bulb before placing it in the infant's mouth or nose. **B,** Once the bulb syringe is in the mouth or nose, release the bulb and allow the fluids to fill the syringe. **C,** Withdraw the syringe and release the contents of the syringe onto a towel. Do not place the tip so far into the mouth that it touches the back of the throat.

BOX 6-1 Normal Respiratory Rates

Adults	12–20 breaths per minute
Children	15–30 breaths per minute
Infants	25–50 breaths per minute

BOX 6-2 Signs and Symptoms of Inadequate Breathing

- A rate that is too slow
    - Less than 8 in adults
    - Less than 10 in children
    - Less than 20 in infants
- Inadequate chest wall movement
- Increased effort of breathing
- Mental status changes
- Shallow breathing
- Bluish (cyanotic), pale, cool, and clammy skin
- Gasping
- Grunting
- Slow heart rate with slow respirations

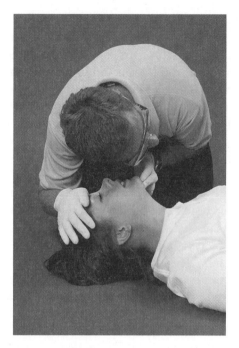

Fig. 6-22 To assess for the presence of breathing, look at the chest, listen for air movement, and feel for exhalation of air against your cheek.

breathing is too shallow to sustain life. Box 6-2 lists the major signs and symptoms of inadequate breathing.

ARTIFICIAL VENTILATION

Previous sections in this chapter described how to maintain the patient's airway by positioning the head, neck, and jaw and how to keep the airway clear of obstructions. These airway management skills help keep the passageways open, but do not deliver oxygen to the lungs. Once the airway has been assured and breathing is assessed, breathing for the patient may be necessary. Patients who are not breathing adequately have only the oxygen in their lungs and bloodstream remaining. Patients who are breathing inadequately, or not at all, must be artificially ventilated in order to stay alive.

There are three methods the First Responder can use to assist patients who are not breathing on their own. Each of these methods has advantages and disadvantages and they are not equally effective for all patients. The three techniques of artificial ventilation used by First Responders are:
1. Mouth-to-mask
2. Mouth-to-barrier device
3. Mouth-to-mouth

REVIEW QUESTIONS

Clearing the Compromised Airway and Assessing Breathing

1. The recovery position should only be used on the _____ patient who is breathing adequately.

2. What are the two reasons that you should not perform blind finger sweeps in infants and children?

    _____

    _____

3. How long can you suction an adult patient?
    A. 5 seconds
    B. 15 seconds
    C. 30 seconds
    D. Until the airway is clear

4. List the normal respiratory rates:

    Adults _____–_____ breaths per minute.

    Children _____–_____ breaths per minute.

    Infants _____–_____ breaths per minute.

1. Uninjured, unresponsive. 2. You could push the obstruction further into the airway or stimulate swelling; 3. B; 4. Adults—12-20, Children—15-30, Infants—25-50

Each of these techniques will be discussed in detail, but there are some principles that apply to all methods of artificial ventilation. Whenever you artificially ventilate a patient, you are pushing air into their airway. This air goes into both the lungs and the stomach. The air that goes to the stomach becomes trapped and will eventually interfere with ventilation and cause the patient to vomit. In order to decrease the amount of air going to the stomach, and increase the amount of air going to the lungs, deliver each ventilation slowly, over $1/2$ to 2 seconds per breath for adult patients. Deliver ventilations to children or infants over 1 to $1^1/_2$ seconds.

Each ventilation must deliver a proper volume of air to the patient. The average adult needs 800–1200 ml per breath. This is about the volume of three to four cans of soda. Unfortunately, it is difficult to measure the exact volume of air you are delivering, so you should ventilate until you see the chest rise. During exhalation, you should be able to hear and feel air escape and observe the fall of the chest. Too large a volume will cause air to enter the stomach and should be avoided. Obviously, children and infants require less volume than adults.

You must also ventilate the patient at the proper rate. For adults, a good rule of thumb is that, each time you feel a need to breathe, the patient needs to breathe also. This will result in a ventilation rate of approximately 10 to 12 breaths per minute. The younger a patient is, the faster they need to breathe, so for infants and children you should ventilate 20 times per minute. Ventilate a newborn patient at a rate of 40 breaths per minute.

Principle 6-2 lists the key principles in ventilating a patient with any technique.

MOUTH-TO-MASK VENTILATION TECHNIQUE

Mouth-to-mask ventilation is the preferred method of ventilating a non-breathing patient for the First Responder. It is a simple technique, and requires a minimal amount of equipment. Resuscitation masks are small, inexpensive, and light. As a First Responder, you should always have a resuscitation mask available. They can easily fit into a first aid kit, the glove compartment of your vehicle, and can even be carried with you.

Mouth-to-mask ventilation is very effective because you use both hands to open the patient's

airway and seal the mask to the face. Although there are a number of different manufacturers of masks, most have similar features (Fig. 6-23).

Each mask has a flexible seal or gasket that creates an airtight seal with the patient's face. Resuscitation masks have an opening into which you exhale to breath for the patient. You should select a mask that has a one-way valve to divert exhaled air or vomit away from the rescuer. Masks should be transparent so you can see any vomit or foreign material inside the mask and avoid blowing it into the patient's mouth. Many masks are designed to be reusable, provided they are cleaned after use.

Masks come in a variety of sizes and are designed to fit from the bridge of the nose and come to just below the bottom lip. If the mask is triangular, the apex of the triangle in placed toward the patient's nose. Selecting the appropriate mask size is very important, since air will leak

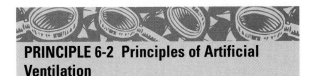

PRINCIPLE 6-2 Principles of Artificial Ventilation

1. Maintain an open airway.
2. Use an oral or nasal airway if indicated.
3. Ensure an airtight seal between the mask or barrier device and the patient's face.
4. Prevent air from going into the stomach. Ventilate slowly and only until the chest rises.
5. Ventilate the patient with an age appropriate rate.
6. Allow for complete, passive exhalation.
7. Deliver the ventilation over $1^1/_2$–2 seconds for adults, 1–$1^1/_2$ seconds for infants and children.
8. If ventilation cannot be delivered, consider the possibility of an airway obstruction.

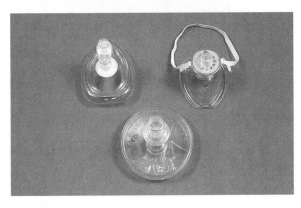

Fig. 6-23 Resuscitation masks.

around a mask that is too large or too small, resulting in inadequate ventilation.

Obtaining a proper seal with the patient's face is the most important part of mouth-to-mask ventilations. This can be particularly challenging for patients with facial hair, facial trauma, or dentures. Seal the mask by placing the heel and thumb of each hand along the border of the mask and compressing firmly around the margin. If there is any leaking of air when you ventilate, it will severely decrease the effectiveness of your ventilation. If you have difficulty obtaining a mask seal, lift the skin of the face up to the mask and continue ventilation. The technique of mouth-to-mask ventilation is described in Technique 6-8.

Some manufacturers have masks specially designed for use on infants and children. To work

effectively, the mask should fit properly. You should size the mask from the bridge of the nose to just below the bottom lip. A mask that is too large will result in inadequate ventilation, primarily due to mask leakage. If you cannot ventilate the patient, you should reposition the head, check the mask seal, and consider the possibility of a foreign body airway obstruction.

MOUTH-TO-BARRIER DEVICE VENTILATION TECHNIQUE

The main advantage of **barrier devices** over mouth-to-mask ventilation is the size of the devices. Barrier devices are even smaller and lighter than masks. They are typically disposable and less expensive than masks. As a First Responder, you should never be in a position in

---

TECHNIQUE 6-8 Mouth-to-Mask Ventilation

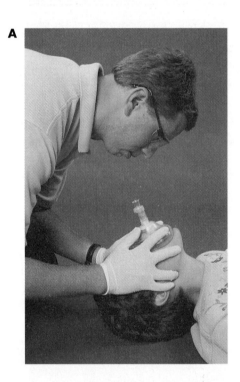
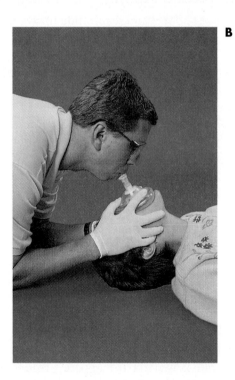

Fig. 6-24 Follow body substance isolation precautions. **A,** Connect the one-way valve to the mask, if it is not already attached. Open the airway by tilting the head back (if no trauma is suspected) and lifting the jaw, and inserting an oral or nasal airway. From a position at the top of the patient's head, place the mask on the patient. **B,** Seal the mask to the patient's face with the heel and thumb of each hand. Place the index fingers on the portion of the mask that covers the chin. Place the other fingers along the bony margin of the jaw and lift the jaw while performing a head-tilt. Take a normal breath, seal your lips over the ventilation port, and exhale slowly and constantly for 1½ to 2 seconds for adult patients, and 1 to 1½ seconds for infants or children. Stop ventilating when the patient's chest rises. Allow the patient to passively exhale between breaths. Ventilate the adult patient once every 5 seconds and infants and children once every 3 seconds.

which you do not have immediate access to either a mask or a barrier device. Although some rescuers prefer to use a barrier device over a mask, the mask has been demonstrated to be more effective for most patients.

There are many designs of barrier devices (Fig. 6-25). Unfortunately, manufacturers are not required to rigorously test these products. You should fully evaluate the effectiveness of each type. Whichever device you choose, make certain it has a low resistance during ventilation. Most barrier devices do not have exhalation valves and tend to leak around the shield. With practice, you can overcome some of these limitations and use a barrier device to effectively ventilate most patients. Technique 6-9 describes the technique of ventilating a patient with a barrier device.

Most barrier devices are designed for use on adult patients. Unless specifically designed and sized for pediatric patients, barrier devices should not be used when ventilating infants and children.

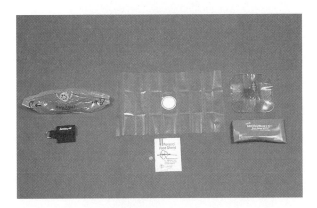

Fig. 6-25 Barrier devices.

MOUTH-TO-MOUTH VENTILATION TECHNIQUE

Mouth-to-mouth ventilation is a quick, effective method of delivering oxygen to the non-breathing patient that does not require any equipment. Mouth-to-mouth ventilation uses the rescuer's exhaled air for ventilation. The rescuer's exhaled air contains enough oxygen to support the patient.

TECHNIQUE 6-9 Mouth-to-Barrier Device Ventilation

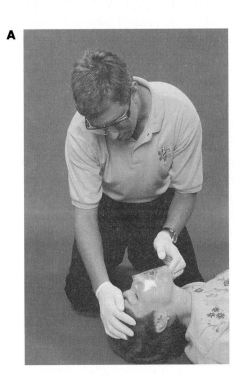

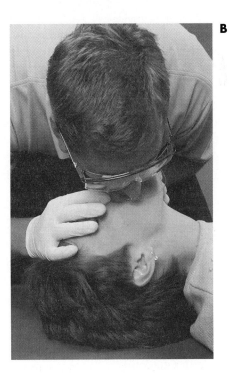

Fig. 6-26 Follow body substance isolation precautions. **A,** Open the patient's airway with the head-tilt, chin-lift and place barrier device over the patient's face. **B,** Pinch the patient's nose, take a normal breath, seal your lips to the barrier device, and exhale slowly and constantly for $1\frac{1}{2}$ to 2 seconds. Stop ventilation when the patient's chest rises. Allow the patient to passively exhale between breaths. Ventilate the adult patient once every 5 seconds.

TECHNIQUE 6-10 Mouth-to-Mouth Ventilation

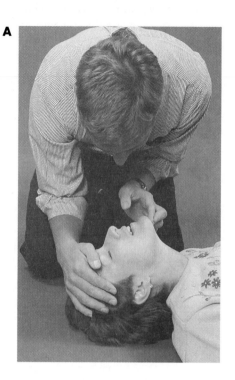 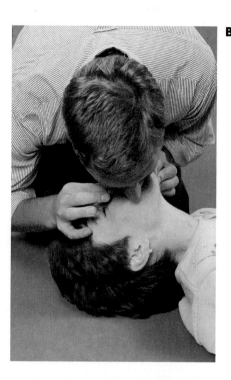

Fig. 6-27 A, Open the patient's airway with the head-tilt, chin-lift. **B,** Pinch the patient's nose, take a normal breath, seal your lips to the patient's lips, and exhale slowly and constantly for $1\frac{1}{2}$ to 2 seconds for adult patients, or 1 to $1\frac{1}{2}$ seconds for infants or children. When ventilating an infant, seal your lips around the infant's mouth and nose. Stop ventilation when the patient's chest rises. Allow the patient to passively exhale between breaths. Ventilate the adult patient once every 5 seconds and infants and children once every 3 seconds.

The decision to perform mouth-to-mouth ventilation is a personal choice, and must be made with the understanding of the implications of your decision. Mouth-to-mouth ventilation requires direct physical contact with the patient, and can place the rescuer at risk for contracting an infectious disease.

Practically, there are situations when you may want to ventilate a patient, and not have a mask or barrier device available. This should not occur in any situation in which you are functioning as a First Responder, but may occur if you ever have to ventilate a friend or family member. For that reason, it is very important that you practice and maintain proficiency in mouth-to-mouth ventilation. Technique 6-10 illustrates the steps of mouth-to-mouth ventilation.

SPECIAL CONSIDERATIONS FOR TRAUMA PATIENTS

Unresponsive trauma patients present a considerable challenge in airway management. In addition to the possibility of bleeding into the airway or facial trauma, spinal injuries require special care. All techniques of ventilation have to be modified so that the head is not tilted. This is accomplished by using the jaw thrust maneuver without head-tilt with each ventilation technique. This can be difficult and tiring, so you should practice these skills often. These modifications are described in Technique 6-11.

ASSESSING THE EFFECTIVENESS OF ARTIFICIAL VENTILATION

Whenever you ventilate a patient, it is very important to assess the adequacy of the artificial ventilation. Regardless of the technique, you must continually evaluate the effectiveness of the ventilation. This is accomplished mainly by watching the rise and fall of the chest, and by hearing and feeling the escape of air from the mouth and nose during exhalation.

Boxes 6-3 and 6-4 list some of the signs of adequate and inadequate ventilation.

BOX 6-3 Signs of Adequate Ventilation

- The chest rises and falls with each artificial ventilation
- The patient is being ventilated at least 12 times per minute for adults, or 20 times per minute for infants and children
- The adult patient is ventilated over a period of $1\frac{1}{2}$ to 2 seconds; infants or children over 1 to $1\frac{1}{2}$ seconds

BOX 6-4 Signs of Inadequate Ventilation

- The chest fails to rise and fall with each ventilation
- No air is felt or heard escaping during exhalation
- The rate is either too fast or too slow
- The abdomen is getting larger

There are a number of causes of inadequate chest rise. The most common cause of poor ventilation results from improperly opening the airway. If you are having difficulty ventilating, the first corrective action is to reposition the airway. Box 6-5 describes other corrective actions to consider if repositioning the jaw fails to correct the situation. If all else fails, consider the possibility of a foreign body airway obstruction.

SPECIAL SITUATIONS IN AIRWAY MANAGEMENT

PATIENTS WITH LARYNGECTOMIES

A laryngectomy is a surgical procedure in which the voice box is removed, usually because of throat cancer. After a laryngectomy, the patient may have a tracheal stoma, which is a permanent artificial opening into the trachea (Fig. 6-29).

If a patient with a tracheal stoma must be ventilated, you can seal the resuscitation mask to the neck, directly over the stoma. You can also ventilate by sealing your mouth around the stoma, but the use of a barrier device is preferred. Ventilate slowly, allowing time for the chest to rise and for the patient to passively exhale. Because you are more directly ventilating the lungs, the head and neck do not need to

TECHNIQUE 6-11 Ventilating Trauma Patients

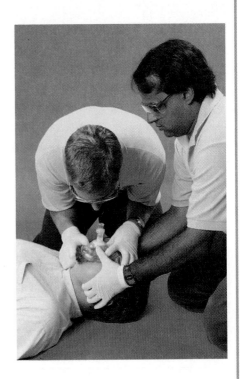

Fig. 6-28 For injured patients, all ventilation techniques are modified to open the airway with the jaw thrust without head-tilt. If at all possible, you should use two rescuers—one to open and maintain the airway and the other to ventilate.

FIRST RESPONDER ALERT

Evaluate the effectiveness of ventilation primarily by:
- observing the rise and fall of the chest
- hearing and feeling the air escape during exhalation

be positioned. If air escapes from the mouth and nose when you ventilate a patient with a stoma, close the patient's mouth and pinch the nose shut.

VENTILATING INFANTS AND CHILDREN

Respiratory emergencies are quite common in children, and you need to be able to artificially ventilate pediatric patients. Because the airway is more pliable, you must pay particular attention to the position of the head. Infants should be ventilated

BOX 6-5 Correcting Poor Chest Rise During Ventilation

Step	Rationale
Reposition the jaw	An improperly opened airway is the most common cause of poor chest rise
Check the mask or barrier seal	Poor seal with the face is the next most common cause of poor chest rise; you can generally hear air leaking through the sides of the mask or barrier device
Check for an obstruction	Foreign body airway obstructions (FBAO) may cause poor ventilation. You may need to perform the age-appropriate FBAO maneuver or suction the patient

REVIEW QUESTIONS

Artificial Ventilation

1. When ventilating the adult, the inspiratory time should be _____–_____ seconds.

2. What is the primary way to assess adequate ventilation?

   _____

3. List two signs of inadequate ventilations.

   _____
   _____

4. Place the corrective actions for ventilation in order:
   A. Check the mask or barrier seal
   B. Check for an obstruction
   C. Reposition the jaw

5. What changes in technique should you make when ventilating an injured patient?
   A. Use the head-tilt only
   B. Only use a barrier device
   C. Mouth-to-mouth ventilation cannot be used
   D. Open the airway without tilting the head

1. 1½–2. 2. By observing the rise and fall of the chest. 3. The chest fails to rise and fall with each ventilation, no air is heard or felt escaping during exhalation, the rate is either too fast or too slow, the abdomen is getting larger; 4. C, A, B; 5. D

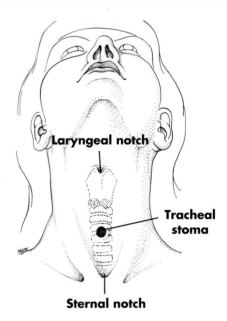

Fig. 6-29 A tracheal stoma is a permanent artificial opening into the trachea.

Laryngeal notch

Tracheal stoma

Sternal notch

far in children or infants. Ventilate children and infants once every 3 seconds.

Excessive pressure causes air to enter the stomach, which severely compromises the effectiveness of ventilation and increases the possibility of vomiting. Gastric distention is more common in infants and children than in adults. You can use an oral or nasal airway to assist in maintaining an open airway in infants and children.

FACIAL TRAUMA

Facial trauma can pose considerable difficulty for managing the airway and ventilating trauma patients (Fig. 6-30). The head and face have a rich blood supply, and injuries to the face cause significant bleeding and swelling.

Be prepared to use suction and positioning (jaw thrust without head-tilt) to keep the airway clear

without flexing or tilting the head. Since infants have a large head in comparison to the rest of their body, placing them on a flat surface causes their head to flex forward. You may need to place your hand or a towel under their shoulders to keep the airway open. Children may need to have their head slightly tilted. Avoid tilting the head back too

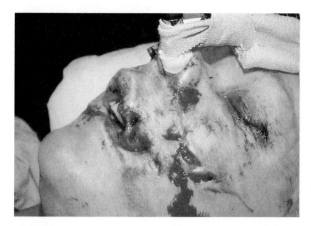

Fig. 6-30 Facial trauma can pose considerable difficulty for managing the airway and ventilating trauma patients.

of blood and vomit. Use an oral or nasal airway to help maximize the airway without tilting the head. Do not use a nasal airway in patients with facial trauma. If there is significant injury to the bones of the skull, it is possible to insert the airway directly into the brain.

If you cannot open the airway in a trauma patient and all else has failed, you must tilt the head back to ventilate the patient. Although moving the neck may cause spinal cord injury, if you do not open the airway, the patient will die.

DENTAL APPLIANCES

Dentures and partial dentures can create a problem for managing the airway. If at all possible, attempt to keep dentures in place when ventilating a patient. They add form and structure to the mouth and make it easier to get a mask seal. If they become dislodged and make it difficult to ventilate the patient, remove them immediately.

FOREIGN BODY AIRWAY OBSTRUCTIONS (FBAO)

In most cases, obstructions to the airway are caused by the tongue of an unresponsive patient contacting the back of the throat. In some situations, foreign objects, such as food, gum, vomit, broken teeth, loose dentures, or blood, can get into the airway and make ventilation difficult or impossible. In these cases, the foreign object must be removed from the airway if the patient is to survive. Trauma to the neck or swelling can also cause an airway obstruction. Airway obstructions can cause cardiac arrest, or can result after a cardiac arrest if the patient vomits

or has dentures that slip out of place. The management of airway obstructions varies according to the degree of obstruction, the patient's age, and if the patient is responsive or unresponsive.

FBAO IN THE RESPONSIVE PATIENT

Foreign bodies that get stuck in the responsive adult's airway are usually caused by a combination of eating too quickly, chewing incompletely, talking while eating, and alcohol consumption. Typically, a piece of food that is too large to swallow becomes lodged in the back of the throat. In the responsive patient, there are three classifications of foreign body airway obstructions: partial FBAO with good air exchange, partial FBAO with poor air exchange, and complete FBAO. You must be able to quickly determine the classification of airway obstruction in the responsive patient, because the management of each is different.

Partial FBAO with good air exchange

If the obstruction is small it will interfere with breathing, but the patient may still be able to get enough oxygen to remain responsive. This is called an airway obstruction with good air exchange. The patient with an airway obstruction that has good air exchange will remain responsive and alert. They may be able to speak and can cough forcefully. You may hear a high-pitched sound, called a **wheeze,** while they breathe or between coughs.

Patients with airway obstruction and good air exchange will be very anxious. This creates an increase in the demand for oxygen and can cause the patient to lose responsiveness. As a First Responder, calm the patient and encourage them to cough forcefully. Hopefully, the patient will be able to clear the obstruction themselves. If you perform any additional interventions, you can cause a partial airway obstruction to become worse. Attempt to resolve an airway obstruction when the partial obstruction results in poor air exchange and in cases of complete airway obstruction.

Partial FBAO with poor air exchange

If the obstruction is large enough, it will be very difficult for the patient to breathe. These patients may have a weak, ineffective cough accompanied with a high-pitched noise on inhalation. Typically, these patients have extreme respiratory difficulty and their skin may have a blue tint.

Complete FBAO

Larger obstructions can prevent any air from being exchanged. As a First Responder, these patients will typically be unresponsive by the time you arrive, but you may witness a complete airway obstruction if you are with someone who chokes in front of you. The patient may clutch the neck with the thumb and fingers. This is an instinctive survival behavior and is often referred to as the **universal distress signal** (Fig. 6-31). With a complete airway obstruction, the patient will not be able to speak, breathe, or cough. Death will follow quickly if prompt action is not taken.

FBAO IN THE ADULT PATIENT
Responsive adult FBAO

The only time you will attempt to relieve an obstruction in a responsive patient is when there is a partial obstruction with poor air exchange or a complete obstruction. Do not attempt any of these procedures on a patient with an obstruction and good air exchange, because of the possibility of making the obstruction worse. Typically, if you respond to an FBAO as a First Responder, the patient will have lost responsiveness prior to your arrival. The most common situation in which you would need to use these skills is if a friend or family member chokes in your presence.

If the patient is still responsive, you should first confirm that they have a complete or partial airway

obstruction with poor air exchange. You should first ask the patient "Are you choking?" If the patient can verbally answer, they have enough air exchange to stay responsive and you should encourage them to cough forcefully to dislodge the object. If the patient cannot speak, or can only make a high-pitched squeaking noise, you must act quickly.

The technique for relieving an obstruction in the responsive adult patient is abdominal thrusts, also called the **Heimlich maneuver,** after its inventor. Abdominal thrusts are very effective because they forcefully raise the pressure in the lungs and can propel the foreign object out of the airway. To perform abdominal thrusts, approach the patient from behind. Inform them that you are going to help them and have them relax as much as possible. Place the thumb side of the fist slightly above the navel and then grab your fist with your other hand. Quickly and sharply pull your hands toward you in an inward and upward fashion (Technique 6-12).

Repeat the abdominal thrusts until the obstruction is relieved or the patient loses responsiveness. If the obstruction is relieved, it is usually with a dramatic exhalation and immediate relief. If the obstruction is not relieved, the patient will lose responsiveness and you should assist them to the floor and initiate the procedure for clearing an obstruction in an unresponsive patient.

Unresponsive adult FBAO

The procedures for dealing with a foreign body airway obstruction in the unresponsive adult combines the use of abdominal thrusts, finger sweeps, and ventilation attempts. In combination, these three techniques are very effective at relieving an obstruction. You may encounter an unresponsive

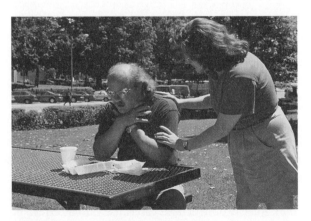

Fig. 6-31 The universal distress signal.

patient with an obstruction as a First Responder, especially when responding to restaurants and nursing homes.

In most cases, you will not realize that the patient has an obstruction until you attempt to ventilate. If the patient has an obstruction, you will meet resistance as you attempt to ventilate. Your first action should be to check to be sure you have properly opened the patient's airway. Perform the head-tilt, chin-lift again to be sure

---

TECHNIQUE 6-12 The Heimlich Maneuver

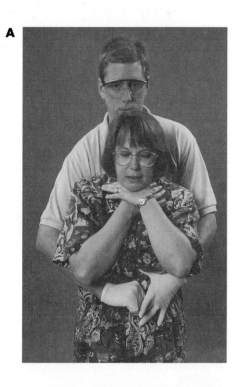

A,

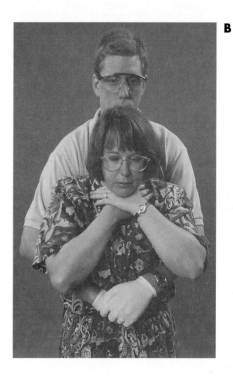

B

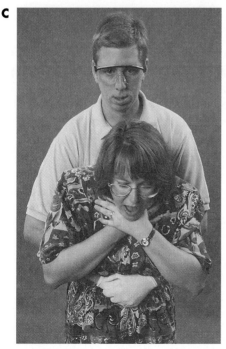

C

Fig. 6-32 Ask the patient "Are you choking?" Inform them that you are going to help them. **A,** Approach the patient from behind and locate the belly button. Place the thumb side of the fist just above the belly button, well below the xiphoid process. **B,** Grasp your fist with your other hand. **C,** Pull inward and upward in discrete sharp blows. Repeat until the object is released or the patient loses responsiveness.

that the airway is open and attempt another ventilation. If you are still experiencing resistance, check the seal of the mask or barrier device you are using. If you are still unable to ventilate the patient, you should proceed to abdominal thrusts.

Straddle the patient and place the heel of one hand slightly above the navel, well below the xiphoid process. Place your other hand on top of the first and interlock your fingers. Be sure that your hands are clear of the rib cage and quickly and sharply thrust inward and upward. Just as in the responsive patient, you are attempting to push the diaphragm up and force air into the lungs to dislodge the object. Technique 6-13 summarizes the steps for performing abdominal thrusts in an unresponsive adult.

After the abdominal thrusts, perform a finger sweep to attempt to remove the object. To perform a finger sweep, kneel next to the patient's shoulders, and turn the head toward you. Place your gloved index finger into their mouth, along the cheek. Insert your finger into the throat and attempt to dislodge any foreign objects you can feel (refer to Technique 6-5).

After the finger sweep, attempt to ventilate the patient. It is possible that the abdominal thrusts and finger sweep dislodged the object from the airway and you may be able to ventilate the patient. If the ventilation is unsuccessful, repeat the sequence of abdominal thrusts, finger sweeps, and ventilations until additional EMS resources arrive. If the ventilation is successful, ventilate the adult patient once every five seconds, the infant or child patient once every three seconds.

Abdominal thrusts are not performed on pregnant patients due to the possibility of injuring the developing baby. In some cases, a patient may be so obese that you cannot get your arms around them. In either of these cases, you should perform chest thrusts instead of abdominal thrusts. To perform chest thrusts on responsive patients, approach them

TECHNIQUE 6-13 Abdominal Thrusts in the Unresponsive Adult

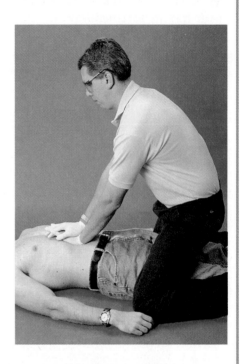

Fig. 6-33 Straddle the patient's thighs. Place the heel of one hand just above the bellybutton and well below the xiphoid process, place your other hand on top of the first and interlock your fingers. Thrust your body weight forward in sharp, discrete blows five times.

from behind, place the flat surface of your fist on the middle of the breastbone and pull sharply inward. In the unresponsive patient, kneel beside the patient. Place the heel of one hand in the middle of the breastbone, being sure to avoid the ribs and the xiphoid process. Place your other hand on top of the first and interlock your fingers. Lock your elbows and sharply push down $1\frac{1}{2}$ to 2 inches. Perform finger sweeps and ventilate as previously described.

FBAO IN INFANTS AND CHILDREN

Anybody who has ever spent time around children knows that they have a tendency to place objects in their mouths. More than 90% of childhood deaths from foreign body airway obstruction are in children below the age of 5, and 65% are infants. Airway obstructions in children are often the result of objects that are not supposed to be eaten, such as toys, balloons, coins, and other small objects that may be lying around. When children are progressing from baby food to solid food, they are prone to airway obstruction from incomplete chewing. Foods such as hot dogs, round candy, nuts, and grapes are common causes of FBAO. Airway obstruction should be suspected in any infant or child who suddenly demonstrates respiratory difficulty with a cough, gagging, **stridor**, or wheezing.

Just as in adults, only attempt to clear a partial FBAO with poor air exchange or complete FBAO. The procedure for clearing an obstruction is slightly different for infants and children than for adults. Also remember that airway obstructions in pediatric patients can be caused by swelling of the airway due to infection. Since stimulation of the throat with you finger could make this situation worse, blind finger sweeps are never performed on infants or children. You should only perform fingers sweeps in infants and children if you see the foreign object causing the obstruction.

FBAO in infants

Since infants are small enough to hold upside down, gravity can be used to help relieve an obstruction. Additionally, the abdominal organs are still developing in infants and could be damaged by abdominal thrusts. Therefore, chest thrusts are used.

Responsive infant FBAO If the infant has a partial FBAO with poor air exchange or a compete FBAO, a combination of chest thrusts and back blows is used. Immediately hold the infant face down with his head lower than his chest. Support the infant on your thigh and use the heel of your other hand to deliver five blows between the shoulder blades (Technique 6-14).

If the obstruction is not relieved, place two fingers on the breastbone, one fingerbreadth below the nipple line. Sharply depress the breastbone $1/2$ to 1 inch, five times (Technique 6-15). Repeat this sequence of five back blows and five chest thrusts until the obstruction is removed, or the infant loses responsiveness.

Unresponsive infant FBAO Once again, you will generally not realize that your patient has an airway obstruction until you attempt to ventilate them after confirming they are not breathing. If you meet resistance during your initial ventilation, reposition the airway to ensure it is open. If you are not able to ventilate, perform five back blows and five chest thrusts. After the five chest thrusts, look into the airway for any obstructions. If you see the object that is occluding the airway,

TECHNIQUE 6-14 Back Blows for FBAO Management in the Infant

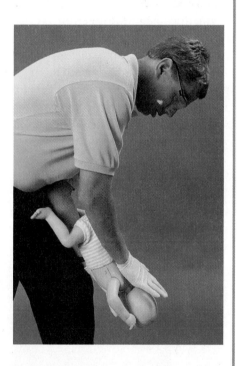

Fig. 6-34 Hold the patient face down with the head lower than the chest, supported on your thigh. Perform firm back blows with the heel of your hand to the area just between the shoulder blades five times.

perform a finger sweep to remove it. If not, attempt to ventilate. Repeat the sequence of back blows, chest thrusts, and inspection of the airway. Continue to ventilate until additional EMS resources arrive.

FBAO in children

Children are too large to be held upside down, so back blows and chest thrusts cannot be performed. Children with airway obstructions are managed in almost the same manner as adults.

Responsive child FBAO Children with complete or partial obstructions with poor air exchange are managed like adults. Approach the patient from behind and place the thumb side of the fist slightly above the navel and well below the xiphoid process. Grab your wrist with your other hand and sharply pull inward until the obstruction is relieved or the patient loses responsiveness.

Unresponsive child FBAO Once you have determined that the patient has an obstruction, reposition the airway and attempt to ventilate. If you are still unsuccessful, straddle the patient's thighs and place the heel of one hand slightly above the navel and well below the xiphoid process. Push inward and upward quickly five times. Look into the mouth for any foreign objects. If you see the object causing the obstruction, perform a finger sweep to remove it. Ventilate and repeat the sequence of abdominal thrusts, inspecting the airway and ventilation until additional EMS resources arrive.

Responsive to unresponsive FBAO management

If you are attempting to relieve an obstruction in a responsive patient and they lose responsiveness while you are treating them, lower them gently to the floor. For an adult, child, or infant, the first step is to manually open the airway with the head-tilt, chin-lift. Since you know they are not breathing, immediately attempt to ventilate. If you are unable to ventilate, go directly to the appropriate technique: abdominal thrusts, chest thrust, or back blows. From this point, the sequence is exactly the same.

FIRST RESPONDER ALERT

If you know that the patient has an airway obstruction, do not waste time checking for breathing or repositioning the airway. Go directly to the appropriate technique after attempting to ventilate.

TECHNIQUE 6-15 Chest Thrusts for FBAO Management in the Infant

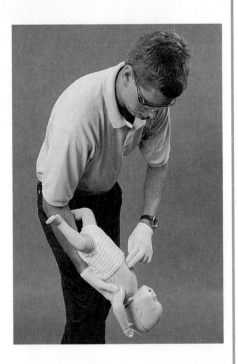

Fig. 6-35 Hold the patient face up with the head lower than the chest, supported on your thigh. Place two fingers on the breastbone, one fingerbreadth below the nipples. Depress the breastbone 1/2 to 1 inch five times.

REVIEW QUESTIONS

Foreign Body Airway Obstruction (FBAO)

1. The most common cause of airway obstruction in the unresponsive adult is the _____.

2. First Responders should not use abdominal thrusts to attempt to relieve an FBAO for an adult patient with good air exchange. True or False?

3. To relieve an obstruction in the unresponsive adult patient, the First Responder should perform _____ abdominal thrusts, then perform a _____ _____, and then attempt to ventilate.

4. Children rarely have airway obstructions serious enough to harm the child. True or False?

5. When attempting to clear the airway of a responsive infant with a complete obstruction, perform 5 _____ _____ followed by 5 _____ _____.

1. Tongue; 2. True; 3. 5, finger sweep; 4. False; 5. Back blows, chest thrusts

CHAPTER SUMMARY

THE RESPIRATORY SYSTEM

The respiratory system maintains the delicate balance of oxygen and carbon dioxide in the body. The airway consists of the passageways from the mouth and nose to the lungs. Airway structures include the nose, nasopharynx, mouth, oropharynx, epiglottis, windpipe (trachea), voice box (larynx), lungs, and the diaphragm. Air is moved in and out of the lungs by the contraction and relaxation of the diaphragm.

OPENING THE AIRWAY

Ensuring an open airway is the most important patient care role of the First Responder. Many circumstances can prevent the free passage of air from the mouth to the lungs. In an unresponsive patient, the base of the tongue resting against the back of the throat can cause an airway obstruction. The head-tilt, chin-lift technique is a simple airway technique that should be performed immediately on any unresponsive, uninjured patient. The jaw thrust without head-tilt should be used on injured patients. Nasal and oral airway devices are very useful in helping to maintain the airway.

CLEARING THE COMPROMISED AIRWAY AND MAINTAINING AN OPEN AIRWAY

The primary method of keeping the uninjured patient's airway open is to place them in the recovery position. This position keeps the tongue away from the back of the throat and allows fluids to drain from the airway. Foreign bodies, such as teeth, gum, and dentures, can create airway problems. They can usually be cleared with finger sweeps. Fluid (such as blood, saliva, vomit) should be suctioned from the airway immediately.

ASSESSING BREATHING

Once you have opened the airway, you should determine if the patient is breathing. If they are breathing, you must then assess the adequacy of breathing. Normal breathing should cause the chest to rise and fall, and the patient must be breathing at an adequate rate and depth.

ARTIFICIAL VENTILATION

Once the airway has been opened, the next priority in patient management is artificial ventilation. First Responders use one of three methods for providing artificial ventilation. Mouth-to-mask ventilations are the preferred method of ventilating a patient. In this technique, the First Responder seals the mask to the patient's face with both hands and exhales into the mask until the chest rises. The next option is to use the mouth-to-barrier technique in which a First Responder exhales through a barrier device into the patient's mouth. The third method of ventilating a non-breathing patient is the mouth-to-mouth technique. Although this technique does not require additional equipment, it may subject the First Responder to infectious diseases.

SPECIAL SITUATIONS IN AIRWAY MANAGEMENT

Special situations present challenges when managing the airway and ventilating certain patients. Patients with stomas can generally be ventilated directly through the stoma. The airways of infants and children are easily compromised by head position, swelling, or fluid. Facial injuries can cause considerable bleeding and swelling. If they remain in place, dental appliances should be kept in place during artificial ventilation.

FOREIGN BODY AIRWAY OBSTRUCTION (FBAO)

Foreign body airway obstructions are common in infants and children, but are immediate life threats to patients of any age. Responsive patients with airway obstructions and good air exchange should be encouraged to cough forcefully to dislodge the object. Responsive patients with an obstruction and poor or no air exchange should be managed immediately. Depending on the age of the patient, a combination of abdominal thrusts, chest thrusts, and back blows may be used to relieve an airway obstruction.

UNITED STATES DEPARTMENT OF TRANSPORTATION NATIONAL HIGHWAY TRAFFIC SAFETY ADMINISTRATION FIRST RESPONDER OBJECTIVES

Check your knowledge. The National Registry of EMTs and many state EMS agencies use the objectives below to develop First Responder certification examinations. Can you meet them?

COGNITIVE OBJECTIVES

1. Name and label the major structures of the respiratory system on a diagram.
2. List the signs of inadequate breathing.
3. Describe the steps in the head-tilt, chin-lift.
4. Relate mechanism of injury to opening the airway.
5. Describe the steps in the jaw thrust.
6. State the importance of having a suction unit ready for immediate use when providing emergency medical care.
7. Describe the techniques of suctioning.
8. Describe how to ventilate a patient with a resuscitation mask or barrier device.
9. Describe how ventilation of an infant or child is different from an adult.
10. List the steps in providing mouth-to-mouth and mouth-to-stoma ventilation.
11. Describe how to measure and insert a oropharyngeal (oral) airway.
12. Describe how to measure and insert a nasopharyngeal (nasal) airway.
13. Describe how to clear a foreign body airway obstruction in a responsive adult.
14. Describe how to clear a foreign body airway obstruction in a responsive child with complete or partial airway obstruction with poor air exchange.
15. Describe how to clear a foreign body airway obstruction in a responsive infant with complete or partial airway obstruction with poor air exchange.
16. Describe how to clear a foreign body airway obstruction in an unresponsive adult.
17. Describe how to clear a foreign body airway obstruction in an unresponsive child.
18. Describe how to clear a foreign body airway obstruction in an unresponsive infant.

AFFECTIVE OBJECTIVES

19. Explain why basic life support ventilation and airway protective skills take priority over most other basic life support skills.

20. Demonstrate a caring attitude toward patients with airway problems who request emergency medical services.
21. Place the interest of the patient with airway problems as the foremost consideration when making any and all patient care decisions.
22. Communicate with empathy to patients with airway problems, as well as with the family members and friends of the patient.

PSYCHOMOTOR OBJECTIVES

23. Demonstrate the steps in the head-tilt, chin-lift.
24. Demonstrate the steps in the jaw thrust.
25. Demonstrate the techniques of suctioning.
26. Demonstrate the steps in mouth-to-mouth ventilation with body substance isolation (barrier shields).
27. Demonstrate how to use a resuscitation mask to ventilate a patient.
28. Demonstrate how to ventilate a patient with a stoma.
29. Demonstrate how to measure and insert an oropharyngeal (oral) airway.
30. Demonstrate how to measure and insert a nasopharyngeal (nasal) airway.
31. Demonstrate how to ventilate infants and children.
32. Demonstrate how to clear a foreign body airway obstruction in a responsive adult.
33. Demonstrate how to clear a foreign body airway obstruction in a responsive child.
34. Demonstrate how to clear a foreign body airway obstruction in a responsive infant.
35. Demonstrate how to clear a foreign body airway obstruction in an unresponsive adult.
36. Demonstrate how to clear a foreign body airway obstruction in an unresponsive child.
37. Demonstrate how to clear a foreign body airway obstruction in an unresponsive infant.

Supplemental Oxygen Therapy

I. Oxygen
II. Equipment for Oxygen Delivery
   A. Oxygen Regulators
   B. Oxygen Delivery Devices

KEY TERMS

Regulator   A device that attaches to an oxygen tank and is used to adjust the flow rate of oxygen to the patient.

Nasal cannula   A low-concentration oxygen delivery device that should be used if the patient will not tolerate a nonrebreather mask.

Nonrebreather mask   A high-concentration oxygen delivery device; the preferred method of administering oxygen in the prehospital setting.

Oxygen is the element of life. A constant supply of oxygen is required by every cell in the body. Our bodies normally get enough oxygen from the air we breathe. In illness or injury, however, the amount of oxygen in the blood may decrease as a result of respiratory difficulty, cardiac failure, or airway obstruction. In these situations, additional oxygen is necessary to decrease the possibility of permanent damage to vital organs. Without exception, the ill or injured patient will benefit from supplemental oxygen. In many EMS systems in the country, First Responders routinely carry and use oxygen.

OXYGEN

The oxygen used by most First Responders is stored in high-pressure tanks. Tanks come in several common sizes (Fig. A-1). Oxygen tanks are usually filled to a pressure of 2000 pounds per square inch. Because this great pressure could be explosive if a tank were damaged, always handle oxygen tanks carefully. The most delicate parts of the tank are the valve and the gauge. Secure oxygen tanks during transport to prevent them from falling or rolling around.

EQUIPMENT FOR OXYGEN DELIVERY

OXYGEN REGULATORS

To deliver oxygen to the patient at the correct pressure and flow rate, an oxygen regulator is used (Fig. A-2). The regulator attaches to the valve of the tank to control the flow of oxygen. Just as with a water faucet, you control the flow rate by adjusting the regulator. Technique A-1 describes how to attach the regulator to the tank.

OXYGEN DELIVERY DEVICES

Once the flow of oxygen is regulated to the desired rate, it can be delivered to the patient. There are many types of oxygen delivery devices available, but only two are generally used by First Responders in prehospital care: nonrebreather masks and nasal cannulas (Fig. A-4). If you work in a setting where another type of mask is used, be sure to learn about it.

Nonrebreather masks

The nonrebreather mask is the preferred prehospital method of delivering oxygen to the patient. This is a high-concentration device that can deliver up to 90% oxygen when the oxygen flow rate is set at 15 L/min. The nonrebreather mask stores oxygen in a reservoir bag. Inflate the reservoir bag with oxygen before you place the mask on the patient. This is done by attaching the tubing to the regulator, setting the flow at 15 L/min, then placing a finger over the one-way valve until the bag is completely inflated (Fig. A-5).

Generally, it is easiest to pull the elastic strap to its full length and place the mask over the patient's head. Position the mask to fit from the

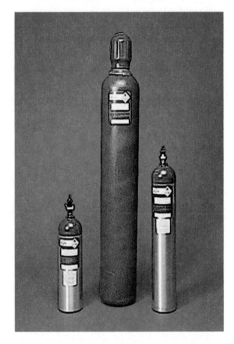

Fig. A-1 Common sizes of oxygen tanks. The D tank is small, the E tank medium, and the M tank large.

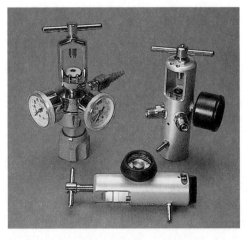

Fig. A-2 Three different kinds of oxygen regulators.

bridge of the nose to the chin and then adjust the strap for a comfortable fit for the patient (Fig. A-6). The reservoir bag should not collapse completely while the patient is breathing.

Nonrebreather masks come in adult and pediatric sizes. The proper mask should fit from the bridge of the patient's nose to just below the bottom lip. Regardless of the mask size, the flow rate should be set at 15 L/min.

In the past, First Responders were instructed to withhold high-concentration oxygen admin-istration for certain patients. The standard has changed, however, for the prehospital setting. Any adult, child, or infant who is in respiratory difficulty should receive high-concentration oxygen.

Some patients become apprehensive when a mask is placed on their face. Usually, if you explain that they are receiving high concentra-tions of oxygen and that this will help them breathe easier, they will calm down. Some patients are more comfortable if they hold the

TECHNIQUE A-1 Attaching Oxygen Regulator to the Tank

A
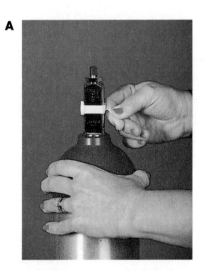

B
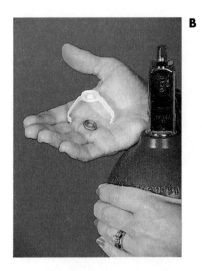

C
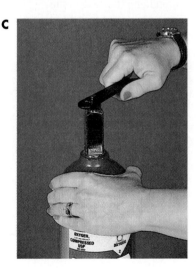

D
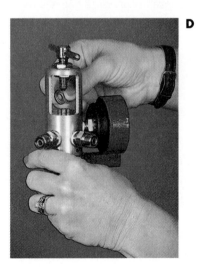

Fig. A-3 A, Remove the protective seal from the valve on the tank. **B,** Attached to the seal is a washer that provides an airtight seal between the regulator and the tank. **C,** Be sure that the valve is facing away from you or anyone else and quickly open and close the valve to blow any dirt or contamination out of the tank opening. **D,** Place the washer over the inlet port on the regulator. **CONTINUED**

TECHNIQUE A-1 CONTINUED

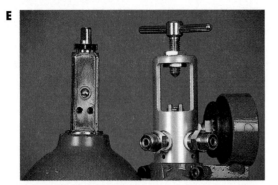

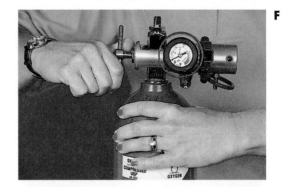

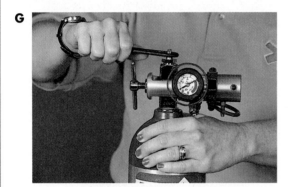

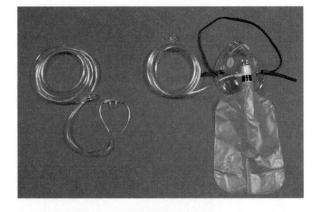

E, Line up the regulator inlet port and pins with the tank opening and holes in the tank valve. The pins are designed so that only an oxygen regulator fits an oxygen tank. Be sure that the flow meter is turned off. **F,** Tighten the screw by hand. **G,** Open the tank valve to test that you have an airtight seal. If oxygen is leaking, tighten the screw until the leak stops. **H,** Adjust the flow meter to the desired setting. When finished, turn off the flow meter and close the tank valve. Release the pressure from the regulator by momentarily opening the flow meter.

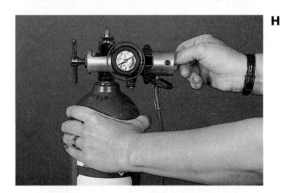

Fig. A-4 A nasal cannula (left) and a nonrebreather mask (right).

mask on their face, instead of having the strap around their head. Having a parent hold the mask close to a child's mouth and nose may help calm a child. If the patient will not tolerate an oxygen mask, you may need to use a nasal cannula.

Nasal cannulas

The nasal cannula is an alternative to delivering oxygen by mask. It is simply a piece of tubing that has holes through which oxygen is blown directly into the patient's nostrils. Nasal cannulas are often used for long-term oxygen therapy in a medical

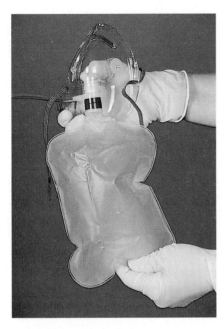

Fig. A-5 Inflate the nonrebreather reservoir bag with oxygen before you place the mask on the patient.

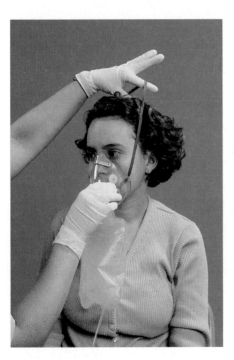

Fig. A-6 Position the mask on the patient, then adjust the strap for a comfortable fit.

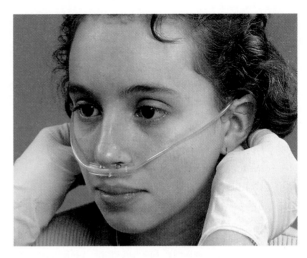

Fig. A-7 Place the prongs of the nasal cannula in the patient's nostrils, then adjust the tubing for comfort.

REVIEW QUESTIONS

Equipment for Oxygen Delivery

1. List the steps necessary to attach a regulator to the oxygen tank.

   _____

   _____

   _____

2. The oxygen delivery device of choice for the patient having severe difficulty breathing is the _____ mask, with the oxygen regulator set at a rate of _____ L/min.

3. What should you do if a patient complains of "being smothered" by an oxygen mask?

   _____

   _____

1. Remove the seal and save the disk, open the tank to blow off any dirt, place the washer over the inlet port of the regulator, attach the regulator onto the tank, tighten the screw, turn the regulator to ensure there are no leaks; 2. Nonrebreather mask, 15; 3. Explain that the patient is getting plenty of oxygen. Use a nasal cannula only if the patient cannot tolerate a mask

facility or at home. To deliver oxygen via nasal cannula, set the flow at a maximum of 6 L/min, then place the prongs into the patient's nostrils (Fig. A-7). Adjust the tubing for the patient's comfort.

In the prehospital setting, nasal cannulas are used only for patients who are still uncomfortable with the nonrebreather mask after you have reassured them that they are getting plenty of oxygen. The nasal cannula is a low-concentration device and is a poor alternative to the nonrebreather mask. It is, however, better than nothing if the patient absolutely will not tolerate the mask.

UNITED STATES DEPARTMENT OF TRANSPORTATION NATIONAL HIGHWAY TRAFFIC SAFETY ADMINISTRATION EMT-BASIC OBJECTIVES

Check your knowledge. Many state EMS agencies use the objectives below to develop First Responder certification examinations. Can you meet them?

COGNITIVE OBJECTIVES

1. Define the components of an oxygen delivery system.
2. Identify a nonrebreather mask and state the oxygen flow requirements needed for its use.
3. Describe the indications for using a nasal cannula versus a nonrebreather face mask.
4. Identify a nasal cannula and state the flow requirements needed for its use.

AFFECTIVE OBJECTIVES

5. Explain the rationale for providing adequate oxygenation through high-inspired oxygen concentrations to patients who, in the past, may have received low concentrations.

PSYCHOMOTOR OBJECTIVES

6. Demonstrate the correct operation of oxygen tanks and regulators.
7. Demonstrate the use of a nonrebreather mask and state the oxygen flow requirements needed for its use.
8. Demonstrate the use of a nasal cannula and state the flow requirements needed for its use.
9. Demonstrate oxygen administration for infants and children.

Advanced First Responder Ventilation Techniques

KEY TERMS

Bag-valve-mask (BVM) A ventilation device consisting of a self-inflating bag, oxygen reservoir, one-way valve, and mask. The BVM is the most common ventilation device used in medicine and is most effectively used with two rescuers.

Flow-restricted, oxygen-powered ventilation device (FROPVD) A ventilation device that attaches directly to an oxygen regulator and delivers a constant flow of oxygen at 40 L/min when the trigger is depressed.

APPENDIX B

Previous sections in this division have described how to ventilate a nonbreathing patient by using the mouth-to-mask, mouth-to-barrier device, and mouth-to-mouth techniques. While these techniques are very effective, they all use your exhaled breath to ventilate the patient. Although exhaled breath contains enough oxygen to sustain life, nonbreathing patients benefit from higher percentages of oxygen.

The following techniques enable you to ventilate a patient with more oxygen than available in your exhaled breath. Unfortunately, they all require additional equipment, which may not be available to you. If you have access to ventilation equipment, you should practice these skills frequently to ensure you are able to perform the skills quickly and effectively in an emergency.

ADVANCED FIRST RESPONDER VENTILATION TECHNIQUES

There are four ventilation techniques you should be familiar with if you have access to the necessary equipment. These techniques are not equally effective, and your system or Medical Director may not approve all of these techniques for First Responders. You should consult your local protocols to determine which, if any, of these techniques are used. The techniques, in decreasing order of effectiveness, are:

1. Mouth-to-mask with supplemental oxygen
2. Two-person bag-valve-mask
3. Flow-restricted, oxygen-powered ventilation device
4. One-person bag-valve-mask

MOUTH-TO-MASK WITH SUPPLEMENTAL OXYGEN TECHNIQUE

Mouth-to-mask ventilation is the most effective method of ventilating a nonbreathing patient. It is a simple technique, and because you can use two hands to create the mask seal, it provides excellent ventilation. Many masks have an inlet port on the mask (Fig. B-1) that enables you to attach oxygen tubing to the device. The constant flow of oxygen enriches the oxygen content of the air you are exhaling into the patient and improves the effectiveness of artificial ventilation.

Mouth-to-mask ventilations with supplemental oxygen are performed exactly as mouth-to-mask ventilations, except that you attach oxygen tubing

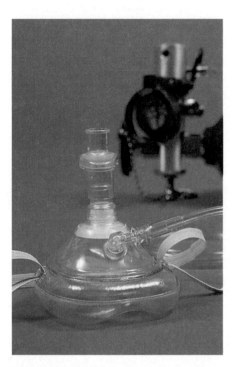

Fig. B-1 Some ventilation masks have a port to attach oxygen tubing to enrich the exhaled breath.

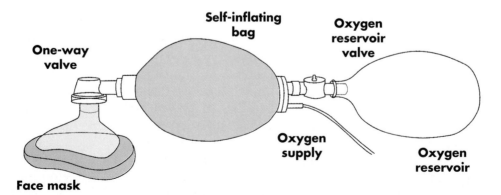

Fig. B-2 The bag-valve-mask device consists of a self-inflating bag, a one-way valve, a mask, and an oxygen reservoir.

to the inlet port on the mask and set the regulator to flow at 15 L/min. Refer to Chapter 6, "The Airway," for a review of the mouth-to-mask ventilation technique. Under normal circumstances, mouth-to-mask with supplemental oxygen will provide the patient with approximately 50% oxygen.

TWO-PERSON BAG-VALVE-MASK TECHNIQUE

The bag-valve-mask (BVM) is a ventilation device commonly used in medicine. The BVM consists of a self-inflating bag, a one-way valve, a mask, and an oxygen reservoir (Fig. B-2). The adult bag has a volume of approximately 1600 ml, which is squeezed to ventilate the patient. The BVM typically delivers less volume than the mouth-to-mask technique.

The BVM is most effective when used with two rescuers. When properly performed, two-person BVM ventilations can deliver 90% to 100% oxygen to a nonbreathing patient when attached to an oxygen source. The BVM can also be used without supplemental oxygen or a reservoir bag, but it only delivers 21% oxygen. The procedure is described in Technique B-1.

A few years ago, a number of BVMs were manufactured with pressure pop-off valves designed to prevent overinflation during ventilating. Research showed that these pop-off valves sometimes resulted in inadequate ventilation. Bag-valve-masks used in emergency situations should not have pop-off valves. Box B-1 lists the features of BVMs.

BOX B-1 Features of the Bag-Valve-Mask

- A self-refilling bag that is either disposable or easily cleaned and sterilized
- A valve that allows a maximum oxygen inlet flow rate of 15 L/min
- Standardized 15/22-mm fittings
- An oxygen inlet and reservoir to allow for a high concentration of oxygen
- A one-way valve that prevents the rebreathing of exhaled air
- Constructed of materials that work in all environmental conditions and temperatures
- Available in infant, child, and adult sizes

TECHNIQUE B-1 Two-Person Bag-Valve-Mask Technique

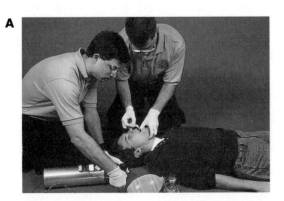
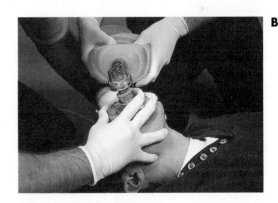

Fig. B-3 A, The first rescuer manually opens the patient's airway from the patient's side. The second rescuer assembles and prepares the BVM (including attaching to oxygen) from a position at the top of the patient's head. The first rescuer then inserts an oral or nasal airway (if tolerated). **B,** The first rescuer holds the bag portion of the BVM with both hands. The second rescuer seals the mask by placing the mask over the bridge of the patient's nose and then lowers the mask over the patient's mouth and upper chin. The second rescuer's thumbs are positioned over the top half of the mask and the index and middle fingers over the bottom half. If the mask has a large round cuff surrounding a ventilation port, the port is centered over the mouth. The first rescuer squeezes the bag slowly and steadily until the chest rises. The second rescuer maintains the airway by using the ring and little fingers to bring the jaw up to the mask and evaluates the chest rise. The first rescuer continues to ventilate the patient at least once every 5 seconds for adults or every 3 seconds for infants and children. The second rescuer maintains the mask seal and open airway and continually monitors the chest rise.

FLOW-RESTRICTED, OXYGEN-POWERED VENTILATION DEVICE TECHNIQUE

The flow-restricted, oxygen-powered ventilation device is an alternative to bag- valve-mask ventilation (Fig. B-4). This device provides 100% oxygen at a peak flow rate of 40 L/min. The valve is designed to prevent over-pressurization of the lungs by an inspiratory pressure relief valve that opens when the pressure exceeds 60 cm of water. Most valves have an audible alarm that sounds when the relief valve is activated. The flow-restricted, oxygen-powered ventilation device should never be used on infants or children because it may cause lung tissue damage and cause air to enter the stomach.

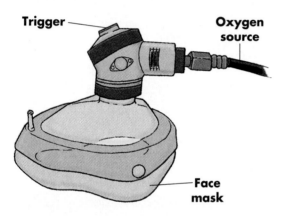

Fig. B-4 A flow-restricted, oxygen powered ventilation device may be used in place of a BVM.

The flow-restricted, oxygen-powered ventilation devices used in the prehospital setting operate in all environmental conditions. The trigger is positioned so that you can maintain the mask seal and airway while ventilating the patient. The main advantage of this technique is that it can be used by one First Responder. The flow-restricted, oxygen-powered ventilation device is preferred over the BVM if only one First Responder is available to ventilate the patient. The procedure is described in Technique B-2.

ONE-PERSON BAG-VALVE-MASK TECHNIQUE

Ventilation with a BVM appears to be a simple skill when practiced on manikins, but on real patients it is very difficult for one First Responder to maintain an open airway, seal the mask, and squeeze the bag. One-person BVM ventilation should be used only as a last resort when no other technique of ventilation is possible. The procedure is described in Technique B-3.

One-person bag-valve-mask ventilation requires a tremendous amount of practice and experience to perform properly.

All techniques for artificial ventilation described in this appendix require that the First Responder maintain an open airway. If the patient is not injured, the head-tilt, chin-lift

---

TECHNIQUE B-2 Flow-Restricted, Oxygen-Powered Ventilation Device Technique

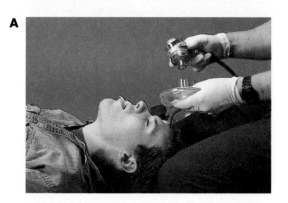
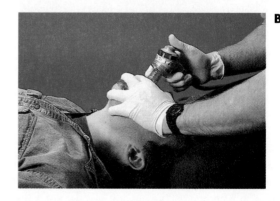

Fig. B-5 Manually open the patient's airway from a position at the top of the patient's head. Insert an oral or nasal airway. **A,** Attach the mask to the flow-restricted, oxygen-powered ventilation device. **B,** Seal the mask by placing the apex of the mask over the bridge of the patient's nose, and then lower the mask over the mouth and upper chin. Position your thumb over the top half of the mask, and the index and middle fingers over the bottom half. Maintain the airway by using the ring and little fingers to bring the jaw up to the mask. Trigger the flow-restricted, oxygen-powered ventilation device until the chest rises. Release the trigger and allow for passive exhalation. Continue to ventilate the patient at least once every 5 seconds for adults. This device should not be used on infants or children.

should be used. The jaw thrust without head-tilt can also be used in conjunction with any of these techniques if the patient has a potential spinal injury.

ASSESSING THE ADEQUACY OF ARTIFICIAL VENTILATION

Whenever you ventilate a patient, it is important to assess the adequacy of the artificial breathing. Especially with advanced First Responder ventilation techniques, everybody attending to the patient must continually evaluate the effectiveness of the ventilation. The signs of adequate and inadequate ventilation are the same with these advanced techniques as the signs listed in Boxes 6-3 and 6-4.

If the ventilation or chest rise is inadequate, you should first check to be sure that you have adequately opened the airway. Next, check the mask seal. Since you now have alternative ventilation

BOX B-2 Correcting Poor Chest Rise During Ventilation When You Have Ventilation Equipment

1. Reposition the jaw
2. Check the mask seal
3. Use an alternative technique (flow-restricted oxygen-powered ventilation device, two-person bag-valve-mask, or mouth-to-mask with supplemental oxygen)
4. Check for an airway obstruction

TECHNIQUE B-3 One-Person Bag-Valve-Mask Technique

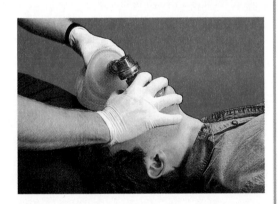

Fig. B-6 Manually open the patient's airway from a position at the top of the patient's head. Insert an oral or nasal airway. Attach oxygen tubing to the oxygen port, and attach the mask to the BVM. Seal the mask by placing the apex of the mask over the bridge of the patient's nose, and then lower the mask over the mouth and upper chin. Make a "C" with your index finger and thumb around the ventilation port. Maintain the airway by using the middle, ring, and little fingers under the jaw to maintain the chin-lift. Squeeze the bag with your other hand slowly and steadily until the chest rises. Allow the patient to passively exhale. Evaluate the chest rise and continue to ventilate the patient at least once every 5 seconds for adults or once every 3 seconds for infants and children.

REVIEW QUESTIONS

Advanced Ventilation Techniques

1. Place the following ventilation techniques in decreasing order of preference.
   A. One-person bag-valve-mask
   B. Flow-restricted, oxygen-powered ventilation device
   C. Mouth-to-mask
   D. Two-person bag-valve-mask

2. List at least four of the desirable features of the bag-valve-mask.

   _____

   _____

   _____

   _____

3. In the two-person bag-valve-mask technique, the EMT at the top of the head is responsible for _____ and

   _____.

4. The flow-restricted, oxygen-powered breathing device provides _____% oxygen at a rate of _____L/min with a pop-off valve set at _____cm of water.

1. C, D, B, A; 2. Self-inflating bag, easily cleaned and sterilized, 15/22-mm fittings/oxygen inlet and reservoir, a valve that prevents rebreathing, works in all environments, available in adult, child, and infant sizes; 3. Holding the mask seal, maintaining an open airway; 4. 100, 40, 60

techniques, you should consider using an alternative ventilation technique if the ventilations are not effective. Remember, not all techniques are equally effective, and one procedure may work while another has failed. If you are still having difficulty in getting an adequate chest rise after you try alternative techniques, you should consider the possibility of an airway obstruction. Box B-2 lists the steps for correcting poor chest rise during ventilation when you have additional ventilation equipment available.

UNITED STATES DEPARTMENT OF TRANSPORTATION NATIONAL HIGHWAY TRAFFIC SAFETY ADMINISTRATION EMT-BASIC OBJECTIVES

Check your knowledge. Many state EMS agencies use the objectives below to develop First Responder certification examinations. Can you meet them?

COGNITIVE OBJECTIVES

1. Describe how to ventilate a patient with a resuscitation mask attached to supplemental oxygen.
2. Describe the steps in performing the skill of artificially ventilating a patient with a bag-valve-mask while using the jaw thrust.
3. List the parts of a bag-valve-mask system.
4. Describe the steps in performing the skill of artificially ventilating a patient with a bag-valve-mask for one and two rescuers.
5. Describe the signs of adequate artificial ventilation using the bag-valve-mask.
6. Describe the signs of inadequate artificial ventilation using the bag-valve-mask.
7. Describe the steps in artificially ventilating a patient with a flow-restricted, oxygen-powered ventilation device.

PSYCHOMOTOR OBJECTIVES

8. Demonstrate how to use a resuscitation mask with supplemental oxygen to artificially ventilate a patient.
9. Demonstrate the assembly of a bag-valve-mask unit.
10. Demonstrate the steps in performing the skill of artificially ventilating a patient with a bag-valve-mask for one and two rescuers.
11. Demonstrate the steps in performing the skill of artificially ventilating a patient with a bag-valve-mask while using the jaw thrust.
12. Demonstrate artificial ventilation of a patient with a flow-restricted, oxygen-powered ventilation device.

Patient Assessment

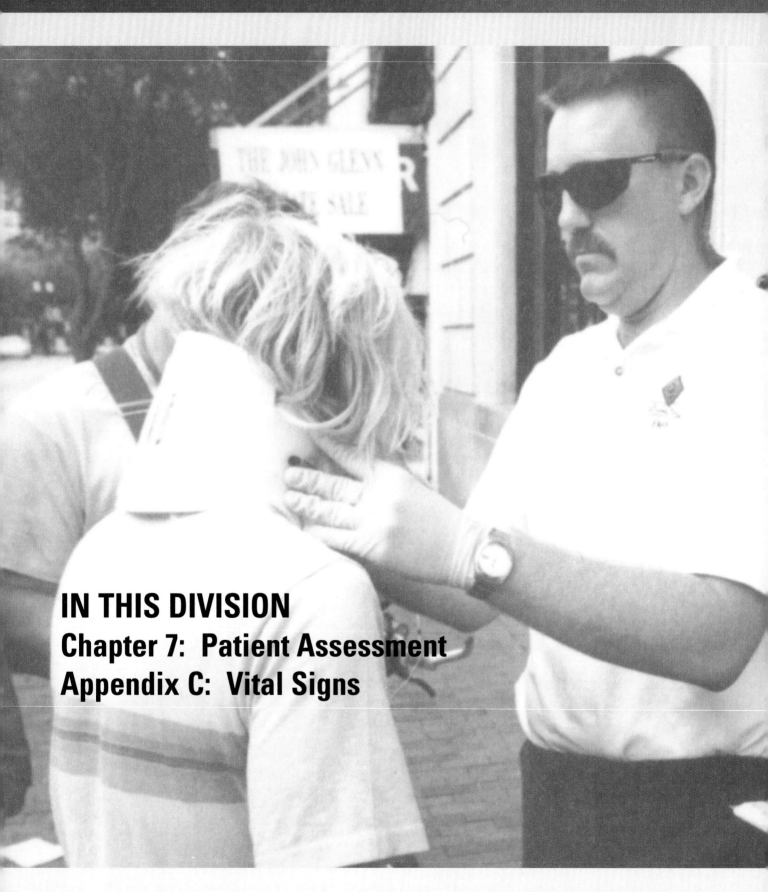

IN THIS DIVISION

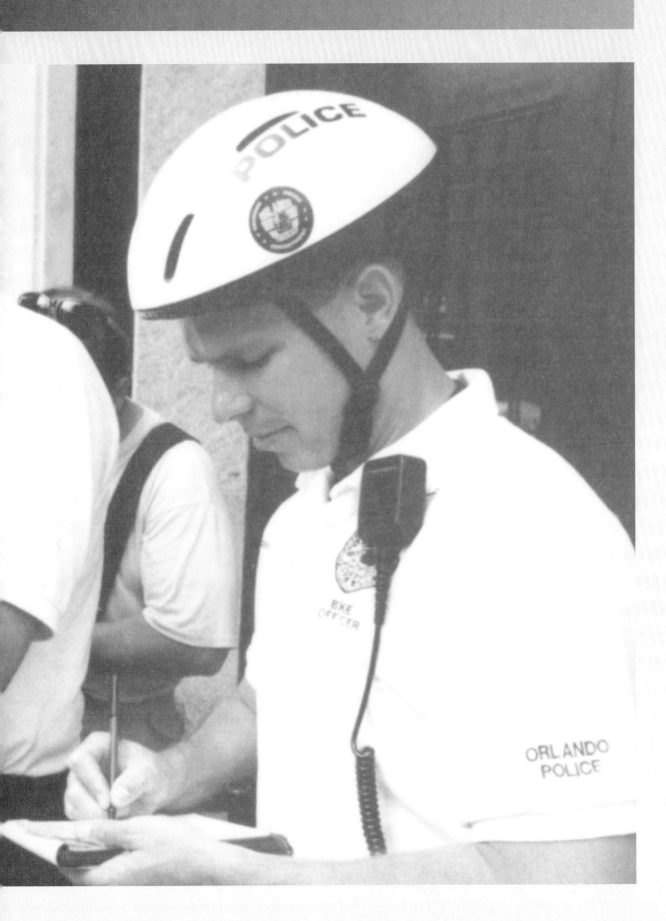

Patient Assessment

SEVEN

I. Scene Size-Up
  A. Body Substance Isolation
  B. Scene Safety
  C. Nature of Illness and Mechanism of Injury
  D. Number of Patients and Need for Additional Help

II. Initial Assessment
  A. General Impression of the Patient
  B. Assess Responsiveness
  C. Assess the Airway
  D. Assess Breathing
  E. Assess Circulation
  F. Report to Responding EMS Units

III. First Responder Physical Exam
  A. Performing a Physical Exam
  B. Medical Patients and Patients With No Significant Injury or Mechanism of Injury
  C. Patient History

IV. Ongoing Assessment

KEY TERMS

Chief complaint   The patient's description of their medical problem.

DOTS   An acronym for the information identified in the First Responder Physical Exam, standing for Deformities, Open injuries, Tenderness and Swelling.

First Responder physical exam   A hands-on evaluation performed by the First Responder to obtain information about the illness or injury.

General impression   The First Responder's immediate assessment of the environment and the patient's chief complaint, accomplished in the first few seconds of the patient contact.

Initial assessment   The first step in the evaluation of every medical and trauma patient used to identify immediate life threats.

Mechanism of injury   The event or force that caused the patient's wounds.

Nature of illness   The event or condition leading to the patient's medical complaint.

Ongoing assessment   The final step of the patient assessment process that involves repeating the initial assessment and continues until patient care is transferred to arriving EMS personnel.

SAMPLE history   An mnemonic for the history of Signs and Symptoms, Allergies, Medications, Pertinent history, Last oral intake, and Events leading to the illness or injury.

Scene size-up   The evaluation of the entire environment for safety, the mechanism of injury or nature of illness, number of patients, and need for additional help.

FIRST RESPONSE

Police officers Dave and Tony, both First Responders, were dispatched to a one car crash on Lexington Drive. They arrived before the ambulance, and immediately began to assess the scene. The scene size-up revealed that one car had crashed head-on into a utility pole. Two patients were in the car, and power lines had fallen across the hood. Dave called dispatch to notify the power company of the situation and to have them respond to the scene immediately. He then called the responding ambulance and gave them preliminary information about the scene.

Recognizing an unsafe scene, they did not approach the car. While waiting for the power company, Tony directed traffic and kept bystanders away from the scene. Although they were unable to assess or begin to care for the patients, their scene size-up kept them from entering a dangerous situation.

Patient assessment is the process by which First Responders gain information about the patient's condition. There are several steps in the patient assessment process: the scene size-up, the initial assessment, the First Responder physical exam, and the ongoing assessment. Each stage of this assessment reveals information that will help the First Responder decide how best to care for the patient. Let's begin by discussing the scene size-up.

SCENE SIZE-UP

The **scene size-up** is the First Responder's first look at the patient and the surrounding situation. Scene size-up incorporates the knowledge, attitude, and skills necessary to stay alive and well. The scene size-up includes checking scene safety, determining the mechanism of injury or nature of illness, finding out how many patients are involved, and determining whether you need additional help.

BODY SUBSTANCE ISOLATION

Before beginning the scene size-up, always consider the need for body substance isolation (BSI) precautions. BSI precautions protect health care professionals from contact with blood and other body fluids (Fig. 7-1). It is your responsibility to take the necessary precautions to protect yourself from contagious diseases. Chapter 2, "The Well-Being of the First Responder," discusses BSI precautions and how and when to use gloves, masks, gowns, and eye protection. Many health care professionals chose to take BSI precautions before they enter the

scene so they are never in a situation in which they are exposed to blood or other body fluids and have not taken precautions.

SCENE SAFETY

The goal of evaluating scene safety is to ensure that you, other First Responders, the patient, or bystanders are not harmed while you are providing care. During the beginning of the scene size-up, evaluate the entire environment for any risks (Fig. 7-2). This size-up provides valuable information to help you stay alive and well. To protect yourself and your crew, use your senses of smell, vision, and sound to evaluate every patient situation.

As a First Responder, your primary responsibility is your own safety. Rushing into a scene before evaluating it for safety may result in personal injury or death. First Responders who do not carefully evaluate situations before entering the scene not only create a danger for themselves but also put their fellow health care professionals at risk. The goal of the First Responder on the scene is to provide early care for the patient. Additional responding personnel should not have to confront a situation in which they have to provide care for both the patient who initially needed EMS and a First Responder who has also become injured. Your responsibility is to ensure your own safety before addressing the safety of the patient or bystanders. Use your good judgment and experience to decide whether a scene is safe. If you decide that a scene is unsafe, do not enter until you can implement safety measures.

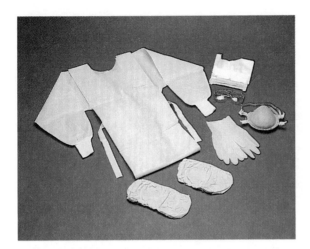

Fig 7-1 Body substance isolation (BSI) precautions protect First Responders from contact with blood and other body fluids.

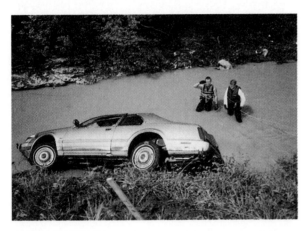

Fig 7-2 First Responders may place themselves at risk by not checking for hazards, such as approaching this unsecured car.

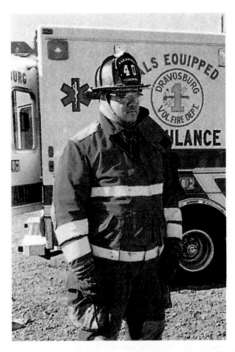

Fig 7-3 First Responders should wear appropriate protective clothing when working around crash scenes.

> **FIRST RESPONDER ALERT**
>
> If the scene is not safe and you cannot make it safe, do not enter.

Everything you see and hear at the scene indicates whether the scene is safe. Trauma scenes with broken glass, torn metal, and spilled hazardous fluids are not the only scenes that can result in injury. Other factors such as dangerous animals or people, fumes or toxic substances, or even overzealous bystanders can place the First Responder in danger. Any First Responder may encounter special situations such as rescue situations, toxic substances, and crime scenes. A simple situation such as an icy street can place the First Responder in danger of being injured. If a dangerous situation is found, take the necessary measures to secure the scene before proceeding. Part of making the scene safe to provide care is wearing the appropriate clothing when working around crash scenes (Fig. 7-3).

After checking that the scene is safe for you and other First Responders to provide care, you are responsible for ensuring the safety of the patient. Your role as a First Responder includes protecting the patient from additional injury that may occur from traffic or other hazards. Bystanders who park their cars inappropriately close to the scene create hazards for themselves, the patient, and you. An approaching vehicle that swerves to miss hitting a bystander might end up in the patient care area. In rescue and extrication operations, protect the patient from metal, flying glass, or sparks created by extrication tools. Patients also require protection from the environment, such as extreme heat or cold.

In some situations you need to ensure the safety of bystanders at the scene after protecting yourself and the patient. Usually law enforcement personnel have this role, but if you are first on the scene you may have to assume this responsibility. Bystanders become so engrossed in the emergency that they fail to watch out for themselves. You should move bystanders away from the immediate area for their safety.

NATURE OF ILLNESS AND MECHANISM OF INJURY

After ensuring safety at the scene, you should evaluate the nature of illness for the medical patient or the mechanism of injury for the trauma patient. The nature of illness is the event or condition leading to the patient's medical condition. The mechanism of injury is the event or force that caused the patient's injury.

To determine the nature of illness, speak with the patient to learn more about the situation (Fig. 7-4). The patient, if responsive, is usually the best source of information. In some cases, the patient is unresponsive or unable to provide information. A family member or a bystander who witnessed the situation or knows the patient's medical history may provide information about the patient.

The appearance of the patient or the clinical signs may make the nature of illness obvious, or you may determine it shortly after your arrival as the patient describes the symptoms. The patient's chief complaint is their description of the medical problem. The nature of illness is the general cause of the problem. For example, the patient may describe their chief complaint as "chest pain." The nature of illness would then be a cardiac problem. If the patient describes the problem as "I can't catch my breath," the nature of illness would be a respiratory problem.

Ask patients about their chief complaint and provide care based on this information and your assessment findings. Ask questions such as: "Why did you call for EMS?" and "How do you feel?"

For trauma patients, after ensuring scene safety and taking BSI precautions, determine the mechanism of injury. The mechanism of injury is determined by looking at the scene to see what forces caused the patient's injury. Sometimes you can tell by looking at the patient and the surroundings. Other times, you will need to get information from the patient. If the patient is unresponsive or cannot provide information regarding the mechanism of injury, ask family, friends, or bystanders who witnessed the incident. The situation may not be what it seems at first. Ask specific questions about the situation, and do not jump to conclusions. The following are examples of questions to consider or ask others when determining the mechanism of injury:

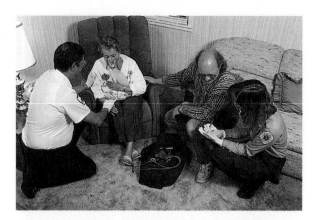

Fig 7-4 Talk to the patient and the patient's family to gain more information about the nature of the patient's illness.

BOX 7-1 Mechanisms of Injury Considered High-Risk for Hidden Injury

- Ejection of driver or passenger from a vehicle
- Driver or passenger in the same passenger compartment where another patient died
- A fall of more than six m (20 ft)
- Vehicle rollover
- High-speed vehicle collision
- Vehicle-pedestrian collision
- Motorcycle crash
- Penetrating trauma to the head, chest, or abdomen

For motor vehicle crashes: How fast was the vehicle traveling? What did the vehicle hit? How much damage was done to the vehicle? Were the occupants wearing seat belts? Were motorcycle drivers wearing helmets? Is the steering wheel bent? Is the windshield cracked? An example of the mechanism of injury to report to arriving EMS personnel could be, "7-year-old female unrestrained front seat passenger of a two-car head-on collision, minor damage to the car, no damage to the windshield."

For falls: How far did the patient fall? What did the patient land on? What part of the patient's body hit the ground first? An example of the mechanism of injury for a patient who has fallen could be, "28-year-old male patient fell three stories, landing feet first on a grassy surface."

For gunfire victims: What kind of gun was used? At what distance was the gun fired? An example of the mechanism of injury for a patient who has been shot is, "17-year-old male shot in the

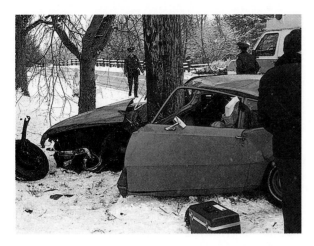

Fig 7-5 You should expect the driver of this car to have significant internal injuries, based on the serious mechanism of injury.

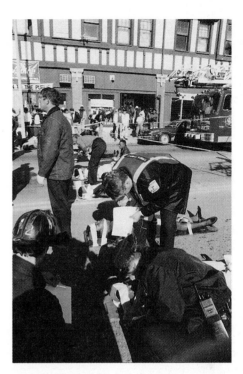

Fig 7-6 Multiple-patient incidents often require additional EMS assistance.

abdomen with a 45-caliber pistol from 5 feet away."

The patient may have sustained injuries besides the ones you first see. Often internal injuries are far more serious than the obvious external injuries to the patient. Evaluating the mechanism of injury helps you know when to suspect hidden injuries and guides you toward providing the most appropriate patient care. First Responders should maintain a high index of suspicion for a patient who seems uninjured, but who has sustained a serious mechanism of injury (Fig. 7-5). Some examples of serious mechanisms of injury are listed in Box 7-1. You should treat any patient who is unresponsive following a traumatic incident as though they have severe injuries, even if you find no injuries on the physical exam.

NUMBER OF PATIENTS AND NEED FOR ADDITIONAL HELP

Calls for individuals with a medical problem usually involve only one patient. However, trauma calls such as motor vehicle crashes often involve more than one patient. When evaluating the scene, you should also determine whether additional patients are present. If you see a car seat in or outside the vehicle, an infant or child patient may be present somewhere on the scene. Gender-specific articles (such as a woman's purse or a man's wallet) may suggest the presence of an unseen patient. Look all around the scene to determine the total number of patients.

If multiple patients are present, you must inform the responding EMS units and request

additional help if necessary (Fig. 7-6). Do not delay the call for assistance. Having the extra help return unneeded is better than to need them and not have them available. If more patients are present than your EMS system can care for, you must begin triage and activate a mass casualty incident plan, as described in Chapter 14, "EMS Operations."

Sometimes you may require additional help for actions other than patient care. You may need help to lift a large patient. You may need law enforcement officials to deal with traffic problems, uncooperative bystanders, or potentially violent scenes. You may need special assistance from fire personnel, rescue personnel, or utility companies. When possible, call for additional help before beginning patient care or when you realize you need assistance. Avoid getting into a situation in which you become so involved in patient care that you do not remember or have time to call for additional help.

INITIAL ASSESSMENT

The first decisions about patient assessment and care are typically made within the first few seconds of seeing the patient. The initial assessment is

REVIEW QUESTIONS

Scene Size Up

1. First Responders should assess_____ _____ before assessing the patient.

2. Before entering the scene, what should you do to protect yourself?

_____

_____

3. If more patients are present than you can handle, what should you do?

_____

_____

1. Scene safety; 2. Assess for danger and take appropriate BSI precautions; 3 Begin triage and request additional help immediately

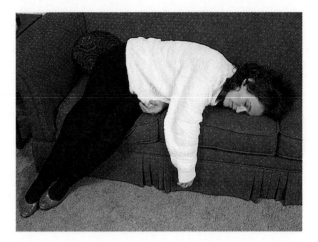

Fig 7-7 The general impression helps you to determine the patient's priority and begin to plan care.

completed to help the First Responder identify immediate threats to the patient's life.

During the initial assessment, you quickly evaluate the patient to form a general impression, assess mental status, assess the airway, assess breathing rate and quality, assess circulation, identify any life-threatening injuries, and provide care based on those findings. After completing the initial assessment, you should report to the responding EMS unit with a brief radio report summarizing the patient information.

Life-threatening injuries include inadequate breathing, major bleeding, inadequate circulation, and a variety of other conditions, which are discussed in later chapters. If you identify a life threat, you must correct it immediately. For example, if blood, vomit, or teeth are present in the airway of a trauma patient, you must clear the airway before performing any other assessment or care. If a patient has no pulse, cardiopulmonary resuscitation (CPR) must begin immediately. By looking at, listening to, and touching the patient, you can identify threats to life.

GENERAL IMPRESSION OF THE PATIENT

After completing the scene size-up and taking appropriate BSI precautions, the first thing to do as you approach the patient is to form a general impression. The **general impression** is your immediate assessment of the environment and the

patient's problem. This process takes place in seconds. The general impression usually allows you to determine the priority of care for the patient. Once you have completed the general assessment, you can form a plan of action for continuing to assess the patient and provide care (Fig. 7-7). During the general impression, you will determine the nature of illness or mechanism of injury, the sex of the patient, and his or her approximate age.

The nature of illness or the mechanism of injury guides your general impression of the patient's general appearance. For example, if a patient was in a rollover car crash that caused severe damage to the car, the patient has potential for serious injury. Even if the patient seems stable or has only minor injuries, you should be suspicious that the patient may have severe internal injuries.

If you are unsure if the patient has a medical problem or an injury, treat the patient as though they have sustained trauma.

ASSESS RESPONSIVENESS

After forming a general impression and before continuing the assessment, you must stabilize or immobilize the spine if the mechanism of injury suggests that a spinal injury may be present. Specific techniques for stabilizing and immobilizing the spine are discussed in Chapter 11, "Injuries to Muscles and Bones." For now, remember that you should not move patients with potential spinal injuries before appropriate immobilization.

To assess the patient's responsiveness, begin by speaking to the patient. Introduce yourself, tell the

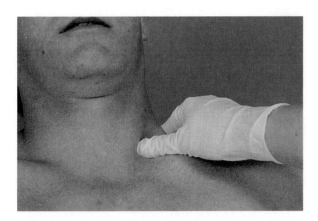

Fig 7-8 Check the patient's response to painful stimuli, such as a shoulder pinch, if the patient does not respond to verbal stimuli.

patient that you are a First Responder, and explain that you are there to help and to provide care until additional help arrives. Note the patient's response.

Patients may be **A**lert; may not be fully alert but still respond to **V**erbal stimuli; may respond only to **P**ainful stimuli; or may be completely **U**nresponsive. The acronym AVPU is a reminder of these four categories, which are described in more detail below. The normal mental status is alert. If the patient is only responsive to verbal or painful stimuli or is unresponsive, they have an altered mental status.

An alert patient is one who interacts with you without prompting. Alert patients know their name, where they are, what time it is, and the reason they called EMS. Some patients may know their name but be unsure of where they are or what time it is. These patients are still alert but are considered disoriented. In a child, alert responses depend on the child's developmental stage. An alert child at almost any age clearly prefers being with their usual caretakers than strangers such as you. Remember that sick and injured children often regress in behavior. For example, children three years of age who can usually say their name may not do so when they are hurt or scared. Assess how well they interact with the environment and their parents.

Some patients may appear to be sleeping but respond when you talk to them. These patients are responsive to verbal stimuli. Some patients may respond only to loud verbal stimuli. Responses in children of any age may range from following a command, to actively trying to find a parent's voice, to crying after a loud noise.

Patients who do not respond to a verbal stimulus may respond to a painful stimulus (Fig. 7-8). Pinching the patient's skin between the neck and shoulder is an adequate painful stimulus. Patients may respond to painful stimuli by making a noise, trying to remove the painful stimulus, or trying to pull away from the stimulus.

If a patient does not respond to verbal or painful stimuli, the patient is unresponsive. Few patients are completely unresponsive. Most patients with decreased responsiveness have some response to pain.

To assess the patient's level of responsiveness, first determine if the patient interacts with you without prompting. If so, the patient is alert. If not alert, will the patient respond to verbal stimuli? If not, will the patient respond to painful stimuli? A patient who does not respond to any stimulus is unresponsive.

Note the responsiveness of the patient in your first interaction and note any later changes. If there is a change in the patient's responsiveness, discuss the trends with the arriving EMS personnel in your verbal report. Be prepared to provide airway support or to treat the patient for signs and symptoms of shock if you note that the patient's responsiveness is deteriorating.

ASSESS THE AIRWAY

You will assess the airway in one of two ways, depending on whether the patient is alert or has an altered mental status. Alert patients may be talking or crying. If they are, the airway is open and you should move immediately to evaluate their breathing. If the patient is responsive to verbal or painful stimuli only and is not talking or crying, you may need to open the airway.

The airway is opened in one of two ways, depending on whether the patient has a medical condition or an injury. For medical patients, perform the head-tilt, chin-lift. For trauma patients, or patients with an unknown nature of illness or mechanism of injury, manually stabilize the spine with your hands and perform the jaw thrust without head-tilt (Fig. 7-9). Refer to Chapter 6, "The Airway," for a review of these procedures.

Once the airway is open, check to be sure it is clear. You may need to use suction, finger sweeps, or position the patient to maintain an open, clear airway. After the airway is open and clear, the next step is to assess breathing.

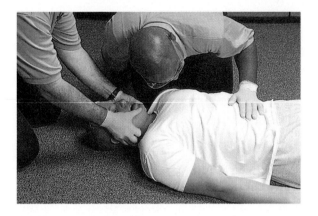

Fig 7-9 Use the head-tilt, chin-lift for medical patients, the jaw thrust without head-tilt for trauma patients.

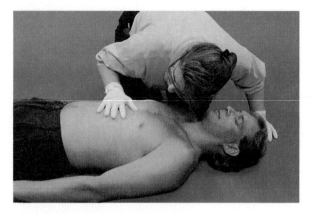

Fig 7-10 Assess breathing by looking for chest rise. Listening for air movement, and feeling the movement of exhaled air against your cheek.

ASSESS BREATHING

Assess the patient's breathing efforts to determine how much effort they are exerting to breathe. Ask the responsive patient if they can speak and assess the effort of breathing. For the unresponsive patient, remember to look, listen, and feel for breathing (Fig. 7-10). Assess the rate and quality of the patient's breathing. Most adults breathe 12 to 20 times a minute and take in a volume of air based on size and weight. You should become concerned if the respiratory rate drops below eight or is greater than 24. A respiratory rate of less than eight per minute or greater than 24 per minute may not provide enough oxygen to support the patient's oxygen demands.

If the patient is responsive, coach them to increase or decrease their respiratory rate. Patients who are breathing too quickly may require oxygen administration. Patients who are breathing too slowly require artificial ventilation. Chapter 6, "The Airway," and Appendix B, "Oxygen Administration Skills," describe the techniques of ventilation and oxygen administration. The First Responder assessing the patient should not stop the assessment to administer oxygen, but should let another crew member perform this task. Not all First Responders have the equipment needed for oxygen administration, so follow your local protocols regarding the use of oxygen and ventilation.

Priorities for assessing breathing and providing necessary treatment are the same for infants and children as for adults. Normal breathing rates depend on the patient's age (see Appendix C, "Vital Signs"). Younger children breathe more quickly than adults. A child who is breathing too slowly is much sicker than one who is breathing too fast. As a child begins to fatigue, their breathing rate begins to slow. This usually represents a child in severe distress. Closely monitor children breathing at a rapid rate. Their rates may begin to drop as fatigue sets in. Provide oxygen and ventilate the patient following your local protocol.

ASSESS CIRCULATION

After evaluating the patient's level of responsiveness, airway, and breathing, and providing interventions as necessary, assess circulation. This assessment involves checking the pulse, looking for major bleeding, and assessing perfusion.

Pulse

For responsive adult patients, assess circulation for rate and quality by palpating the radial artery. If you cannot feel a radial pulse, palpate (feel) the carotid pulse. If the patient is unresponsive upon your arrival at the scene, you should assess the carotid pulse first.

When assessing a responsive child, palpate the brachial or radial pulse first. For the unresponsive child, palpate the carotid or femoral pulse. For infants, responsive or unresponsive, assess the brachial pulse (Fig. 7-11).

When evaluating the pulse, note the rate and quality of the pulse. The pulse rate may be rapid, normal, or slow. The quality can be normal or weak. For patients who have a pulse, palpate the distal (farthest from the trunk of the body — such as the radial or brachial) and central pulses (pulses on the trunk of the body — such as the carotid or femoral) simultaneously (Fig. 7-12). If

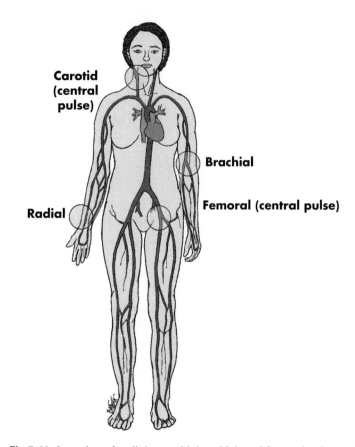

Fig 7-11 Location of radial, carotid, brachial, and femoral pulses.

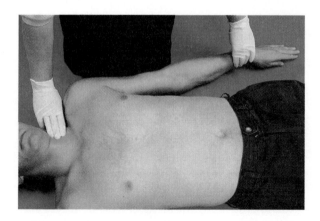

Fig 7-12 Take radial and carotid pulses simultaneously for comparison.

the distal pulse is absent or weaker than the central pulse, the patient is showing a sign of shock.

If no pulse is present, begin CPR. For medical patients who are 12 years of age or older and weigh 40 kg (90 lbs.) or more, an automated external defibrillator (AED) is also used. AEDs and their use are discussed in Appendix D, "Automated External Defibrillation." For medical patients who are less than 12 years of age or less than 40 kg, and for trauma patients, begin CPR and wait for the arrival of additional EMS personnel; AEDs are not used in these cases.

Major bleeding

Next, evaluate the patient for major bleeding. You may have detected major bleeding earlier in the assessment, while you were assessing for life-threatening conditions. As part of assessing the patient's circulation, check again for major bleeding. You may need to expose injured areas by removing clothing to assess for bleeding. For patients with major trauma, you should remove all clothing to properly assess for injury and bleeding. If you see significant bleeding as you assess the patient, treat it as a life-threatening condition as described in Chapter 10, "Bleeding and Soft Tissue Injuries."

Assess Perfusion

By assessing the patient's skin color and temperature, we can assess the patient's perfusion. Perfusion is the process of circulating blood to the organs, delivering oxygen, and removing wastes. Assess the patient's color by looking at the nail beds, inside the lips, or the skin inside the eyelids. Normally, the color of these areas is pink in people of any race. Abnormal colorations include pale, blue-gray, flushed or red, and jaundiced or yellow.

Assess skin temperature by putting the back of your hand against the patient's skin. Normal skin is warm to the touch. Abnormal skin temperatures are hot, cool, or cold. Also note if the skin is dry or moist. Taking the patient's temperature with a thermometer in prehospital settings is not necessary; the basic assessment with your hand is sufficient. If the patient's skin is cool and moist, the patient may be in a state of hypoperfusion (shock). If the skin is hot and dry, the patient may be suffering from a medical condition or having a heat-related emergency.

REPORT TO RESPONDING EMS UNITS

After completing the initial assessment, contact the EMS unit that will be transporting the patient and provide a brief report about the

---

BOX 7-2 Patient Information for Radio Report to EMS Personnel

- Age and sex
- Chief complaint
- Responsiveness
- Airway and breathing status
- Circulation status

REVIEW QUESTIONS

Initial Assesment

1. The general impression guides patient care. True or False?

2. _____Alert   A. Responds to being pinched

   _____Verbal   B. Responds without prompting

   _____Painful   C. Does not respond

   _____Unresponsive   D. Responds to questions

3. Where should you assess the pulse of an infant? _____

1. True; 2. B, D, A, C; 3. Assess the brachial pulse

---

patient's condition. Be sure to speak clearly and provide as much detail as possible concerning your findings (Box 7-2).

Ask the responding EMS personnel to estimate how long it will take them to arrive at the scene. Ask the incoming unit if anything else should be done before their arrival.

FIRST RESPONDER PHYSICAL EXAM

So far we have discussed the scene size-up that takes place before beginning patient care and the initial assessment. Following the initial assessment, your next step is to perform the First Responder physical exam. The goal of the **First Responder physical exam** is to find the patient's injuries or to find out more about the signs and symptoms of their illness, and to begin to manage the condition. All patients receive a First Responder physical exam, but the exam differs depending on whether the patient has a medical or trauma condition. Most patients usually fit into one of these categories. If you are not immediately sure whether the patient has a trauma or medical condition, treat the situation as trauma.

The First Responder physical examination is a methodical head-to-toe evaluation of the patient. To evaluate the patient you will inspect (look) and palpate (feel) for the following signs of injury: Deformities, Open injuries, Tenderness and Swelling. The mnemonic **DOTS** is helpful in remembering the signs of injury. Deformities occur when bones are broken, causing an abnormal position or shape. Open injuries break the continuity of the skin. Tenderness is sensitivity to touch. Swelling is a response of the body to injury that makes the area look larger than usual. Be sure to evaluate the following areas: the head, neck, chest, abdomen, pelvis, and all four extremities.

Alert and responsive adult patients can usually tell you a great deal about the nature of their illness or how they were injured. Infants and children may not describe their symptoms accurately, although their parents may be helpful in explaining their behavior. Some older patients also may not clearly describe their illness or how they became injured. Listen carefully to what all patients tell you, and ask questions to clarify if you are unsure what their responses mean.

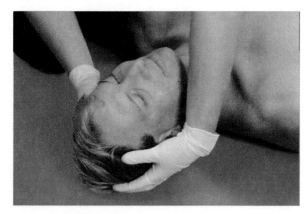

Fig 7-13 Palpate the patient's head.

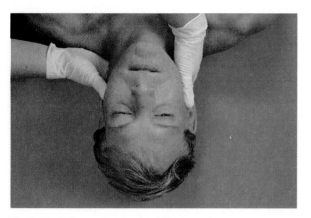

Fig 7-14 Palpate the neck while your partner maintains manual stabilization.

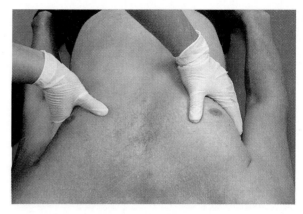

Fig 7-15 Expose and palpate the chest.

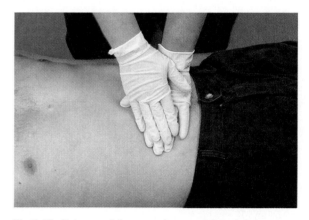

Fig 7-16 Palpate all four quadrants of the abdomen

All patients should receive a physical exam. However, if you are spending all of your time keeping the airway clear or assisting ventilation, do not interrupt care of the airway, breathing, or circulation to perform a First Responder physical exam.

PERFORMING A PHYSICAL EXAM

Beginning at the head, inspect and palpate for DOTS. Palpate the head beginning on the top surface, running your hands toward the back of the head (Fig. 7-13). Bring your hands around to the patient's forehead and feel the face. Note any unstable areas.

Next, evaluate the patient's neck (Fig. 7-14). Remember, for a trauma patient, you must stabilize the spine. Feel around the back, the front, and the sides of the neck for DOTS and look for signs of injury.

Next, evaluate the chest inspecting and palpating for DOTS (Fig. 7-15). An easy way to perform this evaluation is to start at the clavicles

(collar bone) and move to the sternum (breastbone). While inspecting and palpating the ribs, move your fingers as far around the sides toward the back as possible. Ask a responsive patient to take a deep breath. The chest should rise and fall equally on both sides.

Evaluate the abdomen next (Fig. 7-16). Because some patients are particularly sensitive about having their abdominal area touched, inform all patients what you are about to do before you begin. After placing your hand on the abdomen, allow the patient to relax the abdominal muscles so that you can better determine whether the abdomen feels soft or rigid. The abdomen is normally soft. If the abdomen is hard or distended, there may be bleeding into the abdomen caused by an internal injury. While you are evaluating the abdomen, watch the patient's facial expression for grimaces.

If you do not suspect that the patient has a pelvic injury based on the mechanism of injury and the

A

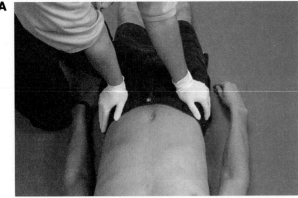

B

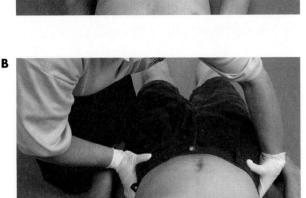

Fig 7-17 Palpate the pelvis by pressing **A**, towards the floor and **B**, towards the midline.

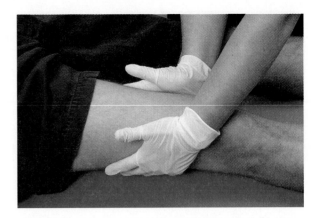

Fig 7-18 Palpate the lower extremities.

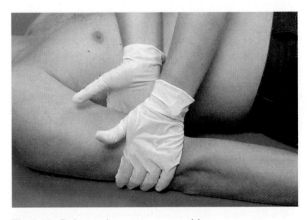

Fig 7-19 Palpate the upper extremities.

patient does not complain of pain, you can also gently palpate the pelvis (Fig. 7-17). Carefully and gently push posteriorly on the patient's hip bone and then to the patient's midline to determine the stability of the pelvis. If motion is present, the pelvis is unstable. If the pelvis is unstable, do not reassess this area. Further movement of the pelvis could aggravate injuries to the spine, nerves, or blood vessels. If the patient complains of pain in the pelvis, or if the mechanism of injury suggests a pelvic injury (for example, a patient who was hit by a truck in the hip), assume an injury is present and do not assess the pelvis.

Finally, check the four extremities. Because you have just evaluated the pelvis, move on to check the lower extremities first. Do not exert pressure with your thumbs only, but use your entire hand to assess the patient's extremities. As you move down the extremity from the pelvis, start high on the thigh of the patient's leg closest to you, and run your hands down the entire extremity (Fig. 7-18), then assess the opposite leg. Continue the assessment by moving to the

patient's upper extremities. Evaluate the arm closest to you, starting at the shoulder and moving to the finger tips. Then check the arm on the opposite side (Fig. 7-19).

After checking each extremity you may check for distal pulse, motor function, and sensation. Pulses can be felt in the feet either on top of the foot or behind the ankle. Motor function is the ability to move and sensation is the ability to feel a touch against the skin. Ask responsive patients if they can wiggle their toes and if they can feel you touching them. You probably cannot assess sensation and motor function in unresponsive patients, because these patients may not react to a touch on the extremities. Make note of the patient's ability or inability to feel or move any of the extremities, and reassess for changes in their condition.

The steps of the First Responder physical examination are the same for infants and children as for adults. You may wish to use a "trunk-to-head" approach, as discussed in Chapter 13, "Infants and Children."

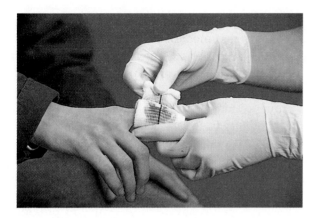

Fig 7-20 A patient with an isolated injury like the one shown here may not need a complete head-to-toe physical exam.

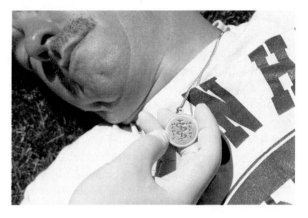

Fig 7-21 The Medic-Alert® tag informs health care providers of the wearer's medical condition if the person is unresponsive or cannot communicate directly.

MEDICAL PATIENTS AND PATIENTS WITH NO SIGNIFICANT INJURY OR MECHANISM OF INJURY

If the patient has a medical complaint, such as chest pain, you may not have to assess the patient from head-to-toe. Ask the patient if any recent trauma may be causing the pain. If they note no trauma, you should inspect and palpate the area involved in the chief complaint.

For patients with a minor injury and no significant mechanism of injury (for example, a patient who cut his finger, or a patient who twisted her ankle while stepping off a curb) begin the physical examination at the site of the injury, using the same components (DOTS) (Fig. 7-20). Remember, however, that if the patient sustained a serious mechanism of injury, there may be underlying injuries of which the patient is not aware. Patients are often aware of only their most painful injury, which is not necessarily the most serious. If you suspect other injuries, or there is a serious mechanism of injury, perform the entire physical exam.

A comparison of two cases will help clarify this principle. In the first case, a patient is in a motor vehicle collision resulting in severe damage to the car and tree. The patient complains only of pain in the right ankle. This patient has sustained a serious mechanism of injury and should receive a head-to-toe physical exam. In the second case, a patient who was jogging suffered a twisted ankle when stepping off a curb. The patient did not fall and complains only of ankle pain. The First Responder physical examination for this patient can be directed toward the ankle only, because the mechanism of injury is not serious.

Remember that the patient evaluation always begins with the scene size-up followed by an initial assessment. You do not need to complete the First Responder physical exam before you begin to treat the patient. Manage any life-threatening conditions when they are found.

Patients experiencing medical emergencies are often scared, anxious, or nervous. Remember that this situation is stressful for the patient and their family. Your role is to care for the patient as a whole person and not just treat their medical condition. Listen carefully to what patients tell you about their illness or injury, and always treat them with respect. Do not be judgmental about the severity of their illness — if they did not feel there was an emergency, they would not have called EMS.

PATIENT HISTORY

Another role of the First Responder is to obtain the patient's pertinent medical history. The history you should obtain is a concise set of information relating to their current medical problem or injury. You should obtain the history from the patient, but you may have to ask family members or friends if the patient can't tell you.

Medical condition identification insignia

When assessing a patient or giving care, you may come across a medical condition identification insignia on a necklace, bracelet, or even ankle bracelet. Its purpose is to inform health care providers of the wearer's medical condition in case the person is unresponsive or cannot communicate directly (Fig. 7-21). Patients wear such devices because they have a potentially serious medical condition such as diabetes, severe allergies, epilepsy, or asthma that requires rapid intervention. A caduceus is sometimes engraved on one side and the patient's medical problem on the other. There may also be an identification number or telephone number for obtaining more information about the patient's medical condition.

The SAMPLE history

When questioning the patient about their medical history, First Responders should take a SAMPLE history. SAMPLE is a mnemonic that stands for six elements of the patient history: **S**igns and **S**ymptoms, **A**llergies, **M**edications, **P**ertinent past medical history, **L**ast oral intake (solid or liquid), and **E**vents leading to the injury or illness.

Signs and symptoms are indications of a possible medical problem. A sign is any medical or trauma condition First Responders can observe in the patient and identify. Examples include information the First Responder can see (such as skin color), information the First Responder can feel (such as pulse rate or skin temperature), and information the First Responder can hear (such as respiratory effort). A symptom is any nonobservable condition described by the patient. For example, patients may state that they feel nauseated, have a headache, or just feel sick. You cannot see these symptoms and can only ask the patient about them. To determine what symptoms the patient has, ask them "How are you feeling?" and "Why did you call for EMS today?" Signs and symptoms are important because they form the basis for patient care.

Ask the patient about any allergies to medications, foods, or environmental factors (e.g., dust, molds, grass), and always look for a medical alert tag. Some people are allergic to certain medications such as penicillin or sulfa drugs. Other people may be allergic to shellfish or other foods. This information may lead you to suspect that an allergic reaction has occurred and to guide appropriate treatment. In addition, if the patient's mental status changes en route to the hospital, you can provide the receiving facility staff with this valuable information.

Identify any medications the patient is taking. Ask the patient if the medications are current or recent and if they have been prescribed by their physician or if they are over-the-counter (OTC). Ask the patient if they have taken their medications as prescribed by their physician.

Ask for pertinent past medical history including recent or past medical problems, surgeries, and injuries. Keep the patient focused on recent or pertinent medical history. Surgery on a patient's ankle 20 years ago, for example, is usually not related to the patient's chief complaint. However, heart surgery five years ago might be important to the patient's current problem. This information may guide you to look for subtle signs and symptoms that may not be obvious at first. In addition, give this information to the medical direction physician, who may request that you provide additional care to the patient. Ask the patient if they are currently seeing a physician for any medical condition. Also ask the patient if they have been in the hospital recently.

Last oral intake includes the time and quantity of both solid and liquid food. Get specific information about any recent change in eating habits or lack of eating. Some patients may intentionally not eat or overeat. Also, consider alcohol intake or ingestion of other non-food substances. The time and

---

REVIEW QUESTIONS

First Responder Physical Exam

1. For a patient with an injured wrist and no significant mechanism of injury, what is the focus of the First Responder physical exam?

2. While evaluating a patient who complains only of pain to her upper arm, the First Responder learns she injured her arm in a car collision. What should the First Responder do?

   _____

3. A _____ is something the patient feels and describes to the First Responder.

4. A _____ is a physical finding that the First Responder can observe.

5. It is important for the First Responder to listen to the patient's history for the last 20 years to avoid hurting the patient's feelings. True or False?

1. Usually just the injured wrist.; 2. The First Responder should perform a head-to-toe exam to evaluate the entire patient. It is always best to err on the side of over-evaluation rather than under-evaluation.; 3. Symptom; 4. Sign; 5. False

quantity of last oral intake is relevant in case the patient needs emergency surgery. Any solids or liquids in the patient's stomach have the potential to cause airway compromise if the patient is unable to protect their own airway. Ask the patient "Have you had anything to eat or drink recently?" If the answer is yes, find out what they ate or drank.

Identify events leading to the injury or illness. Ask the patient what they were doing when the event happened, and any associated symptoms concerning the situation. For example, if the patient complains of chest pain, note if the pain began while the patient was at rest or during exertion. Other symptoms such as dizziness or confusion may also give the receiving facility important information. Sometimes the order in which the symptoms occurred is important. For example, dizziness may be the chief complaint, but the patient may state that it occurred after chest pain began.

For medical patients, the SAMPLE history may be completed before the First Responder physical exam. The information you gather in the SAMPLE history can help you provide care to the patient. Knowing information about past medical problems, allergies, and medications can help the medical direction physician give you guidance. Should a patient become unresponsive after the initial contact with EMS, you will have gained valuable information to help the receiving facility patient care decisions.

ONGOING ASSESSMENT

The purpose of the ongoing assessment is to reevaluate the patient's condition and to check the adequacy of each intervention. Frequent evaluations allow you to notice subtle changes in the patient's condition. The ongoing assessment occurs while you are waiting for additional EMS personnel to arrive at the scene. This allows you to continue to interact with the patient and note changes or trends in the patient's mental status or vital signs. Trends in a patient's status can provide valuable information to the health care professionals who will assume care of the patient.

Once you have responded to a call and have performed the scene size-up, initial assessment, and the First Responder physical exam, continuous evaluation of the patient must take place. The

ongoing assessment repeats the initial assessment (reassess mental status, airway, breathing, and circulation) and the First Responder physical exam. During the ongoing assessment you will also assess the effectiveness of any interventions performed as part of the patient care process (Fig. 7-22). If you are artificially ventilating the patient, make sure the ventilation is adequate by watching the chest rise and monitoring the patient. You must also assess any bleeding control measures that were taken. Any intervention that is no longer meeting the needs of the patient must be corrected immediately. Box 7-3 summarizes the elements of the ongoing assessment.

For stable patients, repeat the ongoing assessment and record the results every 15 minutes. For unstable patients, repeat the assessment and record the results every 5 minutes or less.

Stable patients are those medical or trauma patients who have simple, specific injuries (for example, a patient who injured an ankle playing softball). Unstable patients are those medical

---

BOX 7-3 Components of the Ongoing Assessment

Repeat the initial assessment
- Check mental status
- Check airway patency
- Assess breathing rate and quality
- Assess circulation
  - Pulse rate and quality
  - Skin color, temperature, and condition

Repeat the First Responder physical exam

Evaluate all interventions

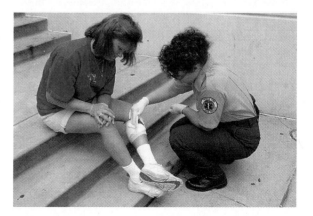

Fig 7-22 Assess interventions to make sure they are still effective.

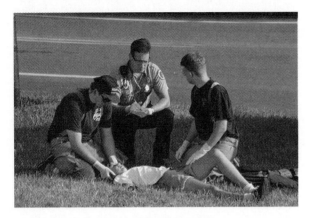

Fig 7-23 When additional EMS personnel arrive, a "hand-off" report will update them about the patient's condition and care provided.

patients in severe distress or trauma patients who have significant injuries or sustained a significant mechanism of injury, even if they seem stable.

Some patients may have life-threatening conditions that require all of your attention. If you are so busy maintaining an open airway by suctioning, you may never have time to assess the patient's skin temperature or color. The ongoing assessment for a patient with life-threatening injuries is almost constant.

An important role we cannot ignore in caring for the patient is calming and reassuring them that you are doing everything you can while additional help is on the way. Do not provide any sense of false hope to the patient or their family if the situation is severe; you are not able to determine outcomes. Remember that the patient is not the only individual who may need reassurance—the family may also require comfort.

Finally, when the transporting EMS personnel arrive on the scene, you should provide a "hand-off" report (Fig. 7-23). The report to arriving EMS personnel is an essential component of your role in the patient care continuum. You will need to give these individuals all the pertinent information obtained concerning the patient as you transfer care to them. Speak clearly and slowly, and provide all information in a logical order. Provide the following information: the patient's name, age, and sex; chief complaint; level of responsiveness; airway and breathing status; circulation status; findings from the physical exam; information from the SAMPLE history; care you have provided and results; and any other information that you believe may be beneficial to assure appropriate continued care.

CHAPTER SUMMARY

SCENE SIZE-UP

First Responders must take precautions to prevent or reduce contact with a patient's blood or other body fluids. Gloves, eye protection, gowns, and masks should be worn as necessary. After taking care of themselves and other First Responders on the scene, First Responders should next protect the patient and then bystanders. Protect patients from further injury from traffic hazards, rescue operations, heat, cold, or any other danger.

If the patient has a medical condition, determine the nature of illness. If the patient has sustained a traumatic injury, determine the mechanism of injury. Determine the number of patients and if additional help is necessary.

INITIAL ASSESSMENT

Form a general impression of the patient during the first few seconds of contact with the patient. Determine the mechanism of injury or nature of illness during the general impression. Identify and correct life-threatening conditions. Determine the approximate age of the patient. Assess the mental status, airway, breathing, and circulation.

FIRST RESPONDER PHYSICAL EXAM

The First Responder physical exam is designed to locate the signs and symptoms of illness and injury, and begin the initial management. All patients will receive a First Responder physical exam; however, you may alter the exam to meet the needs of the patient situation and condition. During the First Responder physical exam, evaluate the head, neck, chest, abdomen, pelvis, and extremities for DOTS (Deformities, Open injuries, Tenderness, and Swelling).

Patients with a minor mechanism of injury and an isolated injury do not always require a complete First Responder physical exam. In these cases, First Responders may evaluate the injury only.

PATIENT HISTORY

When assessing a patient or giving care, you may come across a medical condition identification insignia. Its purpose is to inform health care providers of the wearer's medical condition in case the person is unresponsive or cannot communicate directly. The information you gather in the SAMPLE history can help you provide care to the patient. The mnemonic SAMPLE stands for six elements of the history: **S**igns and **S**ymptoms, **A**llergies, **M**edications, **P**ertinent past medical history, **L**ast oral intake (solid or liquid), and **E**vents leading to the injury or illness.

ONGOING ASSESSMENT

All patients receive an ongoing assessment, which repeats the components of the initial assessment and physical exam. Evaluate stable patients at least every 15 minutes, unstable patients every five minutes or less. The ongoing assessment is also an opportunity to check interventions.

UNITED STATES DEPARTMENT OF TRANSPORTATION NATIONAL HIGHWAY TRAFFIC SAFETY ADMINISTRATION FIRST RESPONDER OBJECTIVES

Check your knowledge. The National Registry of EMTs and many state EMS agencies use the objectives below to develop First Responder certification examinations. Can you meet them?

COGNITIVE OBJECTIVES

1. Discuss the components of scene size-up.
2. Describe common hazards found at the scene of a trauma and a medical patient.
3. Determine if the scene is safe to enter.
4. Discuss common mechanisms of injury/nature of illness.
5. Discuss the reason for identifying the total number of patients at the scene.
6. Explain the reason for identifying the need for additional help or assistance.
7. Summarize the reasons for forming a general impression of the patient.
8. Discuss methods of assessing mental status.
9. Differentiate between assessing mental status in the adult, child, and infant patient.
10. Describe methods used for assessing if a patient is breathing.
11. Differentiate between a patient with adequate and inadequate breathing.
12. Describe the methods used to assess circulation.
13. Differentiate between obtaining a pulse in an adult, child, and infant patient.
14. Discuss the need for assessing the patient for external bleeding.
15. Explain the reason for prioritizing a patient for care and transport.
16. Discuss the components of the physical exam.
17. State the areas of the body that are evaluated during the physical exam.
18. Explain what additional questioning may be asked during the physical exam.
19. Explain the components of the SAMPLE history.
20. Discuss the components of the ongoing assessment.
21. Describe the information included in the First Responder "hand-off" report.

AFFECTIVE OBJECTIVES

22. Explain the rationale for crew members to evaluate scene safety prior to entering.
23. Serve as a model for others by explaining how patient situations affect your evaluation of the mechanism of injury or illness.
24. Explain the importance of forming a general impression of the patient.
25. Explain the value of an initial assessment.
26. Explain the value of questioning the patient and family.
27. Explain the value of the physical exam.
28. Explain the value of an ongoing assessment.
29. Explain the rationale for the feeling that these patients might be experiencing.
30. Demonstrate a caring attitude when performing patient assessments.
31. Place the interests of the patient as the foremost consideration when making any and all patient care decisions during patient assessment.
32. Communicate with empathy during patient assessment to patients as well as with family members and friends of the patient.

PSYCHOMOTOR OBJECTIVES

33. Demonstrate the ability to differentiate various scenarios and identity potential hazards.
34. Demonstrate the techniques for assessing mental status.
35. Demonstrate the techniques for assessing the airway.
36. Demonstrate the techniques for assessing if the patient is breathing.
37. Demonstrate the techniques for assessing if the patient has a pulse.
38. Demonstrate the techniques for assessing the patient for external bleeding.
39. Demonstrate the techniques for assessing the patient's skin color, temperature, condition, and capillary refill (infants and children only).
40. Demonstrate questioning a patient to obtain a SAMPLE history.
41. Demonstrate the skills involved in performing the physical exam.
42. Demonstrate the ongoing assessment.

Vital Signs

Vital Signs
   A. Breathing
   B. Pulse
   C. Skin
   D. Pupils
   E. Blood Pressure
II. Vital Sign Reassessment

KEY TERMS

Accessory muscles The additional muscles used to facilitate breathing in a person in respiratory distress.

Capillary refill The amount of time required to refill the capillary bed after applying and releasing pressure on a fingernail.

Diastolic blood pressure The measurement of the pressure exerted against the walls of the arteries while the heart is at rest.

Labored respirations An increase in the work or effort of breathing.

Noisy respirations Any noise coming from the patient's airway; often indicates a respiratory problem.

Normal respirations Respirations occurring without airway noise or effort from the patient, usually occurs at a rate of 12 to 20 per minute in the adult.

Reactive to light A term referring to pupil constriction when exposed to a light source.

Shallow respirations Respirations that have low volumes of air in inhalation and exhalation.

Systolic blood pressure The measurement of the pressure exerted against the arteries during contraction of the heart.

Trending The process of comparing sets of vital signs or other assessment information over time.

In some systems, First Responders function with a limited amount of equipment, and assessing vital signs is not within their scope of practice. In other systems, First Responders are taught to assess vital signs, and have the necessary equipment. If assessing vital signs is part of your responsibility as a First Responder, read the material in this Appendix and practice the techniques of vital sign assessment often. Check your local protocols regarding vital sign assessment for First Responders.

Listed in this Appendix are the average ranges for respiratory rate, heart rate, and blood pressure listed by age. It is important that you know that these are only average ranges. A patient's heart rate, respiratory rate, or blood pressure measurement may be outside the average range and still be normal for the patient.

VITAL SIGNS

The vital signs you will assess are breathing; pulse; skin color, temperature, and condition; pupil size and reactivity; and blood pressure. They are called vital signs because they can reveal much about the patient's condition and the body's life-sustaining functions. The baseline vital signs are those vital signs you measure or assess when you first encounter the patient; you can use baseline vital signs for comparison with other measurements over time as the patient's condition changes. Baseline vital signs may be assessed by any crew member as time permits. If you are working alone, assess vital signs following the First Responder physical exam.

Vital signs can provide valuable information about the patient's condition. A single set of vital signs does not provide as much information as does a comparison of the patient's vital signs over time. **Trending** is the process of comparing sets of vital signs or other assessment information over time.

Take care to record vital signs accurately. Record the assessment specifics as you take each vital sign, rather than trying to remember all the numbers and recording them later. Be sure to report the baseline vital signs to incoming EMS personnel. This will allow them the opportunity to compare your findings with additional sets of vital signs assessed later in the care of the patient.

BREATHING

The first vital sign to assess is the patient's breathing rate and quality. Observe the patient's breathing by assessing the rise and fall of the chest. One breath is one complete cycle of breathing in and out. Breathing is also called respiration.

Rate

You can determine the patient's respiratory rate by counting the number of breaths in 30 seconds and multiplying by two. If the patient's breathing rate is irregular, count the respirations for one full minute to obtain a more accurate rate. Because patients may subconsciously change their rate of breathing if they know you are monitoring their respirations, do not tell the patient that you are assessing the breathing rate. A good way to avoid telling the patient is to count respirations immediately after you assess the pulse. Keep your hand in contact with the patient's wrist, and the patient generally thinks you are still taking the pulse and will not think about breathing or subconsciously alter respirations.

Factors that affect the patient's respiratory rate include the patient's age, size, and emotional state. Patients often breathe faster than normal when they are ill or injured. The average range of respiratory rates for adults is 12 to 20 breaths per minute. Average ranges by age are listed in Table C-1.

Quality

The quality of breathing is the second part of the respiratory assessment. There are four basic categories for the quality of breathing: normal, shallow, labored, and noisy.

Normal respirations are characterized by average chest wall motion, that is, the chest wall expands with each breath smoothly. The rhythm of normal breathing is regular and even. Normal breathing is effortless. As the patient works harder to breathe, they begin to use accessory muscles. **Accessory muscles** are the additional muscles used to help breathing in a person in respiratory distress. To decide if a patient is using accessory muscles, watch the abdominal, shoulder, and neck muscles for excessive movement. Also look at the muscles between the ribs. If the patient is working hard to breathe, they may be using accessory muscles.

Shallow respirations have slight chest or abdominal wall motion and usually indicate that the patient is moving only small volumes of air into the lungs. Even when the breathing rate is within the average range, patients with shallow respirations may not be receiving enough oxygen with each respiration to support the needs of their bodies.

TABLE C-1	Average Vital Sign Ranges by Age		
AGE	**PULSE**	**RESPIRATIONS**	**BLOOD PRESSURE**
Newborn	120–160	40–60	80/40
1 Year	80–140	30–40	82/44
3 Years	80–120	25–30	86/50
5 Years	70–115	20–25	90/52
7 Years	70–115	20–25	94/54
10 Years	70–115	15–20	100/60
15 Years	70–90	15–20	110/64
Adult	60–100	12–20	120/80

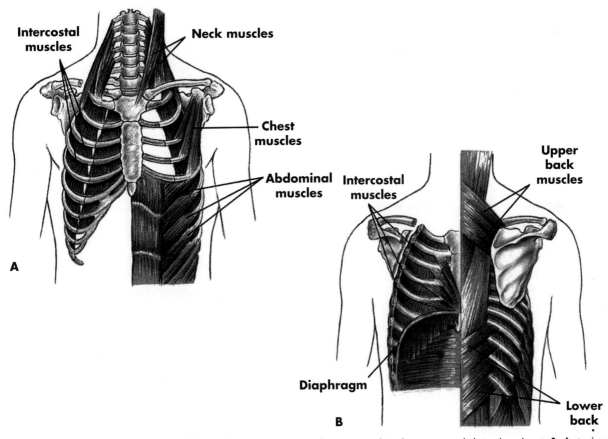

Fig. C-1 When breathing becomes labored, accessory muscles are used to draw more air into the chest. **A,** Anterior view. **B,** Posterior view.

Shallow respirations are common in cases of drug overdose with a depressed respiratory center or in head injury.

Labored respirations indicate a dramatic increase in the patient's effort to breathe. Accessory muscles are commonly used when the patient has

difficulty breathing (Fig. C-1). The patient may be gasping for air. Nasal flaring (the widening of the nostrils during inhalation) and retractions of the supraclavicular muscles (above the clavicles) and intercostal muscles (between the ribs) also indicate labored respirations, especially in infants and

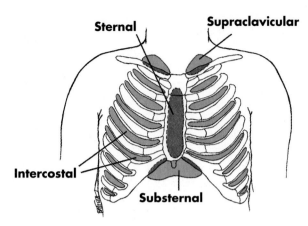

Fig. C-2 Muscle reactions indicate labored respirations, especially in infants and children.

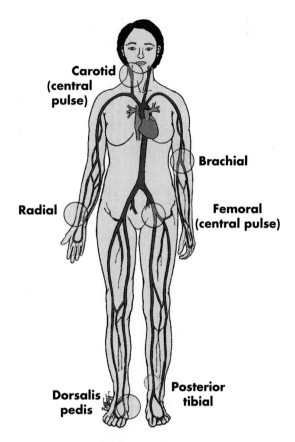

Fig. C-3 Key pulse points in the body.

children (Fig. C-2). Because children and infants normally rely heavily on their diaphragm for breathing, do not assume that the abdominal motion of their breathing automatically indicates labored breathing.

Noisy respirations are abnormal respiratory sounds. Any time you hear noisy breathing, something is obstructing the flow of air. A noisy airway always indicates a respiratory problem.

Any abnormal breathing quality is always an emergency, and you need to intervene to manage the patient's airway and/or breathing. Chapter 6, "The Airway," Appendix A, "Supplemental Oxygen Therapy," and Appendix B, "Advanced First Responder Ventilation Techniques," discuss the techniques to maintain an open airway, administer oxygen, and ventilate the patient.

PULSE

The pulse is the wave of pressure in the blood generated by the pumping of the heart. You can feel the pulse wherever an artery passes over a bone near the surface of the skin. Figure C-3 shows the location of key pulse points in the body. Assess the pulse for both rate and quality.

Rate

The pulse rate is the number of beats in one minute. Assess the pulse rate by counting the number of beats you feel in 30 seconds and multiplying by two. Factors such as the patient's age, physical condition, blood loss, and anxiety can affect the patient's pulse rate. The average range for a resting pulse in adults is 60 to 100. An individual's normal pulse may not fall within this average range, however. For instance, a well-conditioned athlete may have a resting pulse of 50;

although this pulse is outside the average range, it is normal for this patient. When you measure the pulse and obtain low or high rates outside the average range, ask the patient if they know their normal resting pulse rate.

Quality

The quality of the pulse is defined as its strength and regularity. The strength of the pulse can be strong or weak. The rhythm can be regular or irregular.

The pulse should feel strong as you palpate with your fingertips. If the heart is not pumping effectively, or if there is a low volume of blood, the pulse may feel weak. A weak pulse is an early sign of shock (hypoperfusion), which may help you prioritize the patient.

The pulse should also feel regular. A regular pulse does not speed up or slow but has a constant time between beats. If there is not a constant time between beats, the pulse is irregular. An irregular pulse rate may indicate cardiovascular compromise.

Initially, assess the radial pulse in all responsive patients one year of age or older (Fig. C-4). The radial pulse is the pulse in the wrist on the

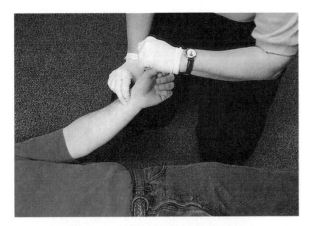

Fig. C-4 Locating the radial pulse.

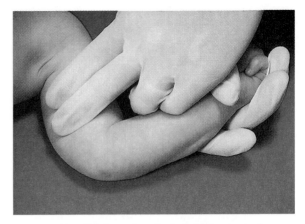

Fig. C-6 Locating the brachial pulse.

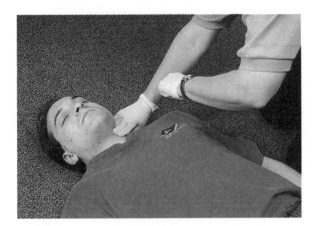

Fig. C-5 Locating the carotid pulse.

thumb side of the forearm. Using two fingers, slide your fingertips from the center of the patient's forearm just to the point where the wrist bends, toward the thumb side of the arm. By applying moderate pressure, you can feel the beats of the pulse. If the pulse is weak, applying more pressure may help you feel a pulse. Too much pressure, however, may occlude the artery, and you will not be able to feel the pulse. If you cannot feel a radial pulse in one arm, try the other arm.

If you are unable to feel a radial pulse in either arm, use the carotid pulse (Fig. C-5). The carotid pulse is felt in the neck along the carotid artery. Locate the Adam's apple in the center of the patient's neck, and slide two fingers toward one side of the neck. Never exert excessive pressure on the neck when feeling for a carotid pulse, especially with geriatric patients. Excessive pressure may dislodge a clot, leading to serious effects. You should never assess the carotid pulse on both sides of the neck simultaneously because this could

cause a drop in the patient's heart rate or occlude blood flow to the brain. For patients less than one year of age, assess the brachial pulse (Fig. C-6). The carotid pulse is normally difficult to locate in these small patients due to the small size of the infant's neck. The brachial pulse is on the inside of the upper arm, between the shoulder and elbow.

To assess the pulse, follow these steps:

1. Locate the radial pulse for patients one year of age or older, and locate the brachial pulse for those less than one year of age.
2. Count the number of beats in 30 seconds and multiply this number by two to determine the pulse rate.
3. Characterize the quality of the pulse as strong or weak and as regular or irregular.

SKIN

The color, temperature, and condition of a patient's skin are assessed because they are good indicators of the patient's perfusion. Assess capillary refill in infants and children younger than six years of age.

Color

Assess skin color in the nail beds, oral mucosa (inside the mouth), and conjunctiva (inside the lower eyelid). These places accurately reflect how much oxygen is in the blood and are easy to assess because the capillary beds run close to the surface of the skin. The normal skin color in these areas is pink for patients of all races.

Abnormal skin colors include pale, cyanotic (blue-gray), flushed (red), or jaundiced (yellow). Poor perfusion (a lack of effective blood flow reaching all body tissues) causes pale skin color. Cyanosis (blue-gray color) indicates inadequate oxygenation (lack of oxygen reaching the cells) or

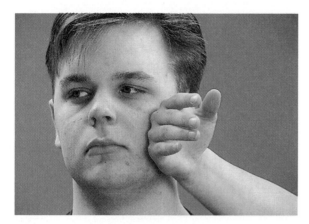

Fig. C-7 Assess skin temperature with the back of your hand.

poor perfusion. Flushed skin may indicate exposure to heat or carbon monoxide poisoning. Finally, a jaundiced or yellow skin color may be an indication that the patient's liver is not functioning properly.

Temperature

Assess skin temperature by placing the back of your hand against the patient's skin (Fig. C-7). The back of your hand is more sensitive to temperature changes than the palm. Assess the skin temperature in more than one location and compare findings. The patient's extremities are more susceptible to environmental changes in temperature than the trunk, so assess the temperature of the skin on the abdomen or back. Normally the skin is warm. Hot skin indicates a fever or exposure to heat. Cool skin indicates poor perfusion or exposure to cold. If the skin is cold, the patient has been exposed to extreme cold.

Condition

The condition of the skin is normally dry — but not so dry that it is cracked. Wet, moist, or extremely dry skin conditions are abnormal. Extremely dry skin may be a sign of dehydration. The term clammy is used to describe cool and moist skin. Clammy skin is a sign of shock (hypoperfusion). For more information on shock, see Chapter 10, "Bleeding and Soft Tissue Injuries."

Capillary refill

Capillary refill is the time it takes for the capillary beds to fill after being blanched (Fig. C-8). Capillary refill is a reliable indicator of hypoperfusion in children. You should assess capillary refill in any patient younger than six years of age.

To assess capillary refill, press on the nail beds, release the pressure, and determine the time it takes for the nail bed to return to its initial color.

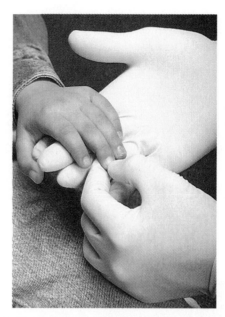

Fig. C-8 Slow capillary refill is an indication of inadequate perfusion in children less than six years of age.

A capillary refill time of less than two seconds is normal. Any capillary refill time longer than two seconds is abnormal and indicates poor perfusion.

PUPILS

The pupils are the dark centers of the eye, which react to changes in the amount of light reaching the eye by constricting (getting smaller) or dilating (getting bigger). The pupils should constrict when exposed to light and dilate when covered from light. Normally both eyes react in the same manner. Sometimes, head injuries or neurological problems can cause the pupils not to be **reactive to light** (termed nonreactive) or cause one pupil to react as expected and the other to be nonreactive (termed unequally reactive). The pupils are normally mid-size, neither constricted nor dilated.

To assess the pupils, follow these steps:

1. Look at the patient's pupils and determine how the pupils look in the ambient light. Note if the pupils are dilated, constricted, or normal.
2. Using a penlight, pass the light across each pupil and note the response. Each pupil should constrict to the same extent (Fig. C-9).

If the area is brightly lighted, such as in bright sunlight, a penlight may not cause the pupils to react. In this case, cover each eye from the light for a few seconds and then uncover it. Note the reaction of the pupils. Head injuries, eye injuries, or drugs can all influence the size and reactivity of the pupils. Note all assessment findings.

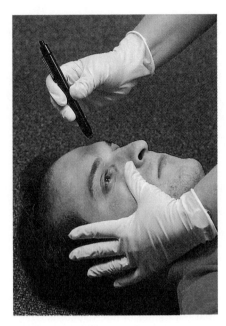

Fig. C-9 Shine a penlight across both eyes to note pupillary reaction.

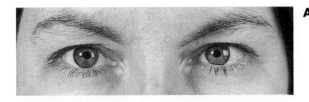

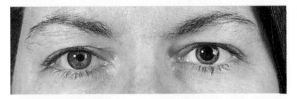

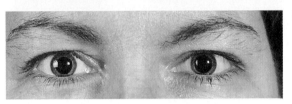

Fig. C-10 The assessment of pupils. Normal pupils are equal and reactive, neither dilated nor constricted. **A,** Constricted pupils. **B,** Uneven pupils. **C,** Dilated pupils.

Figure C-10, A through C, shows constricted pupils, uneven pupils, and dilated pupils.

BLOOD PRESSURE

Blood pressure is a measurement of the force the blood exerts against the walls of blood vessels during the contraction and relaxation phases of the heart. The **systolic blood pressure** is a measurement of the pressure exerted against the walls of the arteries as the wave of blood produced by the contraction of the heart passes that point in the artery. During each contraction of the heart, the pressure rises momentarily as blood is pumped through the arteries. The **dia-stolic blood pressure** is the force exerted against the walls of the blood vessels as the heart relaxes.

Blood pressure is measured in millimeters of mercury (abbreviated mm Hg). Read the blood pressure with the systolic number over the diastolic number. For example: "The patient's blood pressure is 110 over 66"; 110 is the systolic pressure, 66 is the diastolic pressure.

It is important to understand that one blood pressure reading is not valuable, unless it is extremely high or low. Changes in successive blood pressure readings, however, may provide valuable clues about the patient's condition. Document this information on the prehospital care report. Include any values outside the average range or significant changes in your verbal and written report.

There are two methods for obtaining a patient's blood pressure. Auscultation is the preferred method for assessing blood pressure. This method uses a blood pressure cuff and stethoscope (see Technique C-1).

Palpation is an alternate method to measure blood pressure. You measure the systolic blood pressure by feeling for return of the pulse as the cuff deflates. You can use the palpation method in

TECHNIQUE BOX C-1 Measuring Blood Pressure by Auscultation

A

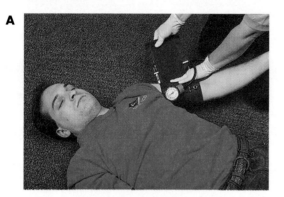

B

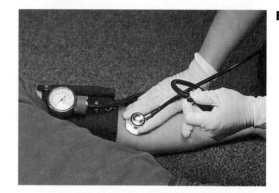

C

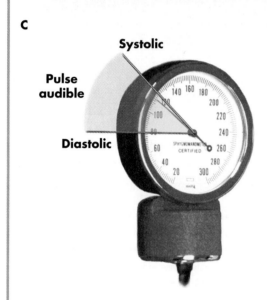

Fig. C-11 Choose a cuff of the appropriate size. Many cuffs have range finders to assist in finding the appropriate size. Apply the cuff so that the center of the bladder is over the brachial artery. The index line should fall between the two range lines when wrapped around the arms. If a range finder is not present, the width of the cuff should go half way around the arm. A cuff that is too large will produce a falsely low reading, while a cuff that is too small will produce a falsely high reading. Palpate the brachial pulse. **A,** Place the blood pressure cuff around the patient's upper arm. The lower edge of the cuff should be about 2.5 cm above the point where you palpated the brachial pulse. **B,** Place the head of the stethoscope over the location of the brachial pulse closer to the wrist than the blood pressure cuff. Close the valve on the blood pressure cuff and inflate it until the pulse disappears, then inflate an additional 30 mm Hg. Slowly release the pressure in the cuff while listening with the stethoscope. **C,** Note the number when you hear the first beat. This is the systolic pressure. Note the number when you hear the beat disappear or become muffled. This number is the diastolic pressure. Record both pressures.

TECHNIQUE BOX C-2 Palpation of Blood Pressure

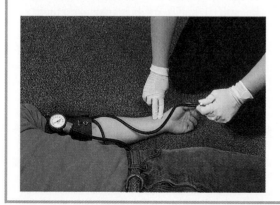

Fig. C-12 Place the blood pressure cuff on the patient's upper arm as for auscultation. Find the patient's radial or brachial pulse distal to the cuff. Inflate the cuff until the radial pulse can no longer be felt, then inflate an additional 30 mm Hg. Slowly release the pressure in the cuff. Note the pressure when the pulse appears. This number is the systolic pressure. The diastolic pressure cannot be measured with this method.

situations when you cannot hear stethoscope sounds well because the patient's pulse is too weak or because the environment is too noisy. Technique C-2 describes how to perform this method.

Measure the blood pressure in all patients more than three years of age. The average ranges of blood pressure for adults and children are listed in Table C-1. Remember that these are only average ranges and that a blood pressure outside these ranges can still be normal for that individual. Ask patients if they know the usual range of their blood pressure.

VITAL SIGN REASSESSMENT

For stable patients, reassess the vital signs every 15 minutes. Stable patients are alert and oriented, with vital signs within the average ranges, and with no signs that their condition is worsening. Reassess the vital signs of unstable patients every 5 minutes as you monitor their condition constantly (Fig. C-13). Patients are unstable when they have mental status changes, vital signs outside average limits, or a worsening condition. Also assess vital signs before and after every intervention.

Remember that your general assessment of the patient comes before vital sign assessment. The initial assessment and First Responder physical exam provide more important information than the vital signs. Notice if the patient appears sick, is in respiratory distress, or is unresponsive. These are better assessments of status than vital signs.

It is also important to remember that the vital sign numbers provided in this chapter are only average ranges. For any individual, a blood pressure, pulse, or respiratory rate not within the average limits can still be appropriate for them. Changes in vital signs allow us to track changes in the patient's condition.

SUMMARY

VITAL SIGNS

A patient's vital signs include: breathing rate and quality; pulse rate and quality; skin color, temperature, and condition; pupils; and blood pressure. Skin colors include pink (normal), pale, cyanotic, flushed, and jaundiced. Skin should be warm and dry. Abnormal skin temperatures include hot, cool, and cold; abnormal skin conditions include wet, moist, and excessively dry. Pupils should be equal in size and reactive to light. Measure the blood pressure for patients more than three years of age. Changes in vital signs can reveal changes in the patient's condition.

VITAL SIGN REASSESSMENT

Evaluate the vital signs of unstable patients every 5 minutes, and every 15 minutes for stable patients. Stable patients are alert and oriented, with vital signs within the average ranges and with no signs that their condition is worsening. Unstable patients have mental status changes, vital signs outside average limits, or a worsening condition.

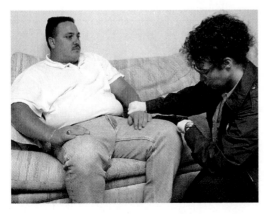

Fig. C-13 Repeat the vital sign assessment every 5 minutes for the unstable patient

REVIEW QUESTIONS

Vital Sign Reassessment

1. List three characteristics of a stable patient.

   _____

   _____

   _____

2. Reassess stable patients every _____ minutes, unstable patients every _____ minutes.

1. A stable patient is alert and oriented, with vital signs within the average ranges, with no signs that their condition is worsening.; 2. 15, 5

UNITED STATES DEPARTMENT OF TRANSPORTATION NATIONAL HIGHWAY TRAFFIC SAFETY ADMINISTRATION EMT-BASIC OBJECTIVES

Check your knowledge. Many state EMS agencies use the objectives below to develop First Responder certification examinations. Can you meet them?

COGNITIVE OBJECTIVES

1. Identify the components of vital signs.
2. Describe the methods to obtain a breathing rate.
3. Identify the attributes that should be obtained when assessing breathing.
4. Differentiate between shallow, labored, and noisy breathing.
5. Describe the methods to obtain a pulse rate.
6. Identify the information obtained when assessing a patient's pulse.
7. Differentiate between a strong, weak, regular, and irregular pulse.
8. Describe the methods to assess the skin color, temperature, and condition (capillary refill in infants and children).
9. Identify the normal and abnormal skin colors.
10. Differentiate between pale, blue, red, and yellow skin color.
11. Identify normal and abnormal skin temperature.
12. Differentiate between hot, cool, and cold skin temperature.
13. Identify normal and abnormal skin conditions.
14. Identify normal and abnormal capillary refill in infants and children.
15. Describe the methods of assessing the pupils.
16. Identify normal and abnormal pupil size.
17. Differentiate between dilated (big) and constricted (small) pupil size.
18. Differentiate between reactive and nonreactive pupils and equal and unequal pupils.
19. Describe the methods of assessing blood pressure.
20. Define systolic pressure.
21. Define diastolic pressure.
22. Explain the difference between auscultation and palpation for obtaining a blood pressure.
23. State the importance of accurately reporting and recording the baseline vital signs.

AFFECTIVE OBJECTIVES

24. Explain the value of performing the baseline vital signs.
25. Recognize and respond to the feelings patients experience during assessment.
26. Defend the need for obtaining and recording an accurate set of vital signs.
27. Explain the rationale of recording additional sets of vital signs.

PSYCHOMOTOR OBJECTIVES

28. Demonstrate the skills involved in assessment of breathing.
29. Demonstrate the skills associated with obtaining a pulse.
30. Demonstrate the skills associated with assessing the skin color, temperature, condition, and capillary refill in infants and children.
31. Demonstrate the skills associated with assessing the pupils.
32. Demonstrate the skills associated with obtaining blood pressure.

Circulation

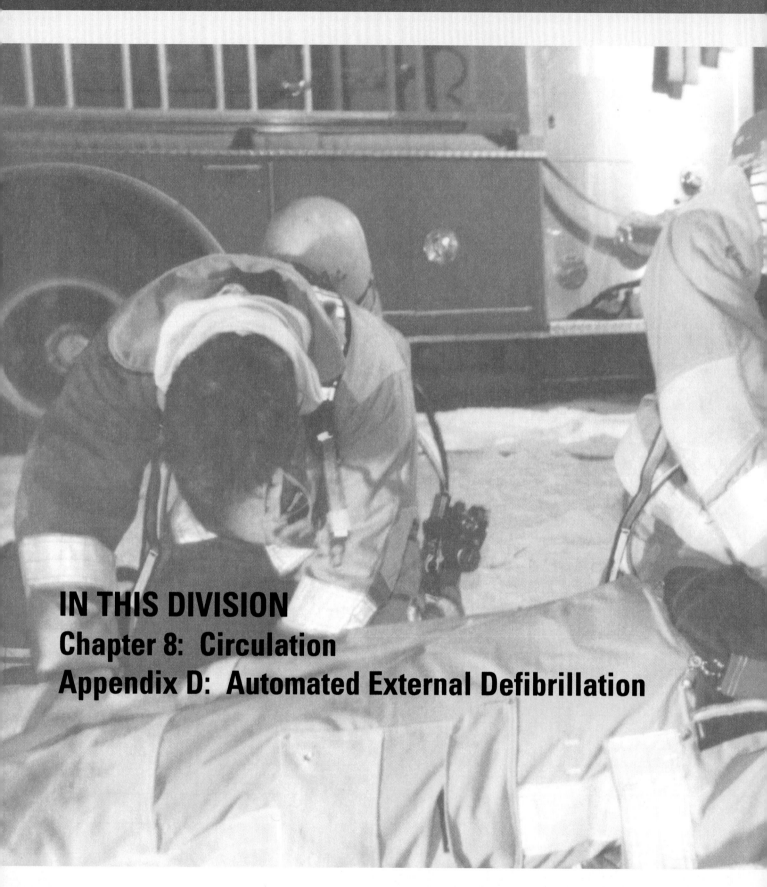

IN THIS DIVISION
Chapter 8: Circulation
Appendix D: Automated External Defibrillation

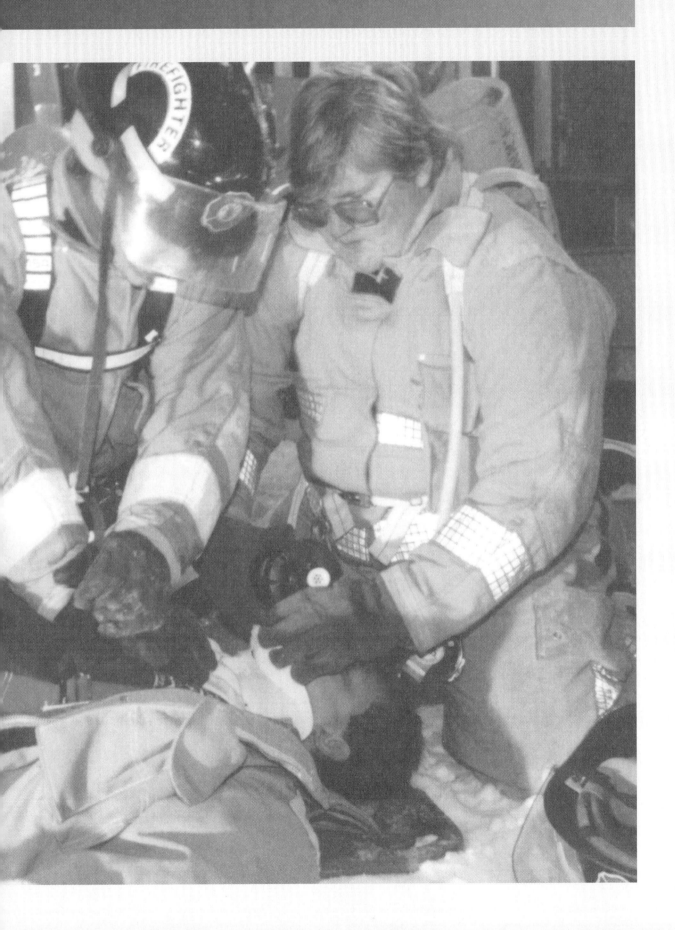

Circulation

KEY TERMS

Automated external defibrillator   Machine used by basic level rescuers to provide an electrical shock to a patient who is not breathing and is pulseless; they are either automatic or semiautomatic.

Cardiopulmonary resuscitation (CPR)   The process of one or two rescuers providing artificial ventilations and external chest compressions to a patient who is pulseless and not breathing.

Chain of survival   The American Heart Association term for the optimum process that should be followed for saving a life. The chain consists of: Early access, Early CPR, Early defibrillation, and Early ACLS.

Cricoid pressure   Pressure exerted by a rescuer to the cricoid cartilage of the patient's neck to close the esophagus, reducing the risk of gastric distention and vomiting.

Defibrillation   The delivery of an electrical shock to the heart to convert a deadly heart rhythm into a normal rhythm.

Rescue breathing   The artificial ventilations provided to a nonbreathing patient by a rescuer during CPR.

Xiphoid process   The bony protrusion that extends from the lower portion of the sternum.

FIRST RESPONSE

When their pagers went off, First Responders Hannah and Marie listened closely to the dispatcher. "Respond to 207 Elm Street for a patient having chest pain." They got into the quick response vehicle and headed for Elm Street.

Upon their arrival, a woman met them at the door and said that her husband, Sam, just collapsed. Hannah rushed to the man and quickly assessed responsiveness by gently shaking him and shouting his name. There was no response. She asked Marie to contact the ambulance and tell them that the patient was unresponsive. Hannah opened Sam's airway and assessed that he was not breathing. She used her pocket mask to administer two rescue breaths. Hannah checked his carotid pulse. There was no pulse.

For the next four minutes, they performed two-rescuer CPR until the ALS unit arrived. Hannah and Marie helped the EMS personnel as they defibrillated the patient and administered medications. Two minutes after the ALS personnel arrived, Sam's pulse returned. The rescuers all knew that if Sam had not received effective CPR when he did, his chance of survival would have been drastically reduced.

Almost 600,000 people die each year from cardiovascular diseases; half of these deaths occur outside the hospital, with sudden death (collapse) being the first sign of cardiac disease in 50% of the cases. Early Cardiopulmonary Resuscitation (CPR), covered in this module, is a major determinant of survival in cardiac arrest.

REVIEW OF THE CIRCULATORY SYSTEM

FUNCTION

The circulatory system functions to deliver oxygen and nutrients to the tissues of the body and removes the waste products from these tissues. Without the continuous beating of the heart, the tissues cannot receive the oxygen and nutrients from the blood that are vital to survival. Later in this chapter, you will learn how chest compressions act to pump the heart and distribute blood to the body, when the heart is not beating on its own.

ANATOMY

The heart has four chambers. The two upper chambers are the atria, and the two lower chambers are the ventricles. The right atrium receives oxygen-poor blood from the veins of the body and pumps it to the right ventricle. The right ventricle pumps the blood to the lungs, where it is oxygenated. The oxygen-rich blood flows from the lungs into the left atrium and is pumped to the left ventricle. The left ventricle pumps the oxygen-rich blood to the body. Valves in the heart between the chambers and major blood vessels prevent the backflow of blood (Fig. 8-1).

Arteries are vessels that carry blood away from the heart to the rest of the body. The aorta is the major artery that originates from the heart; it lies in front of the spine in the chest and abdominal cavities. The carotid arteries are the major arteries in the neck that supply the head with blood. The pulsations of these arteries can be felt on either side of the neck. The artery of the upper arm is the brachial artery. You can palpate its pulsations on the inside of the arm between the elbow and the shoulder. The major artery of the lower arm is the radial artery, and the pulsations can be felt on the thumb side of the wrist. The femoral artery is the major artery of the thigh, and supplies the groin and the lower extremity with blood. You can palpate pulsations from these arteries in the groin (the crease between the abdomen and thigh) on either side of the body (Fig. 8-2).

Capillaries are the tiny blood vessels that connect arteries to veins. They are found in all parts of the body and allow for the exchange of oxygen and carbon dioxide. Veins begin at the capillary beds and carry blood back to the heart from the body. Veins carry unoxygenated blood containing waste

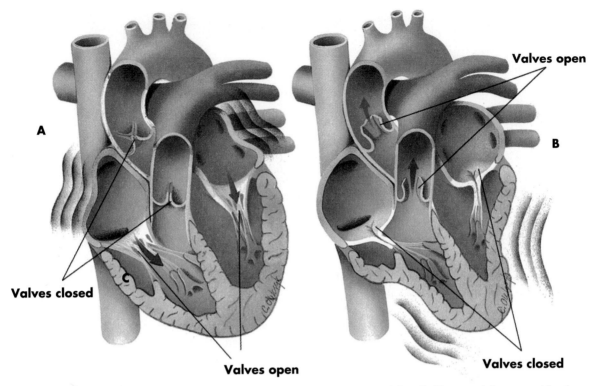

Fig. 8-1 Blood flow through the heart. **A,** The atria pump blood into the ventricles. **B,** The ventricles pump blood to the lungs and rest of the body.

products (such as carbon dioxide) to the heart, and the heart pumps it to the lungs for elimination.

Blood is the fluid portion of the circulatory system, and it carries oxygen and nutrients to the tissues and carbon dioxide from the tissues. Blood also contains cells that fight disease and infection, and cells that help blood clot.

PHYSIOLOGY

When the left ventricle contracts, sending a wave of blood through the arteries, a pulse can be felt. You can palpate the pulse anywhere an artery passes near the skin surface and over a bone. The most common sites for palpating pulses are the carotid artery in the neck, the radial artery in the wrist, the femoral artery in the groin, and the brachial artery in the upper arm.

If the heart stops beating, no blood will flow and the body will not survive. When a patient has no pulse, they are in cardiac arrest. Organ damage begins very quickly without blood flow. Brain damage begins within 4 to 6 minutes after cardiac arrest. Within 8 to 10 minutes, brain damage becomes irreversible. First Responders use a combination of external chest compressions and artificial ventilations to circulate and oxygenate the

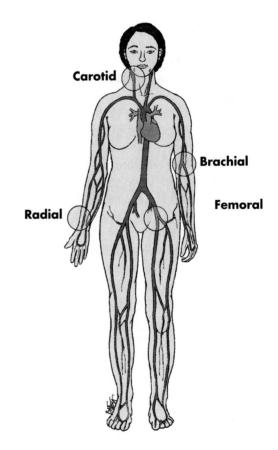

Fig. 8-2 Pulse sites.

blood anytime the heart is not beating. This combination of compressions and ventilations is called cardiopulmonary resuscitation (CPR).

Reasons for the heart to stop beating include heart disease, respiratory arrest (especially in infants and children), drowning, suffocation, congenital abnormalities, electrical shock, trauma, and bleeding. Some medical emergencies, such as stroke, epilepsy, diabetes, allergic reactions, electrical shock, and poisoning, also can result in cardiac arrest. Whatever the reason, First Responders should perform CPR on any patient in cardiac arrest.

CARDIOPULMONARY RESUSCITATION

DEFINITION

Cardiopulmonary resuscitation (CPR) combines artificial ventilation and external chest compressions to oxygenate and circulate blood when a patient is in cardiac arrest. By performing external chest compressions, the rescuer depresses the sternum, or breastbone, to change the pressure in the chest. This causes enough blood flow to sustain life for a short time.

CPR *cannot* sustain life indefinitely and is only effective for a short period. The effectiveness of delivering oxygen to the body decreases the longer CPR is performed. Often, the patient needs an electrical shock to the heart, called **defibrillation,** to survive. By performing CPR, the amount of time that defibrillation will be effective is increased. Therefore, you must start CPR as early as possible. This keeps the heart pumping and the blood circulating until the defibrillator is available.

CHAIN OF SURVIVAL

The successful resuscitation of a patient in cardiac arrest outside the hospital depends on the links in the **chain of survival.** The American Heart Association Chain of Survival consists of: early access, early CPR, early defibrillation, and early advanced cardiac life support (ACLS). Weak links in the chain lower survival rates.

Early access

Early access is dependent upon public education and awareness of cardiac emergencies and the EMS system. The public must be informed of the signs and symptoms of a cardiac emergency and know when and how to contact emergency

---

REVIEW QUESTIONS

Review of the Circulatory System

1. Which of the following arteries can be palpated in the neck?
   A. carotid
   B. radial
   C. brachial
   D. femoral

2. The ventricles of the heart pump blood to the lungs and the body. True or False?

3. The First Responder's emergency medical care for all patients in cardiac arrest is

   _____.

4. CPR is a combination of _____, to circulate blood, and _____, to oxygenate the blood.

5. Of the following, which statement is TRUE?
   A. First Responders can do nothing if the patient is in cardiac arrest.
   B. Organ damage is rare in cardiac arrest patients.
   C. Brain damage begins 4 to 6 minutes after cardiac arrest.
   D. You should only start CPR if you know the cause of cardiac arrest.

1. A; 2. True; 3. CPR; 4. compressions, ventilations; 5. C

BOX 8-1 Signs and Symptoms of a Cardiac Emergency

- Squeezing, dull pressure or pain in the chest that commonly radiates to the arms, neck, jaw, or upper back
- Sudden onset of sweating
- Difficulty breathing
- Anxiety or irritability
- Feeling of impending doom
- Abnormal and sometimes irregular pulse rate (high or low)
- Abnormal blood pressure (different from the patient's normal blood pressure)
- Pain or discomfort in the abdomen (severe indigestion)
- Nausea or vomiting

medical services. Rapid recognition of the emergency and rapid notification of EMS is key to this link in the chain of survival. Box 8-1 lists signs and symptoms of a cardiac emergency. For adult patients, we teach the public to "Phone first"—even before they start CPR—because having advanced life support en route is important. By gaining early access into the system, the caller can also receive 9-1-1 pre-arrival instructions and dispatch-directed CPR. The emergency medical dispatcher may give the caller instructions on how to handle the situation and what they can do to help.

Early CPR

The lay public and First Responders provide early CPR. Public education provides family members, co-workers, and bystanders with the knowledge of how to begin CPR for a patient in cardiac arrest. First Responders trained in CPR are responsible for ensuring that it be done promptly and properly.

Early defibrillation

Early defibrillation is now an EMT-Basic skill. Some areas train First Responders in the use of the automated external defibrillator (AED). An automated external defibrillator is a machine used by basic level rescuers to provide an electrical shock to a patient who is pulseless and not breathing. Including this skill into the scope of practice of the First Responder works well in many communities. Early defibrillation can make the difference between life and death for a patient in cardiac arrest, even more so than early CPR. Check your local protocols to find out if this skill is part of your First Responder curriculum. Refer to Appendix D for details on the use of the automated external defibrillator.

Early advanced cardiac life support

Early advanced cardiac life support (ACLS) is the final element in the chain of survival. The American Heart Association advises that you call 9-1-1 before you start CPR for adult patients. This provides the shortest time between the cardiac arrest and the arrival of personnel trained in ACLS who can use defibrillation and medications to help the patient. If each link in the chain of survival is completed, the better the chance of survival for the patient. The resuscitative effort is a continuum of care beginning at a basic level and progressing toward an advanced level as soon as possible.

In some communities, First Responders are responsible for early access and early CPR, then to call for additional EMS personnel. Some First Responders will also learn the skills of early defibrillation using an AED. As a First Responder, you must learn what responsibilities you have in the chain of survival in your community.

TECHNIQUES OF ADULT CPR

CPR is indicated when the patient is not breathing and does not have a pulse. The performance of CPR is done in various assessment and intervention steps called the "ABCs of CPR." Many techniques of CPR are similar in the adult, child, and infant. When no differences are described, the technique is the same for all patients. The reasons to begin CPR are very specific: the patient must be pulseless and not breathing. There are also specific situations when you can stop CPR once you have started. Refer to Box 8-2 for the reasons to discontinue CPR after you have started.

STEPS OF ADULT CPR

Step 1: Assess Responsiveness and Activate EMS

The First Responder arriving on the scene may be the first person to encounter and care for the patient. Advanced level rescuers should also be en route to the scene. If they are not, the First Responder contacts dispatch to ask for ALS assistance. As always, assure a safe scene before approaching the patient. Be sure to follow body substance isolation precautions while performing CPR.

First the rescuer must determine unresponsiveness in the patient. This can be done by gently shaking the patient and asking, "Are you OK?" If there is no response in an adult patient, activate EMS immediately. If there is only one rescuer, contact EMS before any further assessment of the

---

BOX 8-2 When to Discontinue CPR

CPR started by a First Responder should be continued until:

- Effective circulation and breathing have returned.
- Care is transferred to another provider who is trained to First Responder level or higher.
- Care is transferred to a physician.
- The rescuer is unable to continue CPR because of hazards, exhaustion, or the endangerment of others.

patient is completed (Box 8-3). If there are two rescuers, one can contact EMS while the other continues the assessment. If ALS personnel are already en route, you can skip this step.

If the patient is responsive, monitor the airway and interact with the patient to find out why they need help. Always have an understanding and caring attitude toward patients needing your care. Keep the patient calm and reassure them that an ambulance is on the way. Complete the First Responder physical exam.

Step 2: A is for Airway

The next step in the assessment of the unresponsive patient is opening the airway (Fig. 8-3). The patient must first be lying on their back on a firm surface. If the patient is lying face down, roll the patient onto their back. If you suspect the patient has been injured, take precautions to stabilize the cervical spine as you roll the patient. Move the patient so that the spinal column remains in a straight line. Techniques for moving patients with possible spinal injuries are discussed in Chapter 11, "Injuries to Muscles and Bones."

In a medical situation, the rescuer kneels by the patient's side and uses the head-tilt, chin-lift maneuver to open the airway, as described in Chapter 6, "The Airway."

In situations where trauma is suspected, use the jaw thrust maneuver without head-tilt to open the airway. The jaw thrust without head-tilt is also described in Chapter 6.

Step 3: B is for Breathing

Determine if the patient is breathing adequately on their own or if they need assistance. Once the airway is opened, the rescuer places his or her cheek and ear close to the patient's mouth while looking toward the patient's chest. Look to see if the chest is rising, listen for breathing, and feel any air that may be coming from the patient's mouth (Fig. 8-4). This should be done for 3 to 5 seconds.

If the patient is breathing adequately and there is no trauma, place the patient in the recovery position (Fig. 8-5). Carefully move the patient onto their side without compromising the integrity of the spine. The patient's airway remains open much easier in this position, and fluids drain from the mouth.

If the patient is not breathing at all or not breathing adequately, rescue breathing should be provided (Fig. 8-6). Providing artificial ventilations to a patient who is not breathing is called rescue breathing. Rescue breathing can be accomplished by

BOX 8-3 How to Activate EMS

If EMS has not been activated when you arrive on the scene, dial 9-1-1 or the emergency number in your local area, or the dispatch center, identify yourself as a First Responder, and provide the following information:
- Location of the emergency
- Telephone number
- What happened (medical or trauma and what type)
- How many patients there are
- Condition of the patient (unresponsive, bleeding, etc.)
- What treatment is being provided to the patient(s), if any
- Any other information requested by the operator

Hang up only on the request of the emergency operator to make sure they have all of the information they need.

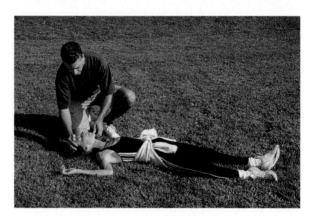

Fig. 8-3 If the patient is unresponsive, the next step is to open the airway.

mouth-to-mouth, mouth-to-barrier device, or mouth-to-mask ventilations. Refer to Chapter 6, "The Airway," for a review of these techniques. If you are trained and have the equipment, you can also ventilate the patient with a bag-valve-mask or flow-restricted, oxygen-powered ventilation device, as described in Appendix B, "Advanced First Responder Ventilation Techniques."

Ventilate the adult patient with approximately 800 to 1200 ml of air, at a rate of 10 to 12 breaths per minute. Each ventilation should take $1^{1}/_{2}$ to 2 seconds. If the air does not go in on the first ventilation attempt, reposition the airway to ensure that it was open. If the air still will not go

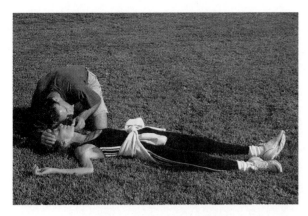

Fig. 8-4 Look, listen, and feel for breathing.

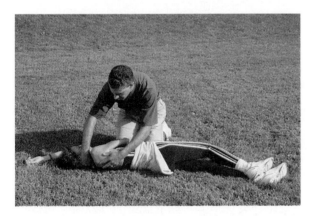

Fig. 8-5 Place the patient in the recovery position if no trauma is suspected and the patient is breathing.

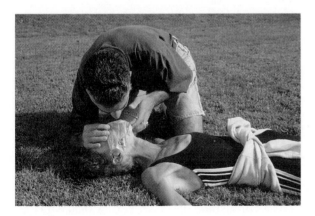

Fig. 8-6 If the patient is not breathing, provide artificial ventilations.

in, refer to the foreign body airway obstruction maneuvers in Chapter 6, "The Airway."

Cricoid pressure can be used if there is a rescuer available who can be designated to perform the skill. This rescuer cannot assist with chest compressions or artificial ventilations. By placing pressure against the cricoid ring, you can compress the esophagus between the cricoid cartilage and the spinal column, which reduces the risk of gastric distention and vomiting during artificial ventilation. Two fingers are placed upon the cricoid cartilage of the patient's neck. To find the cricoid cartilage, first find the patient's Adam's apple (bony prominence in the neck) and slide the fingers down the neck toward the patient's feet. The hard ring felt below the Adam's apple is the cricoid ring. Pressure is exerted toward the spine, using the thumb and index finger on either side of the cricoid ring (Fig. 8-7). Once you begin cricoid pressure, you must continue to hold pressure until an ALS provider can protect the airway by placing a tube into the trachea. This endotracheal tube isolates the airway and will keep vomit from passing through the trachea. Releasing cricoid pressure before the airway is protected would likely cause an airway compromise.

Step 4: C is for Circulation

After the airway is open and breathing assessed, determine the circulatory status. The rescuer checks the carotid pulse in the neck of the adult patient for 5 to 10 seconds. Maintain the head-tilt, chin-lift throughout this process. Find the prominence (Adam's apple) on the patient's neck and place the index and middle fingers on it. Slide the fingers to the side of the neck closest to you until they are in the groove between the trachea and the muscles. This is where you can palpate the carotid pulse (Fig. 8-8).

If a pulse is found, but the patient is not breathing, the rescuer should perform rescue breathing at a rate of 10 to 12 per minute (one breath every 5 seconds) for the adult patient. Stop every few minutes to reassess the status of the patient's breathing and circulation.

If no pulse is found, the patient is in cardiac arrest and you must begin external chest compressions. Again, the patient should be supine on a firm, flat surface for the compressions to be effective. Hand position for chest compressions varies with the age of the patient.

HAND POSITION FOR CHEST COMPRESSIONS IN THE ADULT

To find the correct hand position for chest compressions on the adult patient, the rescuer should locate the edge of the ribs on the side of the patient closest to them. Trace the ribs to the center of the patient until the ribs meet the sternum and the xiphoid process. The xiphoid process is the end of

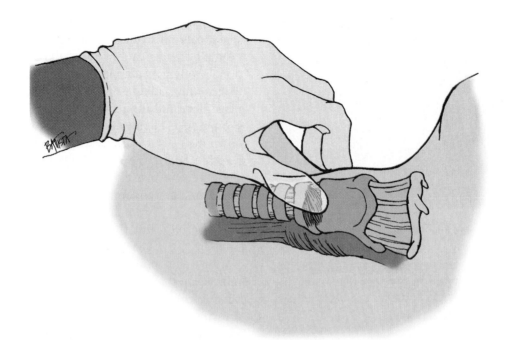

Fig. 8-7 Firm pressure on the cricoid ring collapses the esophagus without compromising the airway.

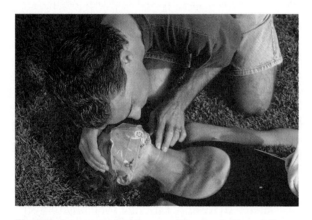

Fig. 8-8 Assessment of the carotid pulse in the adult patient.

the sternum closest to the patient's abdomen. Place two fingers on the xiphoid process with one hand and the heel of the other hand over the lower half of the sternum (beside the two fingers, not on top of them). Then place the heel of the other hand on top of the one placed on the sternum. The fingers may be interlaced or simply rested on one another, but should be off the chest (Fig. 8-9A and B).

To perform compressions, the rescuer leans directly over the patient, so that their shoulders are over the sternum to provide compressions that are straight down. The knees are shoulder-width apart to provide a stable base. The arms are kept straight and locked (Fig. 8-10). Leaning forward and bending at the hip joint, the rescuer should exert

enough pressure to compress the sternum $1\frac{1}{2}$ to 2 inches for the adult patient. Release pressure between each compression to let blood flow to the heart. The compression and relaxation phases should be equal. The hands should remain on the chest at all times so the correct position is not lost. Movement should be rhythmic, rather than jerky or bouncing. The rate of compressions should be 80 to 100 per minute for the adult patient. Box 8-4 lists the steps for adult one-rescuer CPR.

Even when CPR is performed properly, chest compressions can cause broken ribs, bruising, or other injuries. Do not stop CPR even if you suspect that there may be an injury to the ribs or chest wall. If the patient is in cardiac arrest, always perform CPR.

Adult CPR can be performed with one or two rescuers. Two-rescuer CPR is much more efficient and less tiring than one-rescuer CPR (Fig. 8-11). In two-rescuer CPR, one rescuer performs rescue breathing while the other performs chest compressions. Box 8-5 lists the steps for adult two-rescuer CPR. If the rescuer performing compressions becomes fatigued, the rescuers may switch positions at the direction of the rescuer at the chest. During two-rescuer CPR, the rescuer at the airway can palpate for a pulse at the carotid artery while the other rescuer is doing compressions. If the compressions are effective, a pulse should be felt.

Refer to Table 8-1 for a summary of adult CPR.

A

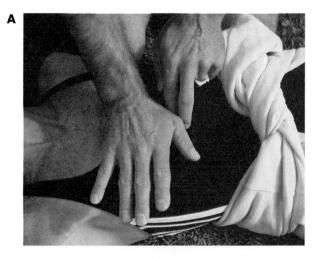

B

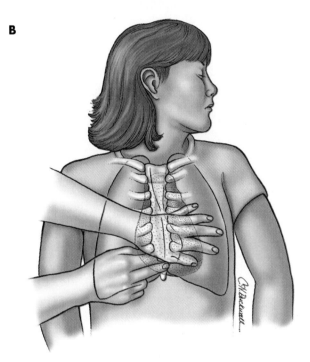

Fig. 8-9 A and **B** Proper hand positioning for compressions in the adult patient.

BOX 8-4 Steps of Adult One-Rescuer CPR

Following the recommendations of the American Heart Association, one-rescuer adult CPR should follow these guidelines:

1. Determine unresponsiveness.
2. Activate EMS.
3. Position the patient and open the airway.
4. Assess breathing for 3 to 5 seconds.
5. If the patient is breathing and there is no trauma, place them in the recovery position. If the patient is not breathing, give two rescue breaths.
6. Assess circulation for 5 to 10 seconds.
   If the patient has a pulse, but is not breathing, perform rescue breathing at 10 to 12 breaths per minute.
7. If the patient does not have a pulse, find hand position and begin chest compressions.
   Perform 15 chest compressions at a rate of 80 to 100 per minute.
   Open the airway and deliver two rescue breaths.
   Begin 15 more chest compressions.
8. Perform four cycles of 15 compressions to two ventilations.
9. Reassess the pulse for 3 to 5 seconds.
   If the patient has a pulse, reassess breathing:
   If breathing is present, keep reassessing the patient and place them in the recovery position.
   If breathing is absent, continue rescue breathing at 10 to 12 per minute.
   If the patient does not have a pulse, begin a cycle of 15 chest compressions.
10. If CPR is continued, stop to reassess the patient every few minutes.

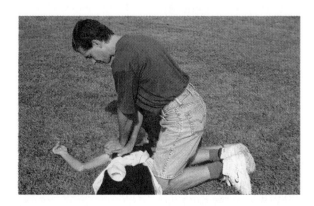

Fig. 8-10 Proper position to perform chest compressions on an adult patient.

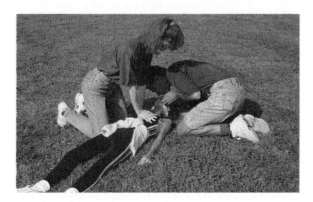

Fig. 8-11 Two rescuer CPR is more efficient and less tiring than one person CPR.

BOX 8-5 Steps of Adult Two-Rescuer CPR

1. Rescuer 1 assesses responsiveness. If the patient is unresponsive, Rescuer 2 activates additional EMS personnel.
2. Rescuer 1 opens the airway and assesses breathing:
   If breathing is present, rescuers place the patient in the recovery position.
   If breathing is absent, Rescuer 1 performs two rescue breaths over $1\frac{1}{2}$ to 2 seconds each.
3. Rescuer 1 assesses circulation:
   If a pulse is present, but breathing is absent, Rescuer 1 continues rescue breathing at a rate of 10 to 12 breaths per minute.
   If a pulse is absent, Rescuer 2 finds hand position and performs 5 chest compressions at a rate of 80 to 100 per minute.
4. After every 5 compressions, Rescuer 1 performs one rescue breath ($1\frac{1}{2}$ to 2 seconds each). Rescuer 2 pauses so air can fill the lungs.
5. Perform twenty cycles of 5 compressions to 1 ventilation then reassess the pulse:
   If there is a pulse, reassess breathing and treat accordingly.
   If there is no pulse, continue with 5 compressions to 1 ventilation. Reassess every few minutes.

TABLE 8-1 Adult CPR

ADULT CPR	One-rescuer CPR	Two-rescuer CPR
Compression	15 compressions	5 compressions
Ventilations	2 ventilations	1 ventilation
Rescue breathing	10-12 per minute $1\frac{1}{2}$–2 seconds each	
Compression rate	80–100 per minute	
Number of initial cycles	4 cycles	20 cycles
Depth of compressions	$1\frac{1}{2}$–2 inches	

FIRST RESPONDER ALERT

Make sure your hands are not placed over the xiphoid process while performing chest compressions. If compressions are done over the xiphoid process, that piece of bone could break off and damage internal organs.

TECHNIQUES OF INFANT AND CHILD CPR

Many of the techniques used in infant and child CPR are similar to those used in adult CPR. In those situations, the adult section will be referenced. Similar to adult CPR, infant and child CPR follows a step-by-step assessment process.

STEPS OF INFANT AND CHILD CPR
Step 1: Assess responsiveness

The rescuer must first assess responsiveness. Tap on the infant or child's shoulder or shout their name.

If the patient is unresponsive, a single rescuer should shout for help and then administer one minute of CPR before activating EMS by phone. Infants and children suffer cardiac arrest primarily from a respiratory problem, whereas adults generally suffer cardiac arrest from a cardiac problem. Because of this, infants and children will benefit from the immediate treatment of opening the airway and providing and circulating oxygen to the tissues. If a second rescuer is available, they should contact EMS while the first rescuer continues the assessment.

Step 2: A is for Airway

Maintaining an open airway is one of the most important aspects of infant and child CPR because the primary reason for cardiac arrest is respiratory arrest. The airway must be opened as soon as possible (Fig. 8-12A and B).

In a medical situation, open the airway with a head-tilt, chin-lift. The technique for infants and children is the same as the non-trauma adult. The rescuer tilts the head back gently to the neutral position. Be careful not to put pressure on the fleshy part of the neck.

If you suspect the patient has traumatic injuries, open the patient's airway using the jaw thrust without head-tilt technique. The procedure is the same as the adult jaw thrust.

Step 3: B is for Breathing

Once the airway is open, the rescuer assesses the patient's breathing in the same manner that

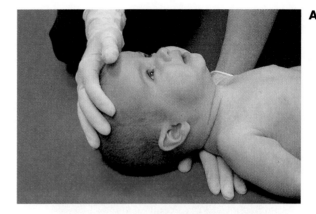

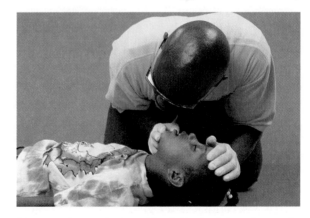

Fig. 8-12 A and **B** After assessing responsiveness, open the airway.

was used for the adult (Fig. 8-13). If the patient is breathing inadequately, perform rescue breathing.

Rescue breathing can be performed by mouth-to-mouth, mouth-to-barrier device, or mouth-to-mouth contact (Fig. 8-14). If a mask is available, it should be used if it fits properly. However, do not delay treatment to find a mask. If the patient is under one year old, the rescuer places their mouth over the mouth and nose of the patient to create a seal. If the patient is over one year old, the rescuer places their mouth over the patient's mouth and creates a seal. Use the index finger and thumb of the hand on the forehead to pinch the nose closed. Administer two slow breaths (1 to 1$\frac{1}{2}$ seconds per breath) and observe the rise and fall of the patient's chest with each breath. The volume of air should be enough to make the patient's chest rise. For the infant and child, the rate of rescue breathing is one breath every 3 seconds (20 breaths/minute).

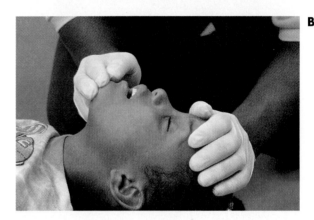

Fig. 8-13 Assess for breathing by looking, listening, and feeling for respiration.

Step 4: C is for Circulation

After assessing airway and breathing, the rescuer assesses circulation.

For patients less than one year old, the pulse is checked in the brachial artery of the upper arm (Fig. 8-15). The rescuer should place his thumb on the outside of the arm between the

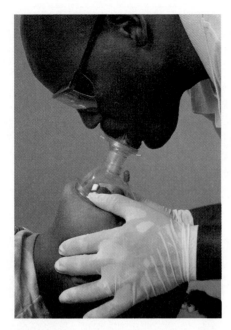

Fig. 8-14 Ventilate the patient if they are not breathing on their own.

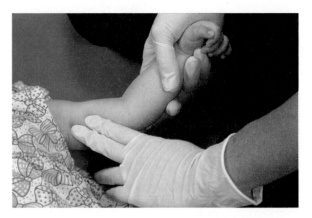

Fig. 8-15 Assess circulation in the infant by palpating the brachial artery.

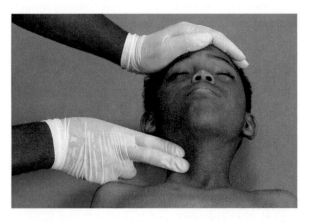

Fig. 8-16 Assess circulation in the child by palpating the carotid artery.

FIRST RESPONDER ALERT

Providing rescue breaths too rapidly or in too large a volume can result in gastric distention and vomiting. Always deliver breaths slowly at 1 to 1½ seconds each.

elbow and the shoulder, and then press the index and middle fingers on the inside of the arm to palpate the pulse. If the infant has a pulse but is not breathing, perform rescue breathing at a rate of 20 per minute (once every 3 seconds). For children over the age of one year, check the pulse in the carotid artery of the neck (Fig. 8-16). If the pulse is present, the rescuer provides rescue breathing at a rate of 20 per minute (once every 3 seconds). After giving 20 breaths, activate the EMS system.

HAND POSITION FOR CHEST COMPRESSION IN THE INFANT

If the infant does not have a pulse, place the infant on a firm surface. Compress on the lower half of the sternum. Keep one hand on the patient's head to maintain a head tilt. Place the index finger of the other hand across the nipples of the patient. The next two fingers are placed beside the index finger. Lift the index finger from the chest; compressions

are done with the middle and ring fingers (Fig. 8-17A and B). Avoid compressing over the xiphoid process. Compress ½ to ⅓ the depth of the chest (about ½ to 1 inch). Perform at least 100 compressions per minute for the infant.

Pause after five compressions to give one ventilation. Perform 20 cycles (about one minute) and reassess the patient. If you are alone, activate EMS at this time. If the patient's breathing and pulse return, place the infant in the recovery position. If only the pulse returns, continue with rescue breathing. If the pulse does not return, continue with compressions and ventilations and reassess every few minutes. Box 8-6 lists the steps of infant CPR.

HAND POSITION FOR CHEST COMPRESSION IN THE CHILD

If the patient does not have a pulse, provide chest compressions. Perform compressions for the child (over one year) on a firm, flat surface. Place the

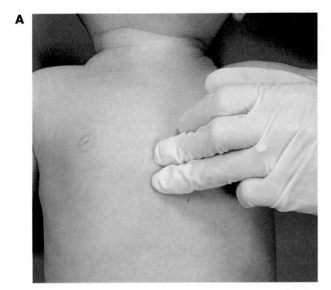

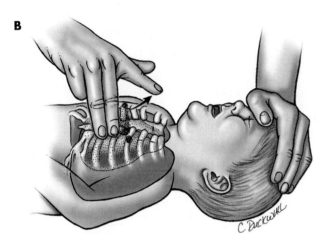

Fig. 8-17 A and **B** Proper finger position for chest compressions on an infant.

BOX 8-6 Steps of Infant CPR

1. Assess responsiveness.
2. Open the airway using the head-tilt, chin-lift for medical patients or the jaw thrust for trauma patients.
3. Assess breathing:
   If the patient is breathing, place them in the recovery position.
   If the patient is not breathing, administer two rescue breaths (1 to 1½ seconds each).
4. Assess circulation using the brachial artery:
   If the patient has a pulse, continue rescue breathing at a rate of 20 per minute (every 3 seconds).
   If the patient does not have a pulse, perform chest compressions at a rate of at least 100 per minute.
5. Perform 20 cycles (about one minute) of 5 compressions to one ventilation and then reassess the patient.
   If the patient has regained pulse and breathing, place them in the recovery position.
   If the patient has regained a pulse only, continue with rescue breathing at a rate of 20 per minute.
   If the patient has not regained a pulse, continue with cycles of 5 compressions to one ventilation and reassess the patient every few minutes.
6. If only one rescuer is present, activate EMS after the initial 20 cycles of CPR.

closest hand on the patient's forehead to maintain the head-tilt throughout the CPR sequence. With the other hand, locate the margin of the rib cage and trace to the sternum, as in adult CPR. Visualize the location of the xiphoid process and place the heel of the hand above that area on the sternum (Figure 8-18A and B). The chest is compressed ½ to ⅓ of its depth (about 1 to 1½ inches) with one hand. The compressions should be smooth and the fingers should not lie on the chest. This hand should remain on the chest so that placement does not have to be found again.

The compressions are done at a rate of 100 per minute. At the end of every fifth compression, pause to perform one rescue breath (1 to 1½ seconds). Perform 20 cycles of 5 compressions to 1 ventilation and then reassess the patient. If a lone

rescuer is performing CPR, EMS should be contacted at this time. Box 8-7 lists the steps of child CPR.

If the patient regains breathing and a pulse, place them in the recovery position. If the patient regains a pulse, but is not breathing, continue with rescue breathing. If the patient does not have a pulse and is not breathing, continue with CPR and reassess every few minutes.

In children, CPR may be performed with two rescuers. One rescuer will ventilate the patient and the other will perform chest compressions, the same as for adult two-rescuer CPR. Infants are too small to effectively perform two-rescuer CPR without interfering with each other, so one-rescuer CPR is performed.

Refer to Table 8-2 for a summary of infant and child CPR.

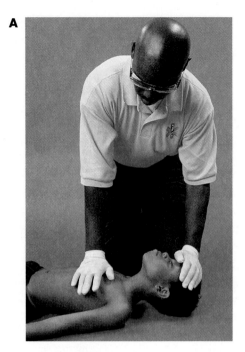

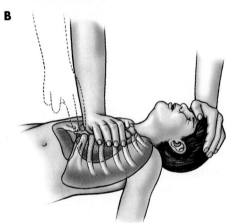

Fig. 8-18 A and **B** Proper hand position for chest compressions on a child.

BOX 8-7 Steps of Child CPR

1. Assess responsiveness.
2. Open the airway using the head-tilt, chin-lift for medical patients or the jaw thrust for trauma patients.
3. Assess breathing:
   If the patient is breathing, place them in recovery position.
   If the patient is not breathing, administer two rescue breaths (1 to 1½ seconds).
4. Assess circulation, using the carotid artery:
   If the patient has a pulse, continue with rescue breathing at a rate of 20 per minute.
   If the patient does not have a pulse, perform chest compression at a rate of 100 per minute.
5. Perform 20 cycles (about one minute) of 5 compressions to one ventilation and then reassess the patient.
   If the patient has regained a pulse and breathing, place them in the recovery position.
   If the patient has regained a pulse, but not breathing, continue with rescue breaths.
   If the patient has not regained a pulse, continue with cycles of 5 compressions to one ventilation and reassess every few minutes.
6. If only one rescuer is present, activate EMS after the initial 20 cycles of CPR.

INTERACTING WITH FAMILY AND FRIENDS

The responsibilities of the First Responder are not limited to care of the patient. The family members and friends of the patient may be experiencing extreme anxiety and fear about the situation. The First Responder should interact with understanding and empathy toward the family. First Responders must not offer diagnosis or advanced level treatment suggestions, but can offer reassurance and a caring attitude.

CHAPTER SUMMARY

REVIEW OF THE CIRCULATORY SYSTEM

The circulatory system functions to deliver oxygen and nutrients to the tissues of the body and removes waste products. The heart has four chambers: two atria and two ventricles. Arteries

TABLE 8-2 Summary of Infant and Child CPR

	Infant	Child
Age	Under one year	1–8 years
Breathing	1–1/2 seconds each : rate 20/minute	
Pulse	Brachial artery	Carotid artery
Compressions	Two fingers on sternum; rate at least 100/minute	Heel of hand on sternum; rate 100/minute
Ratio	5 compressions : 1 ventilation	
Compression depth	½ to 1 inch	1–1½ inches

When the left ventricle contracts, sending a wave of blood through the arteries, a pulse can be felt. You can palpate the pulse anywhere an artery passes near the skin surface and over a bone. When a patient has no pulse, they are in cardiac arrest. Organ damage will begin very quickly. External chest compressions are combined with artificial ventilations to oxygenate and circulate the blood. This is called cardiopulmonary resuscitation.

CARDIOPULMONARY RESUSCITATION

CPR cannot sustain life indefinitely and is only effective for a short time. The effectiveness of delivering oxygen to the tissues decreases the longer CPR is performed. The American Heart Association chain of survival consists of: early access, early CPR, early defibrillation, and early advanced cardiac life support.

TECHNIQUES OF ADULT CPR

CPR is indicated when the patient is not breathing and does not have a pulse. The performance of CPR is done in various assessment and intervention steps called the "ABCs of CPR." The steps consist of assessing responsiveness and activating EMS, opening and monitoring the airway, monitoring breathing and providing artificial respirations, assessing the circulation and providing chest compressions, and reassessing and monitoring the patient. Adult CPR can be performed by one or two rescuers.

TECHNIQUES OF INFANT AND CHILD CPR

Begin the assessment, open the airway, and assess breathing the same as you would for an adult patient. If the patient is not breathing, deliver rescue breaths, then assess the carotid pulse in the child or the brachial pulse in the infant. Perform chest compressions on the lower half of the sternum with two fingers on the infant, with one hand on the child.

INTERACTING WITH FAMILY AND FRIENDS

Although the patient is the primary responsibility of the First Responder, the family and friends of the patient may also need comfort and reassurance.

REVIEW QUESTIONS

Techniques of Infant and Child CPR

1. List the steps of infant and child CPR in order:
   A. Assess the situation
   B. Open airway
   C. Activate EMS
   D. Assess breathing
   E. Determine responsiveness
   F. Perform CPR for one minute

2. For infants and children, the compressions should be at a depth of _____ to _____ of the patient's chest.

3. Two-rescuer CPR is performed on a child in the same way that it is performed on an adult. True or False?

4. Place the terms: "Infant," "Child," or "Both" beside the following skills:
   _____ Compression rate of more than 100 per minute
   _____ Rescue breathing at a rate of 20 per minute
   _____ Use two fingers on the sternum for compressions
   _____ Do not compress over the xiphoid process
   _____ Compress $1/2$ to $1/3$ of the chest depth
   _____ Perform cycles of 5 compressions to 1 ventilation
   _____ Compress at a rate of 100 per minute
   _____ Can use two-rescuer technique

5. For infants and children, perform CPR for one minute before activating EMS because they primarily are in cardiac arrest due to respiratory arrest. True or False?

1. E, B, D, A, F, C; 2. $1/2$, $1/3$; 3. True; 4. Infant, Both, Infant, Both, Both, Child, Both, Child; 5. True

---

carry blood away from the heart and veins carry blood to the heart. Capillaries connect arteries to veins. Blood is the fluid portion of the circulatory system and it carries oxygen to the tissues and carbon dioxide away from the tissues.

UNITED STATES DEPARTMENT OF TRANSPORTATION NATIONAL HIGHWAY TRAFFIC SAFETY ADMINISTRATION FIRST RESPONDER OBJECTIVES

Check your knowledge. The National Registry of EMTs and many state EMS agencies use the objectives below to develop First Responder certification examinations. Can you meet them?

COGNITIVE OBJECTIVES

1. List the reasons for the heart to stop beating.
2. Define the components of cardiopulmonary resuscitation
3. Describe each link in the chain of survival and how it relates to the EMS system.
4. List the steps of one-rescuer adult CPR.
5. Describe the technique of external chest compressions on an adult patient.
6. Describe the technique of external chest compressions on an infant.
7. Describe the technique of external chest compressions on a child.
8. Explain when the First Responder is able to stop CPR.
9. List the steps of two-rescuer adult CPR.
10. List the steps of infant CPR.
11. List the steps of child CPR.

AFFECTIVE OBJECTIVES

12. Respond to the feelings that the family of a patient may be having during a cardiac event.

13. Demonstrate a caring attitude towards patients with cardiac events who request emergency medical services.
14. Place the interests of the patient with a cardiac event as the foremost consideration when making any and all patient care decisions.
15. Communicate with empathy with family members and friends of the patient with a cardiac event.

PSYCHOMOTOR OBJECTIVES

16. Demonstrate the proper technique of chest compressions on an adult.
17. Demonstrate the proper technique of chest compressions on a child.
18. Demonstrate the proper technique of chest compressions on an infant.
19. Demonstrate the steps of adult one-rescuer CPR.
20. Demonstrate the steps of adult two-rescuer CPR.
21. Demonstrate child CPR.
22. Demonstrate infant CPR.

Automated External Defibrillation

KEY TERMS

Automated external defibrillator (AED) A machine used by basic level rescuers to provide an electrical shock to a patient who is not breathing and is pulseless; they are either automatic or semiautomatic.

Defibrillation Delivering an electrical shock to the patient's heart to stop a chaotic heart rhythm.

Joule A unit of energy used to measure the amount of electricity delivered during defibrillation.

Ventricular fibrillation A chaotic heart rhythm in which the patient has no pulse and the heart is simply "quivering" inside the chest; the heart is not pumping so no pulse is produced.

Ventricular tachycardia An abnormal heart rhythm in which three or more beats in a row are generated by the ventricles at a rate of 100 beats per minute or more.

Cardiac emergencies are the most prominent type of emergency in the United States. Each year, the use of the automated external defibrillator saves many lives. The **automated external defibrillator (AED)** is a machine used by basic level providers to analyze the patient's cardiac rhythm and deliver an electrical shock that stops the heart's chaotic rhythm. This electrical shock is called **defibrillation**. For the adult patient in cardiac arrest, defibrillation is the highest priority and should be done even before CPR is started. Defibrillation is the primary intervention that makes the greatest difference in the survival of cardiac arrest patients. Early defibrillation is a vital link in the chain of survival and is an important life-saving technique.

THE AUTOMATED EXTERNAL DEFIBRILLATOR

The steps of defibrillation include the recognition and treatment of a heart rhythm that produces no pulse. Basic level providers are generally not trained in the recognition of cardiac rhythms, and therefore in the past, were not able to defibrillate. Since defibrillation is the intervention that most impacts the survival of adult cardiac arrest patients, the use of an automated external defibrillator will allow more providers to deliver this life-saving intervention.

The longer a person is in cardiac arrest, the less likely that defibrillation will be successful. Therefore, the availability of the AED for First Responders is beneficial.

Many EMS systems across the country have shown that basic level EMS providers can save the lives of some cardiac arrest patients with the use of the AED. These EMS systems have added defibrillation to the role of the EMT-Basic and, sometimes, to the role of the First Responder.

OVERVIEW OF THE AUTOMATED EXTERNAL DEFIBRILLATOR

The AED was developed in the early 1980s and has gained widespread application in the United States. Healthcare providers have been using defibrillation for decades as the primary treatment of life-threatening electrical disturbances in the heart. By combining computer technology with the defibrillator, much of the human decision-making and possibility for error has been reduced. The use of an AED can be learned in a short time. In the future, these machines may be available in every shopping mall, airport, or hotel, and their use taught in advanced CPR courses.

The AED works when two conductive patches are placed on the patient's chest and the machine is turned on. The AED then uses computer circuitry to analyze the patient's cardiac rhythm, and to deliver a shock if appropriate. To administer a shock, the AED's computer must detect a life-threatening electrical disturbance in the heart, which is generally a condition known as ventricular fibrillation. **Ventricular fibrillation** is a chaotic dysrhythmia in which the patient has no pulse or respirations, and the heart is simply "quivering" inside the chest (Fig. D-1). The rhythm has electrical activity but does not cause a mechanical pumping action of the heart to produce a pulse.

The AED will shock other rhythms, but these are seldom present on arrival of EMS. One of them, called **ventricular tachycardia,** is three or more beats in a row at a rate of 100 beats or more per minute that originate in the ventricles (Fig. D-2). This rhythm may or may not produce a detectable pulse. This rhythm occurs frequently at the onset of arrest but generally deteriorates quickly to ventricular fibrillation. An AED can shock both rhythms, but the key is that the patient must be pulseless and not breathing before you attach the machine to the patient.

FIRST RESPONDER ALERT

Attach the AED only to patients who are in cardiac arrest—unresponsive with no pulse and not breathing—to avoid delivering inappropriate shocks to patients who have a pulse. Shocking a patient with a pulse may put that patient into ventricular fibrillation or into other unshockable rhythms.

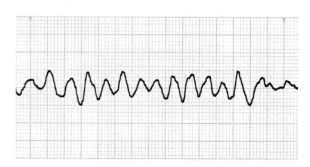

Fig. D-1 Ventricular fibrillation.

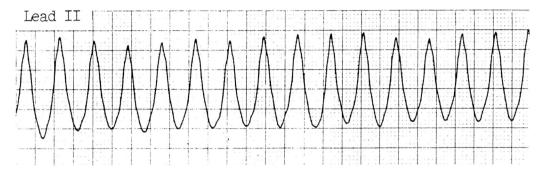

Fig. D-2 Ventricular tachycardia.

There are two types of AEDs: fully automatic and semiautomatic (Fig. D-3). A fully automatic external defibrillator requires the rescuer simply to hook up two defibrillatory patches to the patient's chest, connect the lead wires, and turn on the AED. A semiautomatic external defibrillator requires the rescuer to attach the patches and leads to the patient's chest, turn on the AED, and press a button to analyze the rhythm. The AED's computer-synthesized voice then advises you what steps to take based on its analysis of the patient's cardiac rhythm. Shocks are delivered manually by pressing a button, if advised. Both types of AEDs are designed to deliver up to three shocks in a row.

Depending on whether your AED has a screen that shows the patient's rhythm, you may never know or see the rhythm. Therefore, your primary concerns are the absence or presence of a carotid pulse and following the directions of the AED. Remember that the machine cannot detect pulses, only electrical activity within the heart. The electrical activity may or may not be producing a pulse.

These machines are very accurate in detecting both shockable rhythms and rhythms not needing shocks. A correct and accurate analysis by the AED depends on properly charged defibrillator batteries and proper maintenance of the defibrillator. The few documented cases of inappropriate shocks occurring are attributed to human error, such as using the device on a patient with a pulse or activating it in a moving vehicle, and mechanical error, such as low batteries.

You should stop CPR when the AED is analyzing the patient's heart rhythm or when delivering shocks. Anyone touching the patient or anything attached to the patient may also receive a shock. It is dangerous to be close to the patient when the AED is used. For example, contact with an object that is touching the patient can transmit the high-voltage shock. Do not touch the patient when the

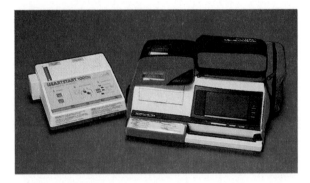

Fig. D-3 Fully automatic (left) and semiautomatic (right) external defibrillators.

rhythm is being analyzed because movement may cause discrepancies in the analysis of the rhythm. You should stop CPR and artificial ventilations, and if the patient is in a vehicle, it should be stopped. Defibrillation is a higher priority than CPR, so it is beneficial to the patient to stop CPR to use the AED. CPR may be stopped for up to 90 seconds when three consecutive shocks are delivered. Resume CPR only after the first three shocks are delivered, or when the AED indicates a "no shock" situation.

ADVANTAGES OF THE AUTOMATED EXTERNAL DEFIBRILLATOR

There are many advantages for the use of the AED. The biggest advantage is that basic level providers who are not trained to read cardiac rhythms can still deliver an electrical shock to the patient's heart.

The speed of operation is very fast—usually the first shock can be delivered to the patient within 1 minute of arrival at the patient's side. The remote defibrillation uses adhesive pads, making it a "hands-off" process. Traditional defibrillators use paddles that the rescuer must hold on the patient's chest, placing the rescuer close to the patient when they deliver the shock. The electrodes are large and easy to place. Some models have an optional rhythm monitoring capability that can be used when personnel knowledgeable in cardiac rhythm interpretation arrive on scene.

The defibrillator will automatically select the energy level of the shock to be delivered, measured in joules (abbreviated J). The AED increases the energy level of each successive shock. The machine will shock the patient the first time at 200 joules, the second time at 200–300 joules, and the third time at 360 joules.

OPERATION OF THE AUTOMATED EXTERNAL DEFIBRILLATOR

When caring for a patient, always take appropriate body substance isolation precautions. On your arrival at the scene, perform the initial assessment, and if appropriate use the AED.

Technique D-1 describes the steps for AED using a common type of semi-automatic external defibrillator.

Figure D-5 illustrates a standardized algorithm for AED use.

To use the fully automatic external defibrillator, follow the same procedure. Once the AED power is turned on, the machine will analyze and shock with no action by the rescuer. After three shocks, check the pulse and continue with the appropriate treatment. The machine will state "clear the patient" before delivering shocks, or will state "no shock indicated" when appropriate.

Not all patients in cardiac arrest will benefit from defibrillation. If the AED does not detect a shockable rhythm, it advises "no shock indicated." Make sure the patient has no pulse and then begin CPR. After one minute of CPR, reanalyze the rhythm.

Because it is vital for the patient to receive defibrillation as soon as possible, pulse checks are not performed after shocks one, two, four, and five. After three shocks, the defibrillator has reached the maximum energy level required. A pulse check should be performed after shock three and after shock six. Follow standard operating procedures in all cases (Box D-1).

The AED generally is not used for patients younger than 12 years of age or patients weighing less than 41 kg (90 lbs). The airway and artificial ventilation are of prime importance in these patients. In young children, cardiac arrest usually results from respiratory compromise, not from cardiac problems. Patients weighing less than 41 kg (90 lbs) may receive too high an electrical

---

BOX D-1

- If no other EMS personnel are on scene, the First Responders should continue CPR and use of the AED until they arrive.
- One First Responder operates the defibrillator, and the other one performs CPR.
- After opening the airway and confirming the patient is in cardiac arrest, defibrillation comes first. Don't delay the analysis of the rhythm or defibrillation. The first shock should be delivered within 60 seconds of arrival at the patient's side.
- All contact with the patient must be avoided during analysis of the rhythm and delivery of shocks. Never analyze the rhythm in a moving vehicle.
- State "clear the patient" before delivering shocks, and verify that everyone is clear.
- No defibrillator can function correctly without properly working batteries. Check the batteries at the beginning of each shift, and carry extra batteries.
- Be familiar with the specific AED used by your service.
- If you are alone when approaching a cardiac arrest patient, use the AED after assessing the ABCs, instead of initiating CPR.

---

charge for their size, resulting in damage to the heart. The AED is also not generally used for patients who are in cardiac arrest due to trauma. If you are unsure if the AED would be appropriate for a patient, contact medical direction.

If the patient does not regain a pulse and there is no available advanced life support back-up, deliver a total of six shocks on scene and then consult medical direction. The medical direction physician may advise you to stay on scene if advanced providers are en route. If you have transport capabilities and additional shocks are ordered en route by the medical direction physician, the vehicle must be stopped completely before the defibrillator can analyze the rhythm. Use of the AED is never safe or appropriate in a moving vehicle. If you are unable to transport the patient, continue with the algorithm under the direct supervision of the medical direction physician until additional personnel arrive.

Do not remove the AED, even after a successful resuscitation. Ventricular fibrillation may recur following successful shocks. If you are with a patient who has been resuscitated but is unresponsive, check pulses every 30 seconds. If at any time the patient becomes pulseless, analyze the rhythm. Deliver up to three stacked shocks if indicated, and continue the resuscitation according to your local protocol.

If you are with a responsive patient having chest pain who becomes unresponsive, is not breathing, and is pulseless, attach the AED, analyze the

TECHNIQUE D-1 Use of the Semiautomatic External Defibrillator

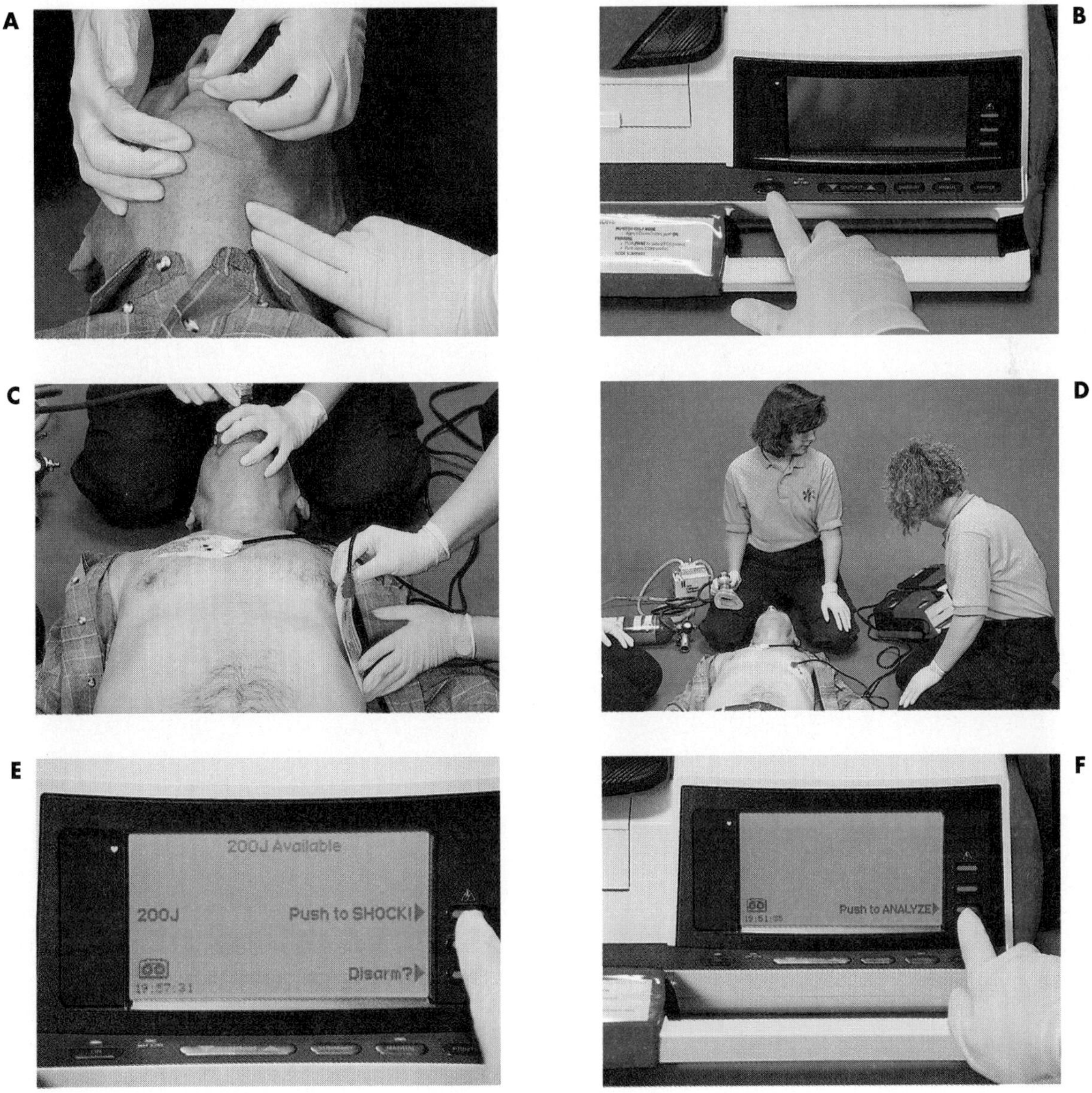

Fig. D-4 Follow appropriate body substance isolation precautions. **A,** Perform the initial assessment and confirm the patient is in cardiac arrest. Stop CPR if it is in progress and verify that the patient is unresponsive, not breathing and pulseless. Resume CPR. If you are the only rescuer present, proceed with the use of the AED. **B,** Turn on the AED's power. If the machine has a tape recorder, turn it on. **C,** Attach the device to the patient. One electrode is placed to the right of the upper portion of the sternum below the clavicle. The other electrode is placed over the ribs to the left of the nipple with the center in the midaxillary line. Most electrodes include diagrams showing correct placement. **D,** Stop CPR, clear everyone away from the patient and initiate analysis of the rhythm. **E,** If the machine advises a shock, deliver the first shock (generally 200 J); if not, go to step L. **F,** Reanalyze the rhythm. **CONTINUED**

TECHNIQUE D-1 CONTINUED

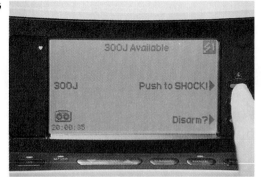

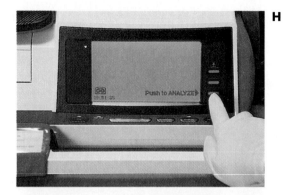

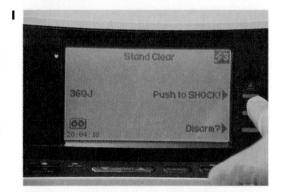

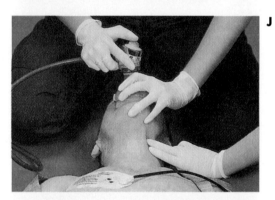

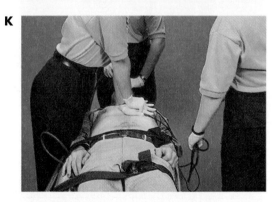

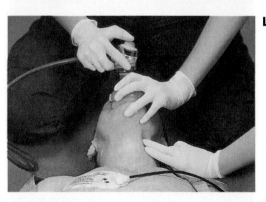

G, If the machine advises another shock, deliver a second shock (at 200–300 J); if not, go to step L. **H,** Reanalyze the rhythm. **I,** If the machine advises another shock, deliver a third shock (at 360 J); if not, go to step L. **J,** Check the patient's pulse. If the patient has a pulse, check breathing. If the patient is breathing adequately, place the patient in the recovery position and monitor the airway and pulse and have the patient transported as soon as possible. If the patient has a pulse and is not breathing adequately, provide artificial ventilations and have the patient transported as soon as possible. If the patient does not have a pulse, resume CPR for 1 minute. At the direction of the AED, deliver one more cycle of up to three stacked shocks (at 360 J), and reassess the pulse. If there is no pulse, continue the stacked shocks. If an ambulance has arrived, consult with medical direction and continue with stacked shocks or have the patient transported. **K,** Have the patient transported as soon as possible. **L,** If the machine advises "no shock," check the patient's pulse. If there is a pulse, check breathing and treat appropriately for adequate or inadequate breathing and have the patient transported. If there is no pulse, perform CPR for 1 minute and then recheck the pulse. Reanalyze the rhythm if there is still no pulse. If "no shock" is again advised and there is still no pulse, resume CPR for 1 minute. Analyze the rhythm a third time. If shock is advised, deliver up to two sets of three stacked shocks separated by 1 minute of CPR, consult the medical direction physician, and have the patient transported. If "no shock" is advised a third time and the patient does not have a pulse, resume CPR and have the patient transported as soon as possible.

Automated External Defibrillation (AED) Algorithm for First Responders

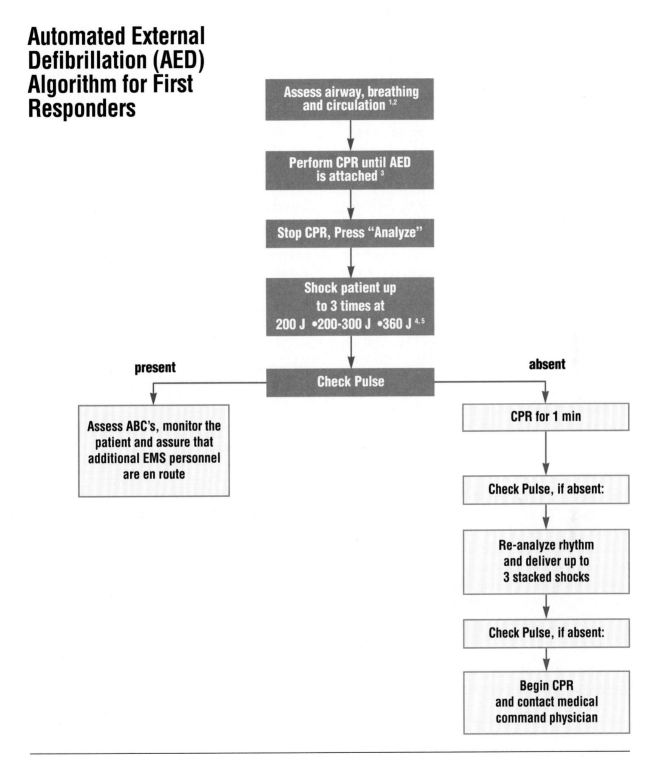

Fig. D-5 Algorithm for AED use.

1. Use appropriate body substance isolation precautions.
2. If CPR was started before your arrival, stop CPR to confirm lack of pulse and breathing.
3. If you are the only rescuer, proceed to the use of the AED.
4. Pulse checks are not required between shocks 1, 2, 4 and 5 unless "no shock" advised.

5. If "no shock indicated" is advised at any time by AED, check pulse. If pulse is absent, perform CPR for 1 minute, recheck pulse and reanalyze the rhythm. After three consecutive "no shock indicated" messages, continue CPR and have the patient transported. Reanalyze the rhythm per your local protocol.

rhythm, deliver up to three shocks if indicated, and continue the resuscitation according to your local protocol. All patients who are experiencing chest pain do not progress to cardiac arrest. Follow the steps in Chapter 8, "Circulation," for the care for a patient who is responsive and has a pulse. The AED should only be attached to patients who are unresponsive and do not have a pulse. **Do not attach the AED to a patient who is responsive or who has a pulse.**

If a situation arises in which you are the only rescuer with an AED, take body substance isolation precautions, and perform an initial assessment to verify that the patient is not breathing and has no pulse. Turn on the AED power, attach the device to the patient, initiate analysis of the rhythm, and deliver a shock if necessary. Follow the local protocol for the remainder of the treatment. Defibrillation should always be the first step before CPR. Do not leave the patient to contact medical direction or to call for assistance until the "no shock indicated" command is given, the pulse returns, three shocks are delivered, or help arrives.

Always follow the local protocol for the use of the AED. Each EMS system has guidelines for continuing education and the use of AED. Use of the defibrillator does not require advanced life support personnel to be at the scene, although they should be notified as soon as possible. It is vital that EMS personnel are contacted and arrive as soon as possible. If there are no advanced life support personnel available in the prehospital setting, the patient should be transported quickly to the nearest facility that has ACLS capabilities. Early ACLS is the final link in the chain of survival.

For safety reasons, do not use the defibrillator near water or in the rain. The defibrillator is an electrical device. If the patient is lying in water or on ice and you are standing in the water beside the patient, the electrical shock will travel from the patient to you through the water. Move the patient to a dry area and remove any wet clothes from the patient. The patient also should not be touching any metal. The electrical discharge from the defibrillator would travel through the patient and through the metal to anyone touching it.

POSTRESUSCITATION CARE

If the patient does not regain a pulse after completing the AED algorithm, follow local protocol regarding whether or not to continue with the use of the defibrillator. If a pulse does return, ensure a patent airway and have the patient transported with basic life support maintained. It is vital that care is maintained after resuscitation of the patient. The patient's airway, breathing, and circulation must be monitored continuously so that the cardiac arrest does not reoccur. Do not remove the defibrillator from the patient if they have been resuscitated. The ALS personnel may remove it when they transport the patient.

Document all findings in your report and inform the advanced life support personnel of all interventions. Be sure to document each step performed, any changes in patient condition, and any responses to interventions. Document all vital signs before and after use of the AED. Document all interactions with bystanders and any information obtained regarding the patient. The prehospital care report is a vital part of the emergency medical care.

AUTOMATED EXTERNAL DEFIBRILLATOR MAINTENANCE

Defibrillators require regular maintenance. The EMS system should have a maintenance schedule for each unit. A checklist, "Operator's Shift Checklist for Automated Defibrillators," must be completed on a daily basis (Fig. D-6). The most common cause of defibrillator failure is improper device maintenance, usually battery failure. Battery replacement schedules should be maintained for each unit.

The American Heart Association publishes a variety of guidelines and additional information on AEDs. Follow these guidelines.

AUTOMATED EXTERNAL DEFIBRILLATOR SKILLS

You must maintain your AED skills. The AED is not a frequently used device in most systems. Therefore, the skills may be forgotten easily if they are not practiced. EMS systems usually require a skill review every 90 days to reassess competency. Medical direction is a required component of systems that use AEDs. Successful learning of automated external defibrillation in a First Responder course does not permit use of the device without approval by state regulations and local medical direction. Every event in which an AED is used

Automated Defibrillators: Operator's Shift Checklist

Date _____ Shift _____ Location _____

Mfr/Model No. _____ Serial No. or Facility ID No. _____

At the beginning of each shift, inspect the unit. Indicate whether all requirements have been met. Note any corrective actions taken. Sign the form.

	OK as Found	Corrective Action/ Remarks
1. Defibrillator Unit Clean, no spills, clear of objects on top, casing intact		
2. Cables/Connectors a. Inspect for cracks, broken wire, or damage b. Connectors engage securely and are not damaged*		
3. Supplies a. Two sets of pads in sealed packages, within expiration date* f. Monitoring electrodes* b. Hand towel g. Spare charged battery* c. Scissors h. Adequate ECG paper* d. Razor i. Manual override module, key, or card* e. Alcohol wipes* j. Cassette tape, memory module, and/or event card plus spares*		

4. Power Supply
 a. Battery-powered units
   (1) Verify fully charged battery in place
   (2) Spare charged battery available
   (3) Follow appropriate battery rotation schedule per manufacturer's recommendations
 b. AC/battery backup units
   (1) Plugged into live outlet to maintain battery charge
   (2) Test on battery power and reconnect to line power		

5. Indicators*/ECG Display a. Remove cassette tape, memory module, and/or event card* b. Power-on display c. Self-test OK d. Monitor display functional* e. "Service" message display off* f. Battery charging; low battery light off* g. Correct time displayed; set with dispatch center		
6. ECG Recorder* a. Adequate ECG paper b. Recorder prints		
7. Charge/Display Cycle a. Disconnect AC plug – battery backup units* b. Attach to simulator c. Detects, charges, and delivers shock for VF d. Responds correctly to nonshockable rhythms e. Manual override functional* f. Detach from simulator g. Replace cassette tape, module, and/or memory card *		
8. Pacemaker* a. Pacer output cable intact b. Pacer pads present (set of two) c. Inspect per manufacturer's operational guidelines		
Major Problem(s) Identified **(Out of Service)**		

*Applicable only if the unit has this supply or capability

Signature _____

Fig. D-6 Example of an AED operator checklist.

must be reviewed by the medical director or designated representative. Reviews of events using the AED may be accomplished by a written report and a review of the voice-electrocardiogram tape recording made by the AED machine or the solid-state memory modules and magnetic tape recordings stored in the device. Quality improvement involves both the individuals using AED and the EMS system in which the AEDs are used.

EMS delivery systems should have all the necessary links in the chain of survival, medical direction, an audit or quality improvement program in place, and mandatory continuing education with skill competency reviews for EMS providers.

APPENDIX SUMMARY

THE AUTOMATED EXTERNAL DEFIBRILLATOR

The automated external defibrillator (AED) allows basic level providers who are not trained in rhythm recognition to deliver an electrical shock to a patient in cardiac arrest. The AED uses computer circuitry to analyze the patient's heart rhythm, and, if appropriate, deliver a shock. AEDs can be fully automatic or semiautomatic. The AED allows for early defibrillation, a vital link in the chain of survival.

If the patient does not regain a pulse after using the AED, follow your local protocol for transport, CPR, and further defibrillation. If the patient does regain a pulse, place them in the recovery position and monitor their airway and breathing until ACLS personnel arrive.

AUTOMATED EXTERNAL DEFIBRILLATOR MAINTENANCE

AED failures are often caused by improper maintenance. The AED should be checked daily. Check the batteries and complete the Operator's Shift Checklist for Automated Defibrillators.

AUTOMATED EXTERNAL DEFIBRILLATOR SKILLS

You must refresh your skills with the AED periodically. A review every 90 days is recommended by many EMS systems. Following an event in which an AED is used, the medical director or a designated representative will review the case for quality improvement.

UNITED STATES DEPARTMENT OF TRANSPORTATION NATIONAL HIGHWAY TRAFFIC SAFETY ADMINISTRATION EMT-BASIC OBJECTIVES

Check your knowledge. Many state EMS agencies use the objectives below to develop First Responder certification examinations. Can you meet them?

COGNITIVE OBJECTIVES

1. List the indications for automated external defibrillation (AED).
2. List the contraindications for automated external defibrillation.
3. Define the role of the First Responder in the emergency cardiac care system.
4. Explain the impact of age and weight on defibrillation.
5. Discuss the fundamentals of early defibrillation.
6. Explain the rationale for early defibrillation.
7. Explain that not all chest pain results in cardiac arrest and the First Responder does not need to attach an automated external defibrillator.
8. Explain the importance of prehospital ACLS intervention if it is available.
9. Explain the importance of urgent transport to a facility with Advanced Cardiac Life Support if it is not available in the prehospital setting.
10. Discuss the various types of automated external defibrillators.
11. Differentiate between the fully automated and the semiautomated defibrillator.
12. Discuss the procedures that must be taken into consideration for standard operations of the various types of automated external defibrillators.
13. State the reasons for assuring that the patient is pulseless and apneic when using the automated external defibrillator.
14. Discuss the circumstances that may result in inappropriate shocks.
15. Explain the considerations for interruption of CPR when using the automated external defibrillator.
16. Discuss the advantages and disadvantages of automated external defibrillators.
17. Summarize the speed of operation of automated external defibrillation.
18. Discuss the use of remote defibrillation through adhesive pads.
19. Discuss the special considerations for rhythm monitoring.
20. List the steps in the operation of the automated external defibrillator.
21. Discuss the standard of care that should be used to provide care to a patient with persistent ventricular fibrillation and no available ACLS.
22. Discuss the standard of care that should be used to provide care to a patient with recurrent ventricular fibrillation and no available ACLS.
23. Differentiate between single-rescuer and multi-rescuer care with an automated external defibrillator.
24. Explain the reason for pulses not being checked between shocks with an automated external defibrillator.
25. Discuss the importance of coordinating ACLS trained providers with personnel using automated external defibrillators.
26. Discuss the importance of postresuscitation care.
27. List the components of postresuscitation care.
28. Explain the importance of frequent practice with the automated external defibrillator.
29. Discuss the need to complete the Automated Defibrillator: Operator's Shift Checklist.
30. Explain the role medical direction plays in the use of automated external defibrillation.
31. Discuss the goal of quality improvement in automated external defibrillation.
32. Define the function of all controls on an automated external defibrillator, and describe event documentation and battery defibrillator maintenance.

AFFECTIVE OBJECTIVES

33. Defend the reasons for obtaining initial training in automated external defibrillation and the importance of continuing education.
34. Defend the reason for maintenance of automated external defibrillators.

PSYCHOMOTOR OBJECTIVES

35. Demonstrate the application and operation of the automated external defibrillator.
36. Demonstrate the maintenance of an automated external defibrillator.
37. Demonstrate the assessment and documentation of patient response to the automated external defibrillator.
38. Demonstrate the skills necessary to complete the Automated Defibrillator: Operator's Shift Checklist.

Illness and Injury

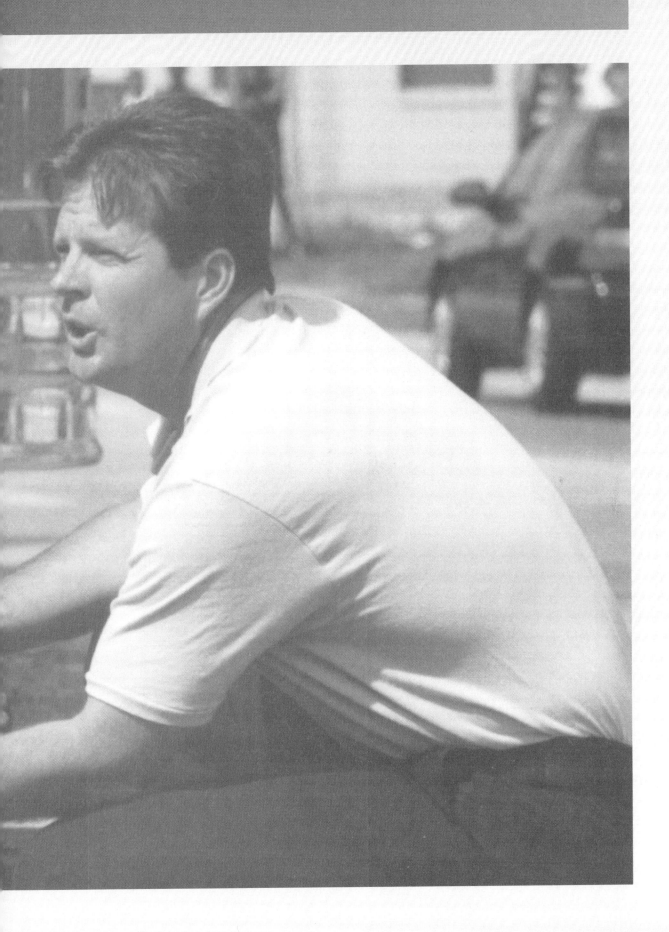

Medical Emergencies

KEY TERMS

Altered mental status A sudden or gradual decrease in the patient's level of responsiveness.

Behavior The manner in which a person acts or performs.

Convulsions Jerky, violent muscle contractions.

Hyperthermia A rise in the body temperature.

Hypothermia A drop in the body temperature.

Seizures A type of altered mental status that may be characterized by convulsions or other sudden changes in responsiveness.

Reasonable force The minimum force necessary to keep the patient from injuring himself or others.

FIRST RESPONSE

Neil and Carlos were detailed for overtime to First Responder Engine Company 53. No sooner had they reported for duty when they were responding to a 64-year-old female with shortness of breath. On the way, Neil admitted to Carlos that he never really liked these medical calls. "I know what to do if they are in cardiac arrest," he confessed, "but I never know what to say to these patients." Carlos smiled and said "I used to feel the same way. Then I realized that just being there and acting professionally is the key. It makes the patient and the family feel so much better if you are just compassionate."

The patient was dripping with sweat as she huffed and puffed to catch her breath. Her husband was very distraught as he watched his wife struggle to breathe. Neil watched as Carlos took control of the situation. He was calm, reassuring, kind, and polite. He held the woman's hand and he looked her in the eye and said, "Everything is under control. The EMTs will be here in about four minutes and they will get you to the hospital in no time." You could see the tension melt off her husband's face when Carlos turned to him and said with a smile, "This is a very good EMS system. We are going to take really good care of your wife."

Carlos got a SAMPLE history and was giving the EMS crew a quick update when Neil realized that he was right. You don't have to be doing CPR or clearing an airway to make a difference.

Most of the patients that you treat as a First Responder call for help because of medical problems. There are, however, many causes of medical problems. Fortunately, as a First Responder you will not have to diagnose what is wrong with the patient. You will gather information and provide care based on your assessment findings. One of the most important roles that you will play in these cases is the ability to provide comfort and reassurance to the patient and family. These situations are very scary to the public. Your calm, professional, and competent demeanor will provide great support in these moments of crisis.

This chapter will cover some of the major medical situations you will encounter. The most common situation will be the patient who has a general medical complaint. The patient is usually awake and your role is to assess the patient, gather information about the patient's history, and make the patient and family comfortable. Altered mental status and seizures are also common problems and your main role will be to perform an assessment and manage the patient's airway. Although environmental problems (i.e., exposure to heat and cold) and behavioral emergencies are less common, there are specific actions you should take. Therefore, considerable attention is paid to them in this chapter.

GENERAL MEDICAL COMPLAINTS

Until now, this book has focused on the treatment of patients with severe, immediately life-threatening conditions. Cases of airway obstruction or cardiac or respiratory arrest are highly critical events that require rapid intervention. However, they represent only a few of the situations that you will encounter as a First Responder. Many patients you see will be responsive, and can tell you about their chief complaint and any associated signs and symptoms (Box 9-1).

Some of these complaints may be the result of very serious medical conditions. Determining the exact cause of these symptoms can be extremely difficult. Fortunately, you do not need to determine the cause of the patient's medical problems to help them. As a First Responder, you will assess each patient to determine their chief complaint, as well as other associated signs and symptoms. You will then provide emergency care based on those findings.

As always, your priority is to assure your own safety. Be sure to complete a scene size-up before approaching the patient. Do not enter a scene that is not safe. The first step in assessing any patient is to complete the initial assessment to determine if any immediate life threats are present. You will next perform a physical exam appropriate for the patient and gather information for the SAMPLE history. You will also continually assess the patient for changes in their condition with the ongoing assessment.

Some First Responders are uncomfortable when caring for patients with general medical complaints. These patients are typically responsive and may be very anxious. It is easy to feel like you are not helping since the patient does not need to have immediate life threats managed. It is very important to appreciate how much you are helping them by being caring and understanding. The most important thing that you can do for patients with general medical complaints and no life-threatening problems is to provide comfort, calm them, reassure them that help is on the way, and that you are going to get them to the hospital quickly.

You should talk to the patient and family and gather as much of the SAMPLE history as you can. This will decrease the time that additional EMS personnel will spend at the scene, and will help you feel confident that you are helping the patient. By approaching the patient with a general medical complaint calmly, professionally, and with compassion, you can provide great comfort and support in

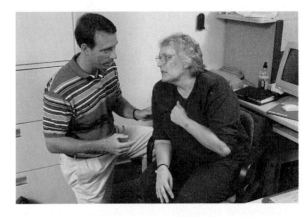

Fig. 9-1 By approaching the patient calmly, professionally and with compassion, you can provide great comfort and support in a stressful situation for the patient and their family.

BOX 9-2 Role of the First Responder - General Medical Complaint

- Complete First Responder assessment
    Scene size-up
    Initial assessment
    Physical exam
    SAMPLE history
    Ongoing assessment
- Comfort, calm, and reassure the family
- Provide a brief report to arriving EMS personnel

FIRST RESPONDER ALERT

If the patient is conscious and has general medical complaints, you do not need to determine the exact cause of their illness. Provide care based on the patient's signs and symptoms.

BOX 9-1 Common Signs and Symptoms in Patients with General Medical Complaints

- Pain (chest, abdominal, back, head, etc.)
- Shortness of breath
- Headache/dizziness
- Disorientation
- Nausea and vomiting

REVIEW QUESTIONS

General Medical Complaints

1. List at least three common signs and symptoms of general medical complaints.

    _____

    _____

    _____

2. Because patients with a general medical complaint are conscious and do not require management of immediate life threats, there is nothing for the First Responder to do. True or False? Why?

1. Pain (chest, abdomen, back, head, etc.), shortness of breath, headache/dizziness, disorientation, nausea and vomiting; 2. False. The First Responder's main role when caring for patients with general medical complaints is to perform a First Responder assessment, including SAMPLE history, care for the patient based on their signs and symptoms, and provide comfort and reassurance to the patient and family.

a highly stressful situation (Fig. 9-1). Box 9-2 lists the steps a First Responder should take when caring for a patient with a general medical complaint.

SPECIFIC MEDICAL COMPLAINTS

There are a few specific medical complaints and situations that require special attention by the First Responder. These are less common than general medical complaints, but require a specific approach. You should treat the patient based on the assessment findings and not worry about the cause of the problem. In all cases, pay particular attention to the airway and maintain a safe environment for the patient.

ALTERED MENTAL STATUS

Altered mental status is a sudden or gradual decrease in the patient's level of responsiveness. This may range from a patient who is slightly disoriented to one who seems asleep and cannot be awakened. Overall, the more unresponsive the patient is, the more critical the situation. Keep in mind, however, that even minor disorientation can signal a serious medical problem and should be considered a true emergency.

Common causes of altered mental status

There are many reasons that a patient may have altered mental status (Box 9-3). Altered mental status may last for any amount of time, from only a few seconds to many years. Remember that determining the cause is not important. You will support the patient, control the airway, and maintain a safe scene while awaiting additional EMS resources. Gather information about the SAMPLE history and calm and reassure the patient and family members.

The role of the First Responder

For a patient with altered mental status, you should complete the First Responder assessment, including the scene size-up, initial assessment, physical exam, and ongoing assessment. If the patient is unable to answer questions, you should obtain the SAMPLE history from a family member, friend, or bystander. Keep in mind that the last sense a patient loses is hearing. Talking to the patient is important even if they are not responding to you. Always assume that the patient can hear you and provide comfort and reassurance.

> **BOX 9-3 Common Causes of Altered Mental Status**
>
> - Fever
> - Infections
> - Poisonings (including drugs and alcohol)
> - Low blood sugar
> - Insulin reactions
> - Head injury
> - Decreased levels of oxygen to the brain
> - Psychiatric conditions

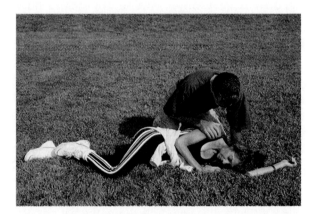

Fig. 9-2 All uninjured patients with an altered mental status should be placed in the recovery position and monitored.

Patients with an altered mental status are at a very high risk for airway problems. Depending on the severity of the altered mental status, the airway may be open or the patient may need airway management and artificial ventilation. Maintain the airway and support ventilation as discussed in Chapter 6, "Airway." Be sure to have suction immediately available.

All uninjured patients with an altered mental status who are breathing adequately should be placed in the recovery position (Fig. 9-2). If the patient is gurgling or snoring with each breath, the tongue or fluids may be obstructing the airway. If the patient is injured, you should suction their airway immediately and consider the use of an oral or nasal airway.

Remember to reassess the airway of a patient with altered mental status frequently. Do not become distracted and forget the basic principles of airway management and patient assessment.

BOX 9-4 Role of the First Responder-Altered Mental Status

- Complete First Responder assessment
  - Scene size-up
  - Initial assessment
  - Physical exam
  - SAMPLE history
  - Ongoing assessment
- Assure airway patency
  - Uninjured patient—place in recovery position
  - Injured or possibly injured patient—consider the use of airway adjuncts and have suction available
- Comfort, calm, and reassure the patient and family

BOX 9-5 Common Causes of Seizures

- Chronic medical conditions (such as epilepsy)
- Fever
- Infection
- Poisoning (including drugs and alcohol)
- Low blood sugar
- Head injury
- Decreased levels of oxygen
- Brain tumors
- Complications of pregnancy

Perform ongoing assessments at least every five minutes. Box 9-4 summarizes the steps of caring for a patient with altered mental status.

SEIZURES

Seizures are a type of altered mental status. There are many types of seizures, but the most dramatic form is characterized by jerky, violent muscle contractions called convulsions. Onset is typically sudden and is usually related to nervous system malfunctions. During the convulsions, patients are usually unresponsive, sometimes stop breathing, and may vomit.

There are other forms of seizures, which can range from an episode in which the patient just seems to stare ahead blankly to convulsions affecting the entire body. Although they can be dramatic, seizures alone are rarely life-threatening emergencies. The biggest dangers of a seizure are the patient injuring himself during a fall, injuring himself during convulsions, or airway obstruction. The length of a seizure may vary tremendously, but it usually lasts less than five minutes. The longer the seizure, the greater the chances of complications, such as vomiting or inadequate respiration.

Common causes of seizures

Many conditions can cause seizures. Be aware, though, that the cause may remain unknown. Spending time trying to decide the cause of the seizure is not important. Box 9-5 lists some common causes of seizures.

Immediately after a seizure, a patient may seem asleep and unresponsive. The brain has suffered a massive discharge of energy, and the body is recovering for a short time after the seizure. After the patient regains responsiveness, they may be agitated or combative. Although a seizure is often a frightening event for bystanders, chronic seizure patients may be familiar with what occurs. They may refuse to let you help them after they become responsive. A seizure is especially frightening for the patient, family, and bystanders when it occurs for the first time or unexpectedly.

The role of the First Responder

Although the patient may be actively seizing, you should still try to perform a First Responder assessment. As always, scene safety is important. Move objects away from the patient so they do not injure themselves during convulsions. If the seizing patient is on a hard surface, try to keep their head from striking the ground or place padding on the floor so they do not cause serious head injuries. Generally, seizures themselves are not particularly dangerous, but the patient can seriously injury himself during the contractions. You should never attempt to restrain the seizing patient. Once you have made the scene safe for you and the patient, perform an initial assessment, physical exam, SAMPLE history, and ongoing assessment.

The most dangerous part of a seizure is the fact that the patient may obstruct their airway. Therefore, you must pay very close attention to the airway of a seizing patient. Often the patient will have significant oral secretions. They should be placed in the recovery position as soon as possible. If the patient's skin appears bluish, they are not breathing adequately, and you must ventilate

---

BOX 9-6 Role of the First Responder—Seizures

- Protect the patient from harming himself
- Complete First Responder assessment
     Scene size-up
     Initial assessment
     Physical exam
     SAMPLE history
     Ongoing assessment
- Assure airway patency
     Place in recovery position
     Have suction available
     Ventilate the patient if necessary
- Comfort, calm, and reassure the patient and family. Protect the patient's modesty.

FIRST RESPONDER ALERT

NEVER place anything into the mouth of a seizing patient. It will likely become an airway obstruction and could cause vomiting.

---

them as soon as possible. The most effective technique is mouth-to-mask ventilation. This can be difficult, but critical to the survival of the patient. Never place anything into the mouth of a seizing patient. Since these patients often vomit, you should have suction nearby.

Remember that seizures can be very alarming to family and bystanders and embarrassing for patients. Provide comfort and reassurance while awaiting additional EMS resources. During the convulsions, the patient may salivate, vomit, and lose control of their bladder and bowels. If possible, you should attempt to protect the patient's modesty by asking bystanders to leave the area.

Since seizures usually last only a few minutes, you may be the only person to witness the seizure. Pay careful attention to what the patient is doing during the seizure. This information can help the receiving facility determine the cause of the seizure. You should report any findings or observations to the transporting EMS personnel.

Box 9-6 summarizes the role of the First Responder for a patient having a seizure.

BOX 9-7 Major Contributing Factors for Generalized Hypothermia

- Cold environment
- Age (very young and the elderly)
- Medical conditions
- Alcohol, poisoning
- Illegal drugs
- Prescription or over-the-counter drugs

EXPOSURE TO COLD

In any locality you may encounter a patient who has been exposed to a cold environment. Even in the tropics, prolonged immersion in water or to night temperatures can cause the body temperature to drop. Many people suffer cold injuries from being around refrigerated food lockers, trailers, or box cars. There are two results of exposure to cold: generalized cold injuries, in which the patient's body temperature drops, and localized cold injuries, in which a specific body part is affected. A single patient can have both generalized and local cold emergencies.

Generalized cold emergencies

Generalized cold emergencies occur when there is a drop in the temperature of the internal organs of the body, a condition known as **hypothermia.** The most common cause of generalized hypothermia is exposure to a cold environment. The temperature does not need to be extraordinarily cold for hypothermia to occur. In fact, the most dangerous temperatures are from 40 to 50°F (5 to 10°C), because people often underestimate the danger of hypothermia and do not dress warmly enough. Other common factors contributing to hypothermia include exposure to water, ice, and snow.

Alcohol use is a complicating factor in many hypothermic patients. Alcohol affects judgment and decision making, often resulting in a patient not seeking shelter from the cold. Alcohol also causes blood vessels in the extremities to dilate, actually increasing heat loss, even though the patient may feel warm.

The old and the young are very susceptible to hypothermia. Older patients lose insulating fat, and the body may not respond as efficiently to an increased need for heat production. Young patients have a large surface area for their small size and very little fat for insulation. Pre-existing medical conditions also increase the likelihood of generalized cold emergencies.

Box 9-7 lists major contributing factors for generalized hypothermia.

Signs and symptoms of a generalized cold emergency

You should consider the possibility of hypothermia whenever the patient has obviously been exposed to the cold. Remember, even in relatively warm conditions hypothermia is possible. Hypothermia occurs in a progression, beginning with a slight drop in body temperature. The early signs and symptoms of hypothermia are very subtle, such as shivering and loss of sensation. The signs and symptoms become more dramatic, such as dizziness and memory loss, as the hypothermia becomes more profound.

Hypothermia may be less obvious in patients with underlying medical conditions, patients who have suffered from overdose or poisoning, or who have spent a long time in a cool environment, such as a home where the furnace may have malfunctioned.

Cool skin in the extremities is not a reliable sign of hypothermia. To determine the patient's internal temperature, place the back of your hand under the patient's clothing against the abdomen. Cool abdominal skin is a sign of a generalized cold emergency.

When the body temperature drops, a normal response is to increase heat production by shivering. Shivering is an effective method of generating body heat, but it is not always present in hypothermic patients. Usually the body stops shivering as the body temperature drops below 90°F (32°C). These patients may have a stiff or rigid posture. Children and infants and many elderly patients have small muscle mass that cannot generate very much heat by shivering.

The most important sign of hypothermia is a decrease in the mental status and motor function of the patient. In hypothermic patients, the level of responsiveness indicates the degree of hypothermia. Hypothermia affects the patient's level of responsiveness and ability to make rational decisions. Some hypothermic patients appear to be intoxicated, may be confused, and may exhibit poor judgment. Some hypothermic patients have become so confused that they remove their clothing in extremely cold weather! Box 9-8 summarizes the signs and symptoms of hypothermia.

BOX 9-8 Signs and Symptoms of Hypothermia

- Cool/cold abdominal skin temperature
- Shivering
- Decreased mental status and motor function
    - Poor coordination
    - Memory disturbances/confusion
    - Reduced or loss of touch sensation
    - Mood changes
    - Less communicative
    - Dizziness
    - Speech difficulty
- Stiff or rigid posture
- Muscular rigidity
- Poor judgment
- Complaints of joint/muscle stiffness

The role of the First Responder

Complete a First Responder assessment, including scene size-up, initial assessment, physical exam, and ongoing assessment. If you suspect that the patient may be hypothermic, you should prevent further heat loss. There is a major difference between rewarming a patient and preventing heat loss. Rewarming some hypothermic patients could cause life-threatening changes in the heart rhythm. You should focus your attention on preventing further heat loss and allow the body to warm itself. The patient should be rewarmed in the hospital under more controlled conditions.

To prevent heat loss, remove the patient from the cold environment. You should remove all wet clothing and cover the patient with a warm blanket. Contrary to popular belief, you should not permit the patient to eat or drink. Coffee, tea, chocolate, cigarettes and other stimulants can worsen the condition. Do not massage the patient's extremities or allow them to exert themselves or walk. Movement of the extremities can cause cold and stagnant blood to return to the heart and cause dangerous changes in heart rhythm. Handle the patient extremely gently.

Unresponsive hypothermic patients may have a very slow and weak heart beat, and may seem dead. Check for a pulse for at least 30 to 45 seconds to confirm that the patient is pulseless. If there is any pulse at all, do not begin chest compressions.

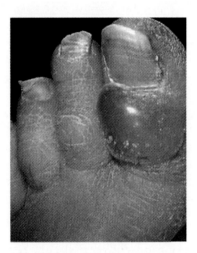

Fig. 9-3 Superficial local cold injury.

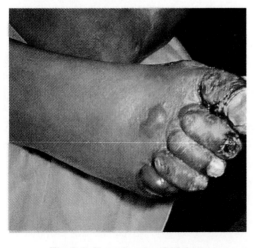

Fig. 9-4 Deep local cold injury.

If the patient has no pulse, begin CPR immediately. Patients can survive long periods of cardiac arrest if they are cold. If the patient is in a cold environment or cold water, and has been in cardiac arrest for less than 60 minutes, begin CPR. Box 9-9 provides a summary of the treatment for a patient with generalized hypothermia.

Local cold emergencies

The generalized cooling of the body is a danger to life, but local cooling can present a danger to the extremities and other body tissues. Local cold injuries result from the freezing or near freezing of a body part. Local cold injuries occur in a gradual progression: the deeper the freezing occurs, the more damage that will result. Local cold injuries are most common in the fingers, toes, ears, nose, and face. These injuries are often called frostbite or frostnip, but these terms can be confusing and should be avoided.

Signs and symptoms of local cold injuries

The signs and symptoms of local cold injuries causing early or superficial injury include (Fig. 9-3):
1. Pale skin that does not return to normal color.
2. Loss of feeling and sensation in the injured area.
3. Skin remains soft.
4. Tingling sensation when rewarmed.

The signs and symptoms of local cold injuries causing late or deep damage include (Fig. 9-4):
1. White or waxy skin.
2. Firm or frozen feeling on palpation.
3. Swelling and blisters.
4. Loss of sensation in the injured area.
5. If the injury has thawed or partially thawed, the skin may appear flushed with areas that are purple, pale, mottled, or cyanotic.

The role of the First Responder

Rewarming of local cold injuries is extremely painful and best performed in the hospital where the patient can be given medication for the pain. The role of the First Responder is to complete the First Responder assessment, including a scene size-up, initial assessment, physical exam, and ongoing assessment. In many cases, the patient will be concerned about permanent damage. Continue to provide comfort and calm the patient while you await additional EMS resources.

First, remove the patient from the cold environment. Protect the cold extremity from further injury. Because the tissues in the cold extremity are susceptible to additional injury, prevent

---

BOX 9-10 Role of the First Responder—Local Cold Injury

- Complete First Responder assessment
    - Scene size-up
    - Initial assessment
    - Physical exam
    - Ongoing assessment
- Assure airway patency - place the patient in the recovery position if they have decreased level of responsiveness
- Remove the patient from the cold environment
- Protect the injured area
    - Remove wet or restrictive clothing
    - Cover with dry, clean clothing or dressings
    - Manually stabilize the injured extremity
- Comfort, calm, and reassure the patient and family

BOX 9-11 Factors Increasing the Risk of Heat Injuries

- High heat and humidity
- Exercise and activity
- Age (very old, very young)
- Preexisting illness and/or condition
- Drugs/medications

---

unnecessary contact with that extremity. The patient often cannot feel pain, so protecting the extremity is important. Remove wet or restrictive clothing and all jewelry to improve blood flow to the area. Manually stabilize the extremity, and cover the injury with clean, dry clothing or a dressing.

There are several actions to avoid:
DO NOT re-expose the area to the cold.
DO NOT break blisters.
DO NOT rub or massage the area.
DO NOT apply heat or rewarm the area.
DO NOT allow the patient to walk on an affected extremity.

As the patient's internal temperature drops, their level of responsiveness decreases. If the patient has any altered mental status, they should be placed in the recovery position. Box 9-10 lists the steps a First Responder should take when caring for a patient with a local cold injury.

EXPOSURE TO HEAT

The body can warm itself more effectively in the cold than cool itself in the heat. Delicate brain tissue is extremely sensitive to high body temperatures; therefore, heat injuries can be a severe life threat. Hyperthermia is a progression of events that occur as the patient's body temperature rises. The terms heat stroke and heat exhaustion have been used to describe the condition of generalized hyperthermia. Because there is considerable

disagreement about the precise meaning of these terms, they should be avoided.

The body eliminates excess heat by sweating and increasing blood flow to the extremities, where heat can be lost from the skin. During exercise or vigorous activity, a person can lose more than 1 liter of sweat per hour! Heat emergencies occur most often when the environment is hot and humid. In these circumstances, the body cannot effectively evaporate sweat or radiate heat to the environment.

The elderly are predisposed to heat emergencies because they have less effective temperature regulation, may be on medications that affect their ability to eliminate heat, and may not be able to get away from a hot environment. Infants and newborns also have less effective control of their body temperature. Infants are not able to get drinking water or remove clothing on their own. Preexisting medical conditions can also predispose an individual to heat injuries. Box 9-11 lists factors that increase the risk of heat injuries.

Signs and symptoms of exposure to heat

Most healthy patients can easily tolerate a small rise in body temperature. If the patient's temperature continues to rise, however, the signs and symptoms of generalized heat emergencies develop.

As in cold emergencies, altered mental status is an important assessment finding in the hyperthermic patient. As body temperature rises, the patient becomes disoriented and confused. If the temperature continues to rise, the patient becomes unresponsive.

The signs and symptoms of heat emergencies are:
1. Muscle cramps
2. Weakness or exhaustion
3. Dizziness or fainting
4. Rapid, pounding heart beat
5. Altered mental status ranging from disorientation to unresponsiveness

REVIEW QUESTIONS

Specific Medical Complaints

1. Why is it NOT important for the First Responder to determine the cause of altered mental status or seizures?

2. How should you manage the airway of an uninjured patient with an altered mental status?

3. The jerky, violent muscle contractions of a patient having a seizure are called _____.

4. What are the two most dangerous complications of a seizure?

5. List six signs or symptoms of generalized hypothermia.

6. You should check the pulse of a hypothermic patient for _____ to _____ seconds before starting CPR.

7. What are the three ways that a First Responder should prevent further heat loss in a hypothermic patient?

8. What is the definition of a local cold injury?

9. List three factors that increase the risk of heat injuries.

10. How should you cool a patient who has been exposed to heat?

   A. Dunk them in cold water

   B. Cover them with rubbing alcohol

   C. Have them drink cold liquids

   D. Remove from the heat and fan them

1. The First Responder will provide care based on the assessment findings, not the cause of the problem.; 2. Place the patient in the recovery position.; 3. Convulsions.; 4. Airway obstruction and injury during a fall or convulsions.; 5. Cool or cold abdominal skin temperature, shivering, decreased mental status and motor function, poor coordination, memory disturbances/confusion, reduced or loss of touch sensation, mood changes, less communicative, dizziness, speech difficulty, stiff or rigid posture, muscular rigidity, poor judgment, complaints of joint/muscle stiffness.; 6. 30-45 seconds.; 7. Remove the patient from the cold environment, remove wet clothing, cover with warm blankets.; 8. The freezing or near freezing of a body part.; 9. High heat and humidity, exercise and activity, age (very old, very young), pre-existing illness and/or condition, drugs/medications.; 10. D

BOX 9-12 Role of the First Responder— Exposure to Heat

- Complete First Responder assessment
  - Scene size-up
  - Initial assessment
  - Physical exam
  - Ongoing assessment
- Assure airway patency - place in the recovery position if decreased level of responsiveness
- Cool the patient
  - Remove the patient from the hot environment
  - Cool by fanning
- Comfort, calm, and reassure the patient and family

The role of the First Responder

First, you should complete the First Responder assessment including the scene size-up, initial assessment, physical exam, and ongoing assessment. Continue to calm and reassure the patient while waiting for additional EMS resources. You should remove the patient from the heat and place them in a cool environment (e.g., an air conditioned vehicle). Cooling the patient by fanning may be effective. Fanning is not effective if the patient is still in a humid environment.

As the patient's internal temperature rises, their level of responsiveness decreases. If the patient has any altered mental status, they should be placed in the recovery position. Box 9-12 summarizes the role of the First Responder when caring for patients exposed to heat.

BEHAVIORAL EMERGENCIES

First Responders encounter many situations involving behavioral emergencies, ranging from reactions to stress to severe mental illness. Some behavioral emergencies result from psychological problems, but many are caused by the use of mind-altering substances such as alcohol, illegal drugs, or prescription medications. Other behavioral emergencies result from a traumatic injury or acute illness.

You must be familiar with behavioral emergencies and know how to handle these delicate situations. Sometimes First Responders approach an apparently safe scene, but then discover that the patient represents a danger to the rescuer. In this case, it is acceptable for First Responders to leave the patient and request law enforcement assistance.

Behavior is the manner in which a person acts or performs. All physical and mental activities of a person are behaviors. Humans behave differently for various reasons. For example, one person may be frightened of something that another person finds humorous. A behavioral emergency results when a person exhibits abnormal behavior in a situation that results in potential harm to himself or others (Fig. 9-5).

A behavioral emergency is a situation in which a patient exhibits behavior that is unacceptable or intolerable to the person, family members, or the community. This behavior might be the result of extreme emotion or mental illness and can lead to acts of violence. Abnormal behavior can also be caused by traumatic injuries or acute illness, such as lack of oxygen or low blood sugar.

BEHAVIORAL CHANGES

Many situational stresses, medical illnesses, and legal or illegal drugs, including alcohol, may alter a person's behavior. Diabetic patients who have low blood sugar may have a change in behavior, such as aggressiveness, restlessness, or anxiety, if they do not stay on a proper diet. Lack of oxygen and inadequate blood flow to the brain are other causes of altered mental status that may result in a behavioral emergency. Behavioral emergencies may also result from head or other trauma with blood loss.

Excessive cold or heat exposure may also produce a reaction in the body that changes a person's behavior. People exposed to a very stressful situation may temporarily panic. Other changes in behavior may result from mental illness and long-term psychiatric illness.

A person experiencing a psychologic crisis, or bizarre thinking or behavior, may panic easily from very little stress, or may become agitated with no apparent or obvious provocation. These patients may be a danger to themselves or to others. They can become violent very easily, and their behavior can change quickly and unpredictably. Treat these patients gently and without sudden moves or actions to prevent scaring and agitating them. Patients in psychological crises may engage in self-destructive or suicidal behavior.

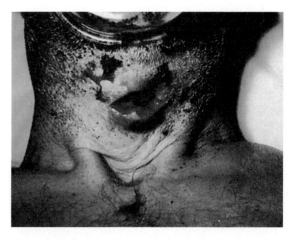

Fig. 9-5 A behavioral emergency resulted in this self-inflicted knife wound.

FIRST RESPONDER ALERT

Use caution! Any object near the patient may become a dangerous object if the patient intends to do harm. Stay near doors and exits. Do not let the patient block your route of escape if the situation becomes out of control.

THE ROLE OF THE FIRST RESPONDER

As with any patient, care begins with the First Responder assessment. Even if the patient is displaying bizarre behavior, you will still need to assess them. When performing the scene size-up, be careful to examine the patient's environment. The initial assessment, physical exam, and ongoing assessment should begin after you are sure the scene is safe for you to enter. The situation may be unsafe, or the patient may have an object that they can use as a weapon. We will discuss how to assess potentially violent situations later in this section.

Providing calm reassurance to the patient experiencing a behavioral emergency is particularly important. Often, a professional demeanor and empathetic approach can significantly defuse a stressful situation. In general, if you are not in danger, do not leave the patient alone. If you think that the patient represents a hazard to themselves or others, ensure that law enforcement assistance is part of the EMS response. In some cases, you may have to involve law enforcement officials and force the patient to be transported against their will.

Assessing behavioral emergency patients

Experienced First Responders have developed a variety of techniques to help them communicate and assess the patient experiencing a behavioral emergency. Using these techniques will help calm the patient and make your assessment more complete and safe. Usually, you should avoid physical contact with the patient or getting so close to them that they perceive you as a threat. You should use your own judgment, but it is acceptable to delay or skip the physical exam if you believe that physical contact with the patient may escalate the situation or place you in danger.

Do not let the patient get between you and the nearest exit route (Fig. 9-6). Stay near doors or exits if possible. If the scene becomes unsafe and cannot be secured after you have entered and begun care, exit as quickly as possible. See Chapter 7, "Patient Assessment," for more detailed information regarding scene safety.

Be sure to introduce yourself and any other strangers to the patient. Explain to the patient why you are there, especially if they are not the one who called for help. Assess the patient for illness or injury to the best of your ability, but do not let the physical exam upset the patient or place you in danger. If there is a medical problem, perform the appropriate interventions while explaining everything to the patient. When you speak to the patient or ask them questions, use a calm, reassuring voice. Be sure to avoid becoming judgmental and allow the patient to explain what happened.

Limit your questions to those that affect your care, as you determine if there is a medical problem that needs to be treated. Too much prying may provoke some individuals into aggressive behavior. Ask basic questions to assess the patient, such as: "What is your name?" "Are you hurt?" "Would you like me to help you with your problem?" Usually the answers to simple questions such as these can help you determine the psychological status of the patient.

When the patient responds, show them that you are listening by rephrasing or repeating what they said. Sometimes patients will tell you how they are feeling (mad, anxious, frustrated,

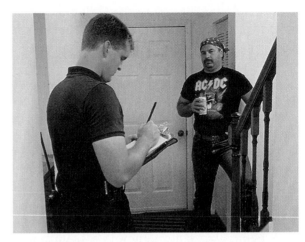

Fig. 9-6 Do not allow any participant in a dispute to position himself between you and the door or exit route.

BOX 9-13 Signs of a Potentially Violent Patient

- History of aggression—check with the family and bystanders if the patient has a history of aggression, combativeness, or violent behavior
- Posture—stands or sits in a position that threatens themselves or others
- Gestures—fists clenched
- Holding objects that can be used as a striking weapon or thrown
- Muscle tension and rigidity
- Yelling
- Verbally threatens to harm self or others
- Use of profanity
- Moves toward care giver
- Carries heavy or threatening objects
- Quick and irregular movements

---

depressed, etc.). You should acknowledge their feelings without judgment. Everybody has different responses to extreme events, and a person's feelings are not right or wrong. Always treat the patient with respect and dignity. Occasionally patients will have disturbed or bizarre thinking. Do not agree with them, but avoid getting into arguments. You can respond in a nonconfrontational, nonjudgmental way such as, "I believe that you hear voices, but I do not hear them."

Observe the patient's appearance, activity, speech, and orientation for time, person, and

TECHNIQUE BOX 9-1

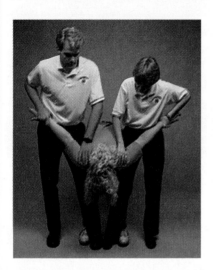

Fig. 9-7 Two responders approach the patient from behind, pull the patient's arms back, and bend the patient forward at the waist to assume the control position.

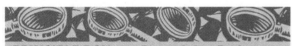

PRINCIPLE BOX 9-1 Restraining Patients

1. Have adequate help, including police assistance if possible
2. Have a plan of action
3. Use only necessary force
4. Stay beyond the patient's range of motion
5. Act quickly
6. Talk to the patient
7. Secure limbs with approved equipment, such as restraints
8. Turning the patient face down on the stretcher may be necessary
9. Cover the patient's mouth with a mask if they are biting or spitting
10. Reassess the patient frequently
11. Document all of your actions

place. If you suspect a drug overdose, collect the drugs or medications found at the scene and give them to the transporting EMS personnel.

Predicting the potential for violence

One of the most important assessment skills you must develop as a First Responder is the ability to predict the potential of a patient becoming violent. This begins in the scene size-up, and must continue throughout your interaction with the patient.

Contact law enforcement if the patient was or is displaying destructive behavior toward self or others. You should also request assistance from law enforcement if you feel threatened or sense that the situation may get out of control. Box 9-13 lists the signs of potential violence

Calming the patient

Try to calm the patient by acknowledging that they are upset and emphasizing that you are there to help them. Do not leave the patient alone unless you are in danger. Ask all questions calmly and reassuringly, and do not be judgmental toward the patient. Repeat the patient's answers to show that you are listening. Recognize how the patient feels, but do not challenge or argue with him. Encourage the patient to tell you what is troubling him.

During questioning, remain a comfortable distance away from the patient, use good eye contact, and do not make sudden movements. You should avoid any unnecessary physical contact. The patient may misinterpret this as a threatening gesture, or as a violation of patient's personal space.

Sit at the same level or lower than the patient. Standing over them and talking down to them may be threatening. It is imperative that you remain calm. Respond honestly to any questions. Never lie about what you are going to do or what will happen to them. Avoid threatening, challenging, or arguing with any disturbed patient. Do not "play along" with visual or auditory delusions. You can use trusted family members or friends to help you calm or communicate with the patient. You should be prepared to stay at the scene for as long as necessary to gain the patient's cooperation.

Restraining the patient

In some situations, you will be unable to calm the patient enough to approach and provide care safely. Family members often insist that the patient be taken to a medical treatment facility, or insist they be treated for their safety or well-being. Patients who do not calm down and are showing destructive behavior toward themselves or others may need to be restrained before treatment and transportation (see Principle 9-1).

Follow your local protocols and laws regarding restraining patients. In many areas, you cannot restrain a patient without the cooperation of law enforcement or without consultation with medical direction.

Restraining patients can be dangerous. If done improperly, you can injure the patient. Suffocation, poor circulation, poor access to the airway or injury, and poor access to the patient are some medical problems associated with restraining patients. You should work with EMS providers and law enforcement personnel. Technique 9-1 demonstrates one method of restraining a violent patient.

If you decide to restrain the patient, you must not use unreasonable force. **Reasonable force** is the minimum force necessary to keep the patient from injuring himself or others. You must not exceed the threshold of reasonable force. Determine reasonable force by looking at all of the variables of the situation, including patient size and strength, type of abnormal behavior, sex of the patient, mental state of the patient, and method of restraint used.

Many patients who are initially aggressive or combative suddenly become calm. In these cases, they are often prone to sudden acts of violence against themselves or others. You may use reasonable force to defend yourself against attack, but be careful not to exceed any force necessary to protect yourself.

Once you restrain the patient, be sure to conduct several assessments. Patients experiencing a behavioral emergency may later claim injury because of the restraints. Be sure that the patient can breathe and use soft leather or padded cloth restraints, not metal handcuffs, so you do not cause soft tissue damage to the patient (Fig. 9-8). Once you apply restraints, do not remove them. The receiving facility or law enforcement personnel should remove the restraints. If the restraints are too tight when you reevaluate them, loosen the restraint, but don't remove them.

To protect yourself against false accusations of excessive force, it is important that you document the patient's condition and behavior before and after restraining them. Be sure to document any abnormal behaviors. If possible, have witnesses present at all times. Some patients have accused First Responders of sexual misconduct while they were restrained. Having First Responders of the same sex as the patient

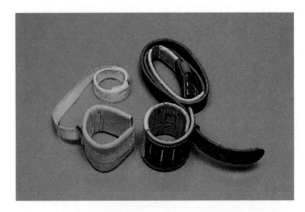

Fig. 9-8 Examples of soft restraints.

BOX 9-14 Role of the First Responder — Behavioral Emergencies

- Complete the First Responder assessment
  Scene size-up
  Initial assessment
  Physical exam and SAMPLE history, if possible
  Ongoing assessment
- Assure airway patency, especially in restrained patients
- Comfort, calm, and reassure the patient and family
- Consider the need to restrain the patient
- Consult with medical direction and law enforcement personnel per local protocol

---

FIRST RESPONDER ALERT

Carefully monitor the restrained patient. Pay particular attention to the active patient who stops struggling.

---

present is beneficial, and never have one person alone with a restrained patient.

Restraining a patient against their will presents a considerable risk of legal action. The likelihood of legal problems is significantly reduced if you can convince the patient to consent to care. Unfortunately, many emotionally disturbed patients resist treatment. To justify restraining a patient, you must have a reasonable belief that the patient will harm himself or others. Whenever possible, make this decision with law enforcement and medical direction.

Patients experiencing behavioral emergencies are typically conscious and able to protect their own airway. If you decide to restrain the patient, be very careful not to block the airway or put pressure on the chest that would prevent the patient from breathing. Continuously perform an ongoing assessment on any restrained patient. Box 9-14 contains a summary of the role of the First Responder when dealing with a behavioral emergency patient.

REVIEW QUESTIONS

Behavioral Emergencies

1. For a patient who is anxious or upset, the First Responder should try to _____ the patient and not leave them alone.

2. Treat the patient with _____, but do not agree with _____ thinking.

3. Contact _____ if a situation becomes out of control or you need help.

4. Involve family and friends when gathering the _____ of the patient.

5. List at least six signs of a potentially violent patient.

   _____   _____

   _____   _____

   _____   _____

6. When are you permitted to restrain a patient?

7. Always have a _____ present when caring for the patient with a behavioral emergency.

8. You must always perform an _____ on a restrained patient.

1. Calm; 2. Respect, disturbed or abnormal; 3. Law enforcement; 4. SAMPLE history; 5. History of aggression, combativeness or violent behavior, threatening position, fists clenched, holding objects that can be used as a striking weapon or that can be thrown, muscle tension and rigidity, yelling, verbally threatens to harm self or others, use of profanity, quick and irregular movements; 6. If the patient is violent and represents a hazard to himself or others and cannot be calmed by any other means; 7. Witness; 8. Ongoing assessment

CHAPTER SUMMARY

GENERAL MEDICAL COMPLAINTS

General medical complaints represent most of the situations you will encounter as a First Responder. The patient may have a variety of signs or symptoms. It is important to provide care to the patient based on the assessment findings and not attempt to determine the cause of the illness. The main role of the First Responder in treating the patient with general medical complaints is to perform a First Responder assessment, including a SAMPLE history, and calm and reassure the patient and their family.

SPECIFIC MEDICAL COMPLAINTS

There are four medical complaints that require specific actions of the First Responder. Altered mental status requires that the First Responder pay particular attention to the airway, perform an assessment to determine life threats, and gather a SAMPLE history. The role of the First Responder in treating seizures is to ensure that the patient does not injure himself during convulsions and maintain the airway. Care for generalized and local cold injuries by assessing the patient and preventing further heat loss. Patients exposed to the heat should be assessed, removed from the hot environment, and cooled by fanning.

BEHAVIORAL EMERGENCIES

Any call can become a behavioral emergency. Behavior is the manner in which a person acts or performs, including all physical and mental activity. A behavioral emergency is a situation in which a person exhibits abnormal or unacceptable behavior that is intolerable to the person, family, or community. Change in behavior may result from mental illness, situational stress, alcohol, drugs, medical illness, or a traumatic injury. Be very cautious when dealing with a behavioral emergency. Emotionally disturbed patients often refuse treatment. You may treat a patient without consent if you believe that the patient will harm himself or others. Document all patient behaviors and witnesses for later verification if needed. Patients may accuse the First Responder of assault or sexual harassment. Always try to have a witness to validate the documentation, and try not to be alone with the patient. It is essential that you know the local protocols and laws regarding treating patients who refuse care.

UNITED STATES DEPARTMENT OF TRANSPORTATION NATIONAL HIGHWAY TRAFFIC SAFETY ADMINISTRATION FIRST RESPONDER OBJECTIVES

Check your knowledge. The National Registry of EMTs and many state EMS agencies use the objectives below to develop First Responder certification examinations. Can you meet them?

COGNITIVE OBJECTIVES

1. Identify the patient who presents with a general medical complaint.
2. Explain the steps in providing emergency medical care to a patient with a general medical complaint.
3. Identify the patient who presents with a specific medical complaint of altered mental status.
4. Explain the steps in providing emergency medical care to a patient with an altered mental status.
5. Identify the patient who presents with a specific medical complaint of seizures.
6. Explain the steps in providing emergency medical care to a patient with seizures.
7. Identify the patient who presents with a specific medical complaint of exposure to cold.
8. Explain the steps in providing emergency medical care to a patient with an exposure to cold.
9. Identify the patient who presents with a specific medical complaint of exposure to heat.
10. Explain the steps in providing emergency medical care to a patient with an exposure to heat.
11. Identify the patient who presents with a specific medical complaint of behavioral change.
12. Explain the steps in providing emergency medical care to a patient with a behavioral change.
13. Identify the patient who presents with a specific complaint of a psychological crisis.
14. Explain the steps in providing emergency medical care to a patient with a psychological crisis.

AFFECTIVE OBJECTIVES

15. Attend to the feelings of the patient and/or family when dealing with the patient with a general medical complaint.
16. Attend to the feelings of the patient and/or family when dealing with the patient with a specific medical complaint.
17. Explain the rationale for modifying your behavior toward the patient with a behavioral emergency.
18. Demonstrate a caring attitude towards patients with a general medical complaint who request emergency medical services.
19. Place the interests of the patient with a general medical complaint as the foremost consideration when making any and all patient care decisions.
20. Communicate with empathy to patients with a general medical complaint, as well as with family members and friends of the patient.
21. Demonstrate a caring attitude towards patients with a specific medical complaint who request emergency medical services.
22. Place the interests of the patient with a specific medical complaint as the foremost consideration when making any and all patient care decisions.
23. Communicate with empathy to patients with a specific medical complaint, as well as with family members and friends of the patient.
24. Demonstrate a caring attitude towards patients with a behavioral problem who request emergency medical services.
25. Place the interests of the patient with a behavioral problem as the foremost consideration when making any and all patient care decisions.
26. Communicate with empathy to patients with a behavioral problem, as well as with family members and friends of the patient.

PSYCHOMOTOR OBJECTIVES

27. Demonstrate the steps in providing emergency medical care to a patient with a general medical complaint.
28. Demonstrate the steps in providing emergency medical care to a patient with an altered mental status.
29. Demonstrate the steps in providing emergency medical care to a patient with seizures.
30. Demonstrate the steps in providing emergency medical care to a patient with an exposure to cold.
31. Demonstrate the steps in providing emergency medical care to a patient with an exposure to heat.
32. Demonstrate the steps in providing emergency medical care to a patient with a behavioral change.
33. Demonstrate the steps in providing emergency medical care to a patient with a psychological crisis.

Bleeding and Soft Tissue Injuries

I. Shock (Hypoperfusion)
    A. Signs and Symptoms of Shock
    B. Role of the First Responder
II. Bleeding
    A. External Bleeding
    B. Internal Bleeding
III. Specific Injuries
    A. Types of Injuries

    B. Role of the First Responder
    C. Special Considerations
IV. Burns
    A. Types of Burns
    B. Role of the First Responder
    C. Special Considerations
V. Dressing and Bandaging

KEY TERMS

Abrasion An open injury involving the outermost layer of skin.

Amputation The loss of an extremity or part of an extremity.

Bandage A nonsterile cloth used to cover a dressing and secure it in place.

Dressing A sterile cloth used to cover open injuries to protect them from further contamination.

Evisceration An open injury in which the internal organs are protruding.

Laceration An open injury of any depth resulting from the force of a sharp object; bleeding may be severe.

Occlusive dressing A dressing that is airtight, such as a petroleum gauze, that is placed over a wound and sealed.

Penetration/puncture wound An open injury resulting from the force of a sharp pointed object in which external bleeding may be limited and internal bleeding may be severe.

FIRST RESPONSE

Martin and Juan were patrolling their route as a call came in for a two-car head-on collision in their area. Turning on their lights and sirens, they headed toward the scene and made sure that EMS, fire, and rescue teams were also dispatched. Arriving on scene first, the police officers quickly assessed the situation: two cars, heavy damage, no fire or liquid hazards noticed. One person was lying on the ground outside the first vehicle and another person was still sitting behind the steering wheel of the other vehicle. Juan went to assess the driver in the car. Martin went to assess the patient lying on the ground.

Martin assessed the patient's airway, breathing, and pulse. He found the airway and breathing to be adequate, but the patient's pulse was rapid and weak. Martin directed another First Responder on the scene to stabilize the patient's head. The patient was responsive to verbal stimuli, but not oriented to what had happened. Martin noticed a large tear in the patient's pants with blood oozing from a wound. After taking appropriate body substance isolation precautions, he quickly retrieved dressings and bandages from his vehicle and placed them over the wound with pressure to control the bleeding. He reassured the patient that EMS was en route to the scene and covered the patient with a blanket to keep him warm. Martin continued to monitor the patient's airway and breathing until additional help arrived.

Martin recognized the early signs of hypoperfusion in this patient and quickly controlled the bleeding, monitored the airway, and prevented further heat loss with a blanket. When EMS personnel arrived, they thanked the officers and transported the patient rapidly to the hospital.

Soft tissue injuries are common and can be very dramatic. Most of these injuries are not life-threatening, but some may result in severe bleeding. Severe bleeding could result in a condition known as shock or hypoperfusion. First Responders must be familiar with the treatment of soft tissue injuries to control bleeding, prevent further injury, and reduce contamination and infection.

SHOCK (HYPOPERFUSION)

Every cell in the body needs a continuous supply of blood to function properly. Each beat of the heart ejects blood into the arterial circulation and moves the blood quickly through the body. As each organ is perfused, the continuous delivery of fresh blood provides oxygen and nutrients, and removes waste.

Any alteration in the body's ability to deliver blood to all of the organs is detrimental. Cell death and organ failure can result from a disruption of blood flow. When patients bleed profusely, they lose blood from within the cardiovascular system. The loss of blood volume decreases perfusion to the many body tissues. This situation of widespread hypoperfusion is called shock.

Shock results when the cardiovascular system cannot adequately deliver oxygenated blood to the body's vital organs. Shock causes delicate tissues to be damaged from a lack of oxygen and a buildup of waste products, and is a life-threatening condition. Hypoperfusion easily damages the brain, heart, lungs and kidneys. The key to effective shock management is to recognize the early signs and symptoms of shock and to ensure that the patient is transported to the hospital before late shock develops.

Shock can be caused by a loss of blood volume. Shock can also be the result of the inability of the heart to effectively pump oxygenated blood to the body, or an abnormal dilation of the vessels. In all cases, recognition and requesting rapid transportation are the priorities for First Responders caring for patients in shock.

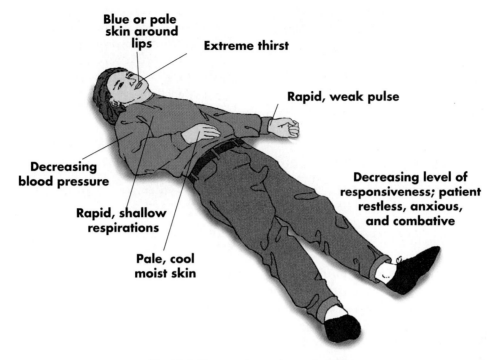

Fig. 10-1 Signs and symptoms of shock.

SIGNS AND SYMPTOMS OF SHOCK

The earliest and most subtle signs and symptoms of shock result from minute changes in blood flow to the brain. Even small changes in the blood flow to the brain can cause a change in the patient's mental state. These changes are generally seen as restlessness, anxiety, and combativeness. It is very easy to dismiss these signs as normal stress for injured patients. The perceptive First Responder recognizes that a change in mental status can be an early sign of shock. Recognizing a change in mental status is especially important for a patient with internal bleeding, because this may be the only indication that the patient is experiencing a life-threatening blood loss. You need not determine whether the patient actually is in shock; you should care for the patient based on whether the signs and symptoms of shock are present (Fig. 10-1).

Many signs and symptoms of shock are related to the body's attempt to maintain perfusion following blood loss. When a patient bleeds significantly, hormones are released into the blood that cause blood vessels to constrict. Blood flow to the skin is decreased, and blood is diverted to vital organs such as the heart, lungs, brain, and kidneys. Decreased blood flow causes pale, cool, and clammy skin. You may also notice that the patient's skin looks pale or blue around the lips or fingers, due to a lack of oxygen in the blood. As the vessels in the body constrict, blood flow to the arms and legs decreases. Decreased blood flow causes weak pulses in the patient's extremities.

Another sensitive sign of early shock is an increase in heart rate. When a patient loses blood, the heart rate increases so that the remaining blood pumps faster. Any time a patient's pulse is faster than normal, you should consider the possibility of early shock. Some patients, especially older adults, may be receiving medications that prevent their heart rates from increasing in shock. Do not ignore other signs of shock even if the patient has a normal heart rate.

If you assess the patient's blood pressure, you may notice a drop as the patient develops late

---

BOX 10-1 Signs and Symptoms of Shock

- Mental status changes, including restlessness or anxiety
- Pale, cool, and moist skin
- Rapid, weak pulse
- Low blood pressure
- Rapid, shallow respirations
- Extreme thirst

BOX 10-2 Emergency Treatment of Patients with Signs and Symptoms of Shock

- Maintain airway/ventilation
- Stabilize the spine if necessary
- Prevent further blood loss
- Keep the patient calm and place them in a position of comfort
- Keep the patient warm
- Do not give food or drink
- Provide care for specific injuries

---

shock. Decreased blood pressure is a late sign of shock and signals that the patient's condition is life-threatening.

You may also notice an increase in the respiratory rate as the patient attempts to oxygenate the remaining blood. As shock progresses, breathing may become shallow, labored, and irregular.

Because blood loss triggers the body's thirst mechanism, patients in shock may ask for something to drink. Because many of these patients will require surgery, do not allow them to eat or drink anything. Box 10-1 summarizes the signs and symptoms of shock.

A patient does not need to have all these signs and symptoms for you to suspect they may be developing shock. A change in mental status or an increased heart rate may be enough for you to suspect that the patient is in an early stage of shock.

ROLE OF THE FIRST RESPONDER

The First Responder should complete a scene size-up before initiating emergency medical care. Take appropriate body substance isolation precautions for the situation. You should perform an initial assessment on all patients and then the physical exam.

After following body substance isolation precautions, the first step in treating the patient with signs and symptoms of shock in the emergency setting is to ensure that the patient has an open airway and good ventilation. The treatment of shock and external bleeding is important, but proper airway management is always the priority.

The next step is to stop or slow the bleeding. Methods for controlling blood loss will be described later in this chapter. Keep the patient calm and allow them to remain in a position of comfort if you do not suspect that they have a spinal injury. If you do suspect a spinal injury, stabilize the spine and monitor the airway closely. If

---

REVIEW QUESTIONS

Shock (Hypoperfusion)

1. List three signs and symptoms of shock.

   _____

   _____

   _____

2. Which of the following is true?

   A. Patients in shock often have slow, strong pulses.
   B. Patients in shock often become very warm and must be cooled.
   C. Pale, cool, moist skin results from poor blood flow to the skin.
   D. Blood flow is diverted away from the brain for patients in shock.

3. List three reasons a patient may be in shock

   _____

   _____

   _____

1. Mental status changes; pale, cool or moist skin; rapid, weak pulse; low blood pressure; rapid, shallow respirations; extreme thirst. 2. C; 3. Blood loss, abnormal blood vessel dilation, inability of the heart to pump effectively

---

the patient is unresponsive and not injured, place them in the recovery position.

Preventing body heat loss for patients in shock is very important. The best way to prevent this problem is to cover the patient with a blanket. You should cover the patient even in warm weather, because injuries decrease the body's ability to generate heat. In cold weather also place

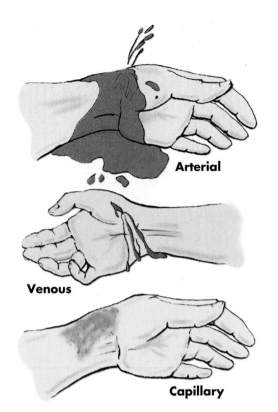

Fig. 10-2 Arterial, venous, and capillary bleeding.

blankets under a patient who is lying on the ground or a cold surface. Attempt to maintain the patient's normal body temperature.

Do not give the patient food or drink because they may need to undergo surgery in the hospital. Provide care for any specific injuries that the patient may have.

Complete an ongoing assessment every five minutes until the transporting EMS personnel arrive. Comfort and reassure the patient that an ambulance is on the way. Box 10-2 summarizes the emergency care of patients with the signs and symptoms of shock.

BLEEDING

Before beginning care for any patient, the First Responder must be aware of the risk of infectious disease from contact with blood or other body fluids. When treating a patient with obvious external bleeding, take appropriate body substance isolation precautions before you approach the patient. Several infectious diseases are transmitted by blood, so protect yourself. Because blood can spurt or splash, you should wear gloves, eye protection,

and a mask. Gowns may be worn in situations where there is a lot of blood. Hand washing after each transport also helps decrease the possibility of spreading diseases. Refer to Chapter 2, "The Well-Being of the First Responder," for a detailed discussion of body substance isolation precautions.

The First Responder should be aware of the body's response to bleeding. The body normally responds to bleeding by contracting the affected blood vessels and clotting. A serious injury with active bleeding may prevent effective clotting from occurring. Uncontrolled bleeding with significant blood loss can lead to shock and possibly to death.

Bleeding may be external or internal. Both types can result in blood loss severe enough to result in shock and subsequent death. You can estimate the severity of the blood loss based on the patient's signs and symptoms. For external bleeding, you should also try to estimate how much blood the patient has lost by looking around the scene.

EXTERNAL BLEEDING

External bleeding can come from three sources: arteries, veins, or capillaries. Each type of bleeding has a slightly different presentation (Fig. 10-2).
Arterial bleeding

Blood in the arteries is under high pressure. External arterial bleeding is characterized by large amounts of bright red, oxygen-rich blood that spurts from the injury. Arterial bleeding is the most difficult to stop because of the high arterial pressure, though, as the patient's blood pressure drops, the spurting may also drop. You must act quickly to reduce significant bleeding from an artery.
Venous bleeding

In contrast to arterial bleeding, venous bleeding is dark red, oxygen-poor blood and flows in a steady stream from the injury. Venous bleeding may be profuse and dangerous, but it is usually easier to control because it is under much lower pressure than arterial bleeding.
Capillary bleeding

Capillary bleeding is usually dark red and oozes from the injury. Capillary bleeding is the least dangerous type of bleeding and normally clots by itself. The most common form of capillary bleeding occurs when the top layers of skin are scraped away.
Bleeding control techniques

Before assessing or caring for the patient, you should always take appropriate body substance isolation precautions. Perform the scene size-up

TECHNIQUE 10-1 Fingertip Pressure

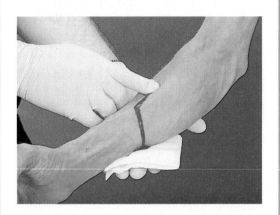

Fig. 10-3 Find exactly where the bleeding is coming from. (This is often one major vessel.) Apply pressure to this point with a gloved finger and continue until you can apply a dressing that will keep pressure on the injury.

TECHNIQUE 10-2 Hand Pressure

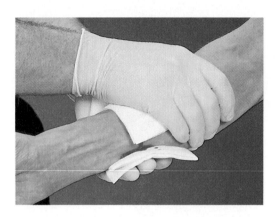

Fig. 10-4 Apply hand pressure with a gloved hand and absorbent dressing. If blood soaks through the dressing, place more dressings on top. Continue to apply manual pressure until you apply a dressing that will keep pressure on the injury.

TECHNIQUE 10-3 Extremity Elevation

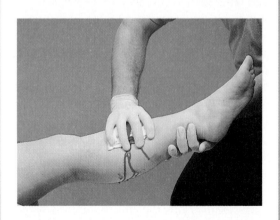

Fig. 10-5 Attempt to control bleeding by direct pressure. Check the entire extremity for other injuries; if there are signs or symptoms of skeletal injuries, do not elevate the extremity until it is splinted. Elevate the extremity above the level of the heart to slow external bleeding.

before entering the scene to begin care. Complete the initial assessment and the physical exam as needed for each patient. Make sure the patient has an open airway and is breathing adequately, then control any bleeding.

Most major bleeding originates from damage to one main artery or a large vein. The most effective method of controlling this type of bleeding is fingertip pressure. To apply fingertip pressure, use the flat part of your fingertip to press directly on the bleeding point. Ideally, do this with sterile gauze. If you do not have immediate access to gauze, simply apply pressure with your gloved finger. If fingertip pressure fails to stop the bleeding, remove the gauze and be sure you are applying pressure to the correct bleeding point. If more than one site of bleeding is found, apply additional pressure. Technique 10-1 lists the steps for fingertip pressure.

If the injury is large or the bleeding is not coming from one spot, more diffuse pressure is required. Hand pressure works by decreasing the blood flow through the arteries and veins leading to the injury. To apply hand pressure, place sterile gauze pads on the injury and apply pressure with your entire hand. If blood soaks through the dressings, do not remove them, but simply place more dressings on top. For gaping wounds with severe bleeding, pack the injury with sterile gauze. Technique 10-2 lists the steps for hand pressure.

When an extremity is injured, there are two additional techniques used as needed when fingertip or hand pressure alone does not stop the bleeding: extremity elevation and pressure points.

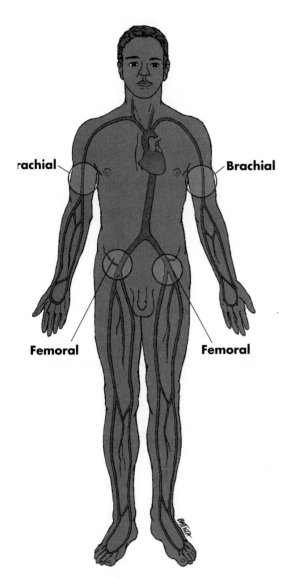

Fig. 10-6 Pressure on arteries can be used to control bleeding in the extremities.

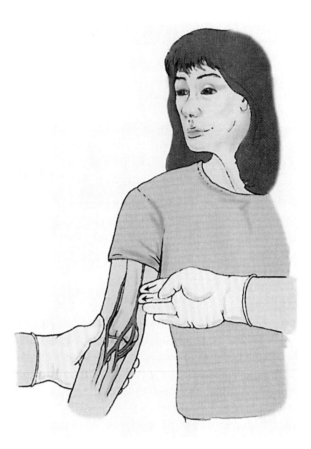

Fig. 10-7 Pressing on a pressure point decreases blood flow to the extremity.

If there is no pain, swelling, or deformity, you should elevate the extremity. Elevation above the level of the heart will decrease blood flow and help to slow all three types of bleeding. Never move an extremity that is painful, swollen, or deformed, because there may be skeletal injuries present and this would aggravate the injury. Technique 10-3 lists the steps for elevating the extremity.

Another technique to decrease bleeding is to use pressure points (Fig. 10-6). If the injury is to the arm, the pressure point is the brachial artery. If the injury is to the leg, the pressure point is the femoral artery. Pressing on the pressure point decreases blood flow to the extremity (Fig. 10-7).

TECHNIQUE 10-4 Pressure Points

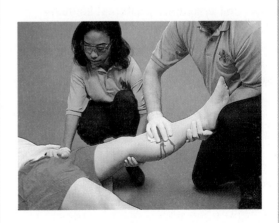

Fig. 10-8 Attempt to stop the bleeding with direct pressure and elevation if possible. Apply manual pressure to the brachial artery or the femoral artery to decrease bleeding in the extremity. Continue to apply pressure while transporting the patient, beacuse release may cause bleeding to resume.

Because no extremity is supplied by a single artery, and venous bleeding is usually also present with arterial bleeding, a pressure point will slow bleeding but rarely stop it. Technique 10-4 lists the steps for controlling bleeding with a pressure point.

A combination of direct pressure, elevation, and pressure points will stop almost all bleeding. After you control the bleeding, complete ongoing assessments every five minutes. Monitor the patient's airway, breathing, and circulation, and reassess bleeding control measures. Comfort the patient and reassure them that an ambulance is on the way.

INTERNAL BLEEDING

Although external bleeding is dramatic and obvious, internal bleeding can be deceptive. Injured or damaged internal organs or painful, swollen, deformed extremities can lead to extensive bleeding that is concealed. Not only is internal bleeding more difficult to recognize, but it is much more difficult to stop. Severe internal blood loss can quickly result in profound shock and death.

A patient can lose huge quantities of blood into cavities of the body, such as the chest, abdomen, and the upper legs. Often, there is no external indication of the bleeding. Any patient who has the signs and symptoms of shock should be assumed to have internal bleeding, treated for shock, and transported immediately.

Signs and symptoms of internal bleeding

Signs and symptoms of internal bleeding include discolored, tender, swollen, or hard tissue such as a large bruise. Increased respiratory and pulse rates, along with pale, cool skin suggest shock and internal bleeding. Nausea, vomiting, thirst, and changes in mental status may also indicate internal blood loss.

Box 10-3 lists the signs and symptoms of internal bleeding.

Role of the First Responder

The First Responder should complete a scene size-up before entering the scene. Perform an initial assessment on all patients and a physical exam and ongoing assessment as needed. If additional EMS resources are en route, comfort, calm and reassure the patient while waiting.

As always, be sure to follow body substance isolation precautions in all cases of bleeding. Ensure that the patient has a patent airway and

provide artificial ventilation if necessary. Manage any external bleeding and reassure the patient. Keep the patient calm. If spinal immobilization is not necessary, the patient may be placed in a position of comfort. Keep the patient warm by placing a blanket over him or her. If a patient has signs and symptoms of shock, treat appropriately.

REVIEW QUESTIONS

Bleeding

1. Place the correct type of bleeding beside the description (arterial, venous, capillary):

_____ Blood oozes from the wound

_____ Blood is bright red

_____ Blood flows as a steady stream

_____ Blood spurts from the wound

_____ Blood often clots spontaneously

2. Place the following steps of bleeding control in order:

A. Pressure points
B. Fingertip pressure
C. Elevation

3. Which of the following statements is correct regarding the management of internal bleeding?

A. The patient should be kept cool so that the blood flows slower.
B. Direct pressure should be placed over the injury site.
C. The patient should be kept calm and treated for shock.
D. Gloves do not need to be worn because there is no external bleeding.

4. If bleeding continues through the dressing while providing diffuse pressure, the dressing should be removed and then replaced with another clean one. True or False?

1. capillary, arterial, venous, arterial, capillary; 2. B, C, A; 3. C; 4. False, the new dressing should be placed over the used one

Above all, if the patient has signs and symptoms of internal bleeding, they need immediate transport! Internal bleeding is extremely difficult to control and must be evaluated at the hospital. Little can be done in the field to stop the bleeding, so the First Responder must rapidly assess, recognize the signs and symptoms of internal bleeding, and ensure rapid transport. Box 10-4 summarizes the management of internal bleeding.

SPECIFIC INJURIES

First Responders will encounter patients with many types of soft tissue injuries. These injuries are frequently painful and may look more serious than they actually are. Trauma to soft tissues may cause closed or open injuries. With a closed injury, the skin remains intact and there is no external bleeding. Open injuries cause a break in the skin and there is usually external bleeding.

TYPES OF INJURIES
Abrasion
An **abrasion** is an open injury that occurs when shearing or scraping forces damage the outermost layer of skin. Abrasions are painful, but rarely life-threatening. The injury is superficial and involves very little, if any, oozing of blood (Fig. 10-9).
Laceration
A **laceration** is any break in the skin that forceful impact with a sharp object has caused, such as a knife or a piece of broken glass. A laceration may be superficial or deep. This may occur in isolation or with other soft tissue injuries. The bleeding may be severe, depending on the location and depth of the wound (Fig. 10-10).
Penetration/Puncture
A **penetration or puncture wound** is caused by a sharp pointed object, such as a knife or a bullet, forced into the body (Fig. 10-11). There may be little external bleeding, but internal bleeding can be severe. Sometimes, there may be an exit wound. Gunshot wounds may involve erratic paths through the body and cause vast amounts of internal damage.

ROLE OF THE FIRST RESPONDER
The role of the First Responder includes performing a scene size-up and then an initial assessment. Care for any life-threatening conditions first, such

BOX 10-3 Signs and Symptoms of Internal Bleeding

- Signs and symptoms of shock, including increased respiratory and pulse rates, pale, cool skin and changes in mental status
- Discolored, tender, swollen or hard tissue
- Nausea and vomiting
- Thirst
- Mental status changes

BOX 10-4 The Management of Internal Bleeding

- Follow body substance isolation precautions
- Maintain an open airway and provide artificial ventilation
- Manage external bleeding
- Keep the patient calm and reassure them
- Place in position of comfort if not immobilized
- Keep the patient warm and treat for shock

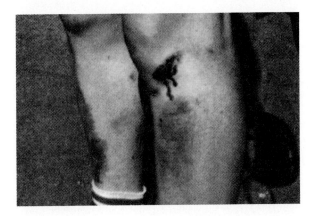
Fig. 10-9 Abrasions caused by a fall from a bicycle.

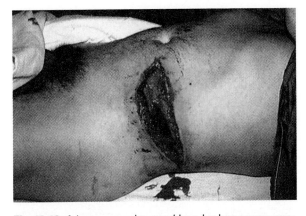
Fig. 10-10 A large wound caused by a broken power saw.

PRINCIPLE 10-1 Emergency Medical Care for Patients with Soft Tissue Injury

1. Take appropriate body substance isolation precautions.
2. Ensure an open airway. Provide artificial ventilation if the patient is not breathing adequately.
3. Treat for shock as described earlier in this chapter.
4. Manage the injury by exposing the wound. Control the bleeding and reduce contamination by placing a dry sterile dressing over the wound and bandaging it in place. Refer to the steps for dressing and bandaging later in this chapter. For serious bleeding, refer to the bleeding control techniques described previously in this chapter.

as an airway obstruction or difficulty breathing. Soft tissue injuries often involve bleeding, so be sure to take appropriate body substance isolation precautions. Provide care for the soft tissue injuries as described in Principle Box 10-1.

Complete ongoing assessment every five minutes. Comfort and calm the patient, and reassure them that an ambulance is on the way.

SPECIAL CONSIDERATIONS

Some injuries require special considerations for emergency medical care. Examples of special injuries include penetrating chest injuries, patients with impaled objects, patients with an evisceration, and amputations.

Penetrating chest injuries

For penetrating chest injuries, apply an **occlusive dressing** to the wound. An occlusive dressing keeps air out of a wound. The dressing is placed over the wound and sealed only on three sides. Leaving one side open will allow the air

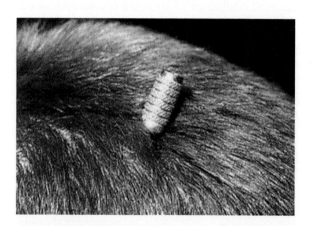

Fig. 10-11 A dart partially embedded in the head.

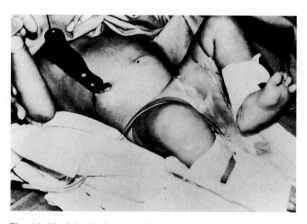

Fig. 10-13 A knife impaled in a child's abdomen.

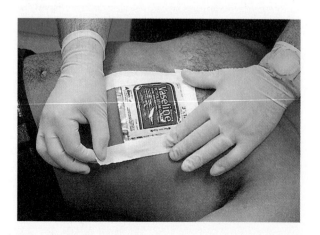

Fig. 10-12 For an open chest wound, use an occlusive dressing taped on three sides, leaving one side open to allow air inside the chest to escape but to prevent more air from entering. The packaging can be taped over the Vaseline gauze to secure the dressing.

inside the chest to escape but will prevent more air from entering through the wound (Fig. 10-12). If no spinal injury is suspected, the patient may assume a position of comfort.

Impaled objects

Any object that is still in the wound when you reach the patient is an impaled object (Fig. 10-13). The care you give depends on the site of the object. Impaled objects are typically left in place, since removal of the object may cause uncontrolled bleeding. You may remove an object through the cheek if it could interfere with the airway. After removing the object, dress the cheek on both sides. You may also remove an object that would interfere with chest compressions or transportation. Objects in other sites should be left in place and stabilized there, including an object in the cheek that does not pose a threat to the airway or an object in the chest that does not interfere with chest compressions. If you can cut off or shorten the protruding portion of the object, stabilize it and cut or break that portion off rather than removing the whole object and risking further damage. Secure the object in place following the steps described in Technique 10-5.

Do not remove objects lodged in the eye, ear, or nose. Stabilize the object and transport the patient. You should stabilize and bandage an impaled object in the eye. Place a protective covering, such as a cone or a cup, over the injured eye and the protruding object. Also cover the other eye, because both eyes move together. Covering the uninjured eye will help minimize the movement of the injured eye.

Eviscerations

An **evisceration** is an open injury in which the organs are protruding through the wound, exposed to the outside environment (Fig. 10-15). Do not attempt to replace the protruding organs. Technique 10-6 lists the steps of care for an evisceration.

Amputations

An **amputation** is the loss of an extremity or part of an extremity (Fig. 10-17). An amputation of an extremity requires special considerations. There may be massive bleeding from the amputation

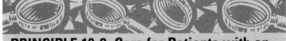

PRINCIPLE 10-2 Care for Patients with an Amputation

1. Follow body substance isolation precautions.
2. Control the bleeding, place sterile dressings over the wound and secure them in place.
3. Take special care to locate and preserve the amputated part. Place the part in a plastic bag. Place that bag in a larger bag and into a container of ice and water. Do not use ice alone and do not use dry ice. Keep the part cool, but do not freeze it.
4. Make sure the amputated part is transported to the hospital with the patient.

TECHNIQUE 10-5 Care for Patients with an Impaled Object

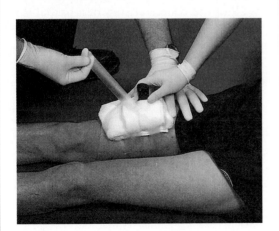

Fig. 10-14 Follow body substance isolation precautions. Manually secure the object in place. Expose the wound area, and control bleeding. Use a bulky dressing to stabilize the object. Secure the dressing in place with tape or bandages.

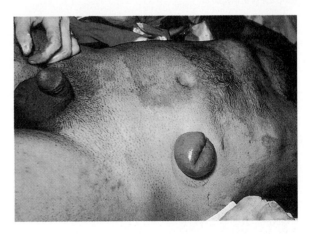

Fig. 10-15 An evisceration caused by a stabbing knife wound.

TECHNIQUE 10-6 Care of Patients with an Evisceration

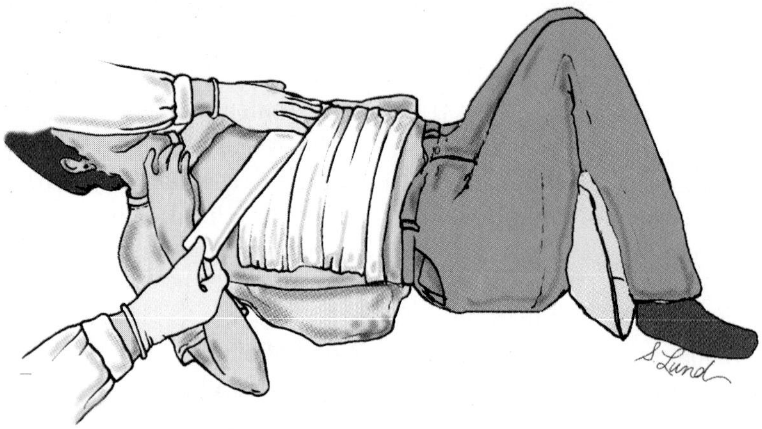

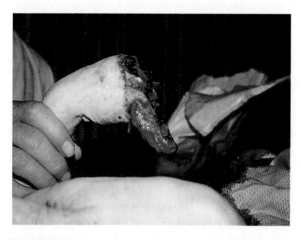

Fig. 10-16 Follow body substance isolation precautions. Do not touch or try to replace the exposed organs in the body. Cut clothing away from the injured area. Next, cover the organs with a thick, moist dressing and secure it in place.

Fig. 10-17 A hand with a nearly amputated thumb and amputated fingers.

site, or bleeding may be limited. Not only does the patient require emergency medical care, but the amputated part (if salvageable) also requires appropriate care to prevent damage and ensure the success of reattachment. Refer to Principle 10-2 for the care of an amputation.

BURNS

TYPES OF BURNS

Burns are another type of soft tissue injury. Burns are classified according to the depth of injury. A superficial burn involves only the outer layer of skin. The skin appears red and there is pain and swelling at the burn site (Fig. 10-18A). A partial-thickness burn involves both the outer and middle layers of skin. There is intense pain at the site, and blisters form. The skin is white to red in color and moist or mottled (Fig. 10-18B). A full-thickness burn extends through all layers of skin to the underlying tissue and may involve the muscle, bone, or other organs (Fig. 10-18C). It has all of the characteristics of a partial thickness burn, but may also include charred skin at the burned area that feels leathery or hard to the touch. The patient may feel little pain at the site of the burn because of loss of sensation from nerve damage.

ROLE OF THE FIRST RESPONDER

The First Responder should perform a scene size-up before providing emergency medical care. All patients should receive an initial assessment and the physical exam. Take appropriate body substance isolation precautions.

Stop the burning process with water or saline. Remove any smoldering clothes or jewelry from the patient. Clothing may have melted to the skin. If this is the case and resistance is met, the clothing should be left in place.

Because the airway may swell anytime after the patient inhales hot air, you must continually

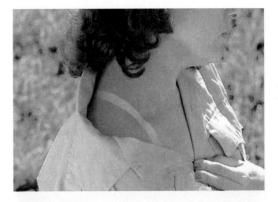

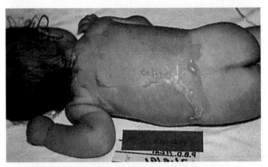

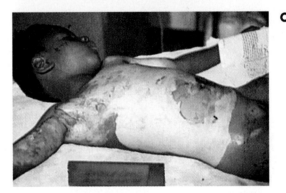

Fig. 10-18 A, A superficial burn. **B,** A partial-thickness burn. **C,** A full-thickness burn.

REVIEW QUESTIONS

Specific Injuries

1. Fill in the blank with the appropriate soft tissue injury (abrasion, laceration, penetration):

   _____ Only the outermost layer of skin is damaged.

   _____ An example would be a stab wound.

   _____ Very little or no external or internal bleeding.

   _____ Caused by a forceful impact with a sharp object and bleeding can be severe.

   _____ Usually caused by a sharp, pointed object with little external bleeding, but possible severe internal bleeding.

2. To prevent further contamination of soft tissue injuries the First Responder will place a sterile _____ over the wound.

3. List the steps for managing an impaled object in order:

   A. Expose the wound area.

   B. Use bulky dressing to secure the object.

   C. Manually stabilize the object.

   D. Control bleeding.

4. The care of a patient with an amputation includes care of the amputated part by placing the part in plastic and freezing it. True or False.

1. abrasion, penetration, abrasion, laceration, penetration; 2. dressing; 3. C, A, D, B; 4. False, never freeze an amputated part, place it in a plastic bag on ice and water.

---

monitor the airway for difficulty breathing or closure. Be prepared to ventilate the patient.

Burns are an open injury and are prone to infection. To prevent further contamination, you should cover the burned areas with a dry sterile dressing. Do not use any type of ointment, lotion, or antiseptic on the wounds. Do not break any blisters.

Perform ongoing assessments every five minutes, and comfort and reassure the patient.

SPECIAL CONSIDERATIONS

Chemical burns are another type of burn, occurring not from heat or fire, but from a chemical reaction. Take appropriate precautions for protection against

A

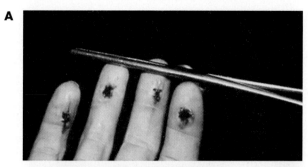

B

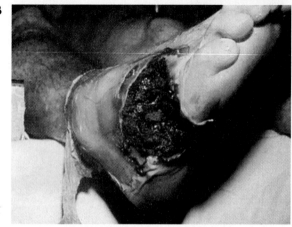

Fig. 10-19 An electrical burn. **A,** The entrance wound. **B,** The exit wound.

any hazardous material. Wear gloves, eye protection, and a gown. Make sure the scene is safe. An industrial facility should have information on all chemicals used at the site. This documentation describes the first aid care for that particular chemical. If the chemical's container is at the scene, check the label for instructions for managing contact burns. For a patient with a burn caused by a chemical powder, in most cases you can brush the dry powder off and flush the skin with large amounts of water. Dry lime should be brushed from the site, but the burn should not be flushed with water because the reaction will cause further damage. For other chemical burns, flush the site immediately. Try not to contaminate the area that is being flushed or any uninjured area; burns are open wounds that may be infected very easily. Consider the possibility of an eye burn if there was any splashing involved. If the chemical was ingested, contact the local poison control center for instructions.

An electrical burn results from exposure to an electrical source. Do not attempt to remove patients from the source unless you have been

educated in how to do so. Do not touch patients until they have been removed from the electrical source. Once the danger has been removed, monitor the patient continuously for respiratory and cardiac arrest. Damage from an electrical burn is often more severe than it appears externally. The electric current may have produced only small entrance and exit wounds (Fig. 10-19, A and B), but could have traveled a long route

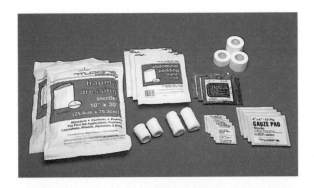

Fig. 10-20 Different sizes of dressings are used for different sizes of soft tissue injuries including large universal dressings and Vaseline gauze. Tape and bandages secure dressings in place.

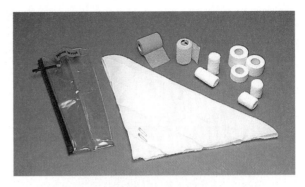

Fig. 10-21 Different types of bandages include adhesive tape, triangular bandages, gauze rolls, self-adherent bandages and an air splint.

inside the body. Treat the injuries as you would any soft tissue injury, but suspect internal and cardiac injury.

Take extra care and precaution when dealing with an infant or child with a burn. These patients have greater surface area in relationship to the total body size than an adult. This results in greater fluid and heat loss. These patients are at a greater risk for shock (hypoperfusion), airway problems, and hypothermia. Make sure you cover the patient to maintain adequate body temperature.

Burns are a common form of child abuse. With burned children, always consider this as a possibility. Child abuse is discussed in greater detail in Chapter 13, "Infants and Children." Any suspicion of abuse must be documented and reported to the receiving facility.

DRESSING AND BANDAGING

To manage soft tissue injuries, you will use dressings and bandages. The purpose of the dressing is to stop the bleeding and prevent further damage to the wound. **Dressings** are made of sterile material and protect the wound from further contamination and infection. The dressing is used to stop bleeding and prevent further damage to the wound. The **bandage** is the material that secures the dressing in place.

Dressings come in many shapes and sizes (Fig. 10-20). There are universal dressings, dressings classified according to size (2 x 2, 4 x 4, 5 x 9, etc.), and adhesive and occlusive types of dressings. An

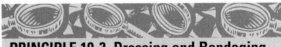

PRINCIPLE 10-3 Dressing and Bandaging

1. Follow body substance isolation precautions.
2. Expose the injured area.
3. Place a sterile dressing over the entire injury.
4. Maintain pressure to control bleeding.
5. Use a bandage to secure the dressing in place with some pressure.
6. If the dressing becomes saturated with blood, add another dressing over it and secure in place.

occlusive dressing is made of nonporous material to prevent the entry of any air and usually contains an ointment that seals the dressing; a piece of plastic wrap or foil can be used as a seal. The appropriate size dressing should be used to completely cover the wound, with about 2.5 cm (1 in.) extra on each side. All dressings should be sterile.

Bandages are used to secure dressings in place. Bandages do not have to be sterile and should be chosen based on the size of the injury and the type of dressing used (Fig. 10-21). Some bandages are self-adherent and sticky. Others are not self-adherent and require the use of adhesive tape that is placed directly over the bandage or dressing with some pressure to help control bleeding. Gauze rolls may be wrapped around the dressing and injured extremity. A triangular bandage may also be used in this manner. Principle 10-3 summarizes the steps for dressing and bandaging soft tissue injuries.

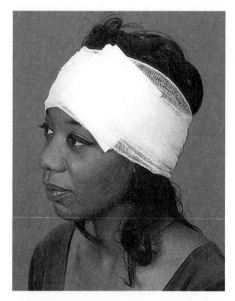

Fig. 10-22 Wrap the bandage around the head to secure the dressing.

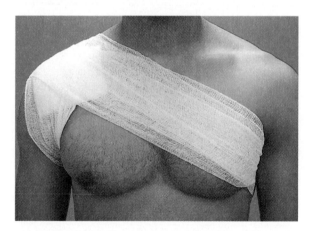

Fig. 10-23 For an injured shoulder, wrap the bandage around the armpit and shoulder to secure the dressing.

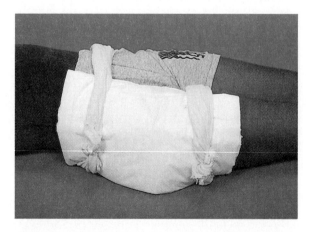

Fig. 10-24 To bandage a hip wound, secure the dressing with bandages wrapped around the waist and leg.

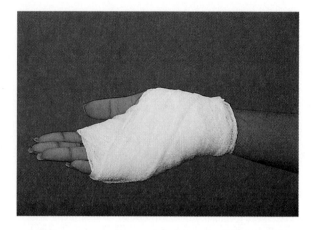

Fig. 10-25 Use a "figure 8" pattern to bandage a hand wound.

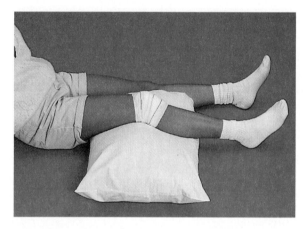

Fig. 10-26 With a wounded elbow or knee, wrap the bandage around the extremity to secure the dressing. Be sure to support the joint and stabilize it in the position found.

The following are examples of how to dress and bandage some specific injured areas.

1. Forehead: If there is no accompanying skull injury, place a dressing over the wound and wrap the bandage around the head to secure the dressing (Fig. 10-22).
2. Shoulder: Wrap the bandage around the armpit and shoulder (Fig. 10-23).
3. Hip: Secure the dressing by wrapping the bandage around the body and around the leg on the injured side (Fig. 10-24).
4. Hand: Wrap the bandage around the hand and the wrist in figure-8 pattern (Fig. 10-25).
5. Joint (elbow or knee): Wrap the bandage around the extremity to secure the dressing. Attempt to stabilize the extremity in the position found (Fig. 10-26).

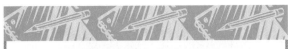

REVIEW QUESTIONS

Dressing and Bandaging

1. The _____ must be sterile because it comes into direct contact with the injury. (Dressing or Bandage)

2. Of the following, which is a type of bandage?
   A. 2 X 2
   B. Universal
   C. Triangular
   D. Occlusive

3. The purpose of the dressing is to secure the bandage in place over the injury. True or False.

4. Choose the correct statement:
   A. The bandage should be sterile because it is placed over the wound.
   B. Dressings protect the wound from further contamination and infection.
   C. The dressing and bandaging will not help to control bleeding.
   D. Dressing and bandaging can only be used on the extremities.

5. List the following statements in order regarding how to use dressings and bandages:
   A. Expose the area.
   B. Use a bandage to secure the dressing in place.
   C. Follow body substance isolation precautions.
   D. Place a sterile dressing over the entire wound.

1. dressing; 2. C; 3. False, the purpose of the bandage is to secure the dressing in place.; 4. B; 5. C, A, D, B

CHAPTER SUMMARY

SHOCK (HYPOPERFUSION)

Shock results when the cardiovascular system cannot adequately deliver oxygenated blood to the body's vital organs. Shock can be the result of a failure of the heart to provide oxygenated blood, abnormal dilation of the vessels, and/or blood volume loss. Signs and symptoms of shock include extreme thirst, restlessness, anxiety, rapid and weak pulse, rapid and shallow respirations, mental status changes, and pale, cool, moist skin.

BLEEDING

The First Responder must be aware of the risk of infectious disease from contact with blood or other body fluids. The severity of the blood loss must be based on the patient's signs and symptoms. Internal and external bleeding can result in severe blood loss with resultant shock and subsequent death.

Arterial bleeding is under high pressure, is bright red and spurts from the wound, and can be difficult to control. Venous bleeding is dark red blood that flows steadily from the wound. Capillary bleeding is dark red blood that oozes slowly from the wound.

SPECIFIC INJURIES

An abrasion affects the outermost layer of skin. It is painful, but will have little or no oozing of blood. A laceration is a break in the skin caused by a forceful impact with a sharp object and bleeding can be severe. A penetration or puncture wound is caused by a sharp pointed object. There may be little external bleeding, but internal bleeding can be severe.

An open chest injury requires the application of an occlusive dressing to the injury. An impaled object must be stabilized, bleeding controlled, and a bulky dressing applied. An evisceration involves a protruding organ and should be covered with a thick moist dressing. A patient with an amputation must be cared for, along with the amputated part. The part should be placed in plastic and then into ice and water.

BURNS

Burns are classified according to their depth. A superficial burn involves only the outermost layer of skin and will be red and painful. A partial-thickness burn involves the outermost and middle layers of skin and will be red with pain and blisters. A full-thickness burn extends through all the layers and will look like the partial-thickness burn along with some charred skin. Chemical burns usually should be flushed with water. Electrical burns often produce severe internal damage with little external damage.

DRESSING AND BANDAGING

Dressings are used to stop bleeding, protect the wound, and prevent further contamination. Dressings come in various styles and sizes and are sterile. Bandages also come in various types and are used to hold the dressings on the wound with pressure.

UNITED STATES DEPARTMENT OF TRANSPORTATION NATIONAL HIGHWAY TRAFFIC SAFETY ADMINISTRATION FIRST RESPONDER OBJECTIVES

Check your knowledge. The National Registry of EMTs and many state EMS agencies use the objectives below to develop First Responder certification examinations. Can you meet them?

COGNITIVE OBJECTIVES

1. Differentiate between arterial, venous, and capillary bleeding.
2. State the steps in the emergency medical care for external bleeding.
3. Establish the relationship between body substance isolation and bleeding.
4. List the signs of internal bleeding.
5. List the steps in the emergency medical care of the patient with signs and symptoms of internal bleeding.
6. Establish the relationship between body substance isolation (BSI) and soft tissue injuries.
7. State the types of open soft tissue injuries.
8. Describe the emergency medical care of the patient with a soft tissue injury.
9. Discuss the emergency medical care considerations for a patient with a penetrating chest injury.
10. State the emergency medical care considerations for a patient with an open wound to the abdomen.
11. Describe the emergency medical care for an impaled object.
12. State the emergency medical care for an amputation.
13. Describe the emergency medical care for burns.
14. List the functions of dressing and bandaging.

AFFECTIVE OBJECTIVES

15. Explain the rationale for body substance isolation when dealing with bleeding and soft tissue injuries.
16 Attend to the feelings of the patient with a soft tissue injury or bleeding.
17. Demonstrate a caring attitude towards patients with a soft tissue injury or bleeding who request emergency medical services.
18. Place the interests of the patient with a soft tissue injury or bleeding as the foremost consideration when making any and all patient care decisions.
19 Communicate with empathy to patients with a soft tissue injury or bleeding, as well as with family members and friends of the patient.

PSYCHOMOTOR OBJECTIVES

20. Demonstrate direct pressure as a method of emergency medical care for external bleeding.
21. Demonstrate the use of diffuse pressure as a method of emergency medical care for external bleeding.
22. Demonstrate the use of pressure points as a method of emergency medical care for external bleeding.
23. Demonstrate the care of the patient exhibiting signs and symptoms of internal bleeding.
24. Demonstrate the steps in the emergency medical care of open soft tissue injuries.
25. Demonstrate the steps in the emergency medical care of a patient with an open chest wound.
26. Demonstrate the steps in the emergency medical care of a patient with open abdominal wounds.
27. Demonstrate the steps in the emergency medical care of a patient with an impaled object.
28. Demonstrate the steps in the emergency medical care of a patient with an amputation.
29. Demonstrate the steps in the emergency medical care of an amputated part.

Injuries to Muscles and Bones

KEY TERMS

Cardiac muscle   The muscle found only in the heart.

Closed injury   An injury that does not produce a break in the continuity of the skin.

Direct injury   The result of force applied to a part of the body.

Indirect injury   The injury affecting an area that results from a force applied to another part of the body.

Involuntary muscle   Smooth muscle found in the digestive tract, blood vessels, and bronchi. They are not under control of the individual.

Open injury   An injury that produces a break in the continuity of the skin.

Twisting injury   The result of a force applied to the body in a twisting motion.

Voluntary muscle   Muscle that is attached to bone. Voluntary muscle is under direct control of the individual.

FIRST RESPONSE

"**T**wo alarm fire at 929 Glenarm Avenue, all units respond!!" As Juan and Bill responded in the truck to the fire, dispatch called them with an update, "One person has jumped from a third story window onto the front lawn, bystander report. EMS contacted." As First Responders, Juan and Bill were prepared for the emergencies that came with the job of firefighting.

As they entered the scene, they looked around for any hazards. Finding none, they approached the patient as the other engine responding sized up the fire. Juan immediately initiated manual stabilization of the patient's head and Bill began asking the responsive patient what had happened and if there were any other victims. The patient stated that he jumped from the window when he realized he could not get out of the house. Bill assessed the patient's airway and pulse. The patient said he felt some tingling in both hands, but couldn't move his feet. Both responders kept the patient calm by talking and asking questions, but did not allow him to move.

After EMS personnel arrived and immobilized the patient to the backboard, Juan could release manual stabilization of the patient's neck. Juan and Bill turned toward the house to help fight the fire.

REVIEW OF THE MUSCULOSKELETAL SYSTEM

The following sections briefly review the musculoskeletal system. For more detailed information, see Chapter 4, "The Human Body."

THE SKELETAL SYSTEM

The skeletal system, along with the muscular system, helps provide body shape, protect internal organs, and assist in body movement. The skeletal system consists of the bones of the skull, the face, the spinal column and thorax, the pelvis, the lower extremities, and the upper extremities. The skull houses and protects the brain. The thorax is made up of the ribs and the breastbone (sternum). The lower end of the breastbone extends into the xiphoid process, which is the landmark for finding the position for chest compressions during CPR. The lower extremities are composed of the upper leg (femur), the knee cap (patella), the lower leg (tibia and fibula), the ankle, feet, and toes. The shoulder is part of the upper arm, and consists of the collarbone (clavicle) and shoulder blade (scapula). The upper extremities are composed of the shoulder, the upper arm (humerus), the forearm (radius and ulna), the wrist, hand, and fingers.

Muscles and bones, together with other connective tissue, allow for body movement. Extremities move at the joints where bones are connected to other bones. Refer to Figure 11-1 for a diagram of the skeletal system.

THE MUSCULAR SYSTEM

No movement in the body could occur without muscles. Every physical activity, from riding a bike to turning the pages of this book, occurs with the contraction of muscles. Muscles, along with the skeletal system, give the body shape, protect internal organs, and assist movement. There are three different types of muscle (Fig. 11-2).

Voluntary muscles are attached to bones. These muscles form the major muscle mass of the body and are controlled by the nervous system and brain. They can be contracted and relaxed at will and are responsible for movement. Voluntary muscles are also called skeletal muscles.

Involuntary muscles are found in the walls of the hollow structures of the gastrointestinal tract and urinary system, as well as the blood vessels and bronchi. Involuntary muscles control the flow of blood, body fluids, and other substances through these structures, and there is generally no conscious control of these muscles. Involuntary muscles are also called smooth muscles.

Cardiac muscle exists only in the heart. Cardiac muscle has the unique ability to contract on its own. Cardiac muscle is involuntary muscle that has its own supply of blood. This muscle can tolerate only short interruptions of blood supply.

REVIEW QUESTIONS

Review of the Musculoskeletal System

1. The _____ is used to determine the correct hand position for chest compressions during CPR.

2. Which of the following statements is correct?
   A. The musculoskeletal system provides for body shape and movement, but does not protect internal organs.
   B. The musculoskeletal system provides protection for internal organs only.
   C. The musculoskeletal system provides for body shape and movement, along with protecting internal organs.
   D. The musculoskeletal system provides protection from germs and gives the body shape.

3. The skull houses and protects the _____.

4. Place the correct type of muscle in each blank (voluntary, involuntary, cardiac):
   _____ Attached to bones
   _____ Found in the heart
   _____ Can tolerate only very short interruptions of the blood supply
   _____ Found in the gastrointestinal tract and urinary system
   _____ Can be contracted by the will of the individual

5. Where bones attach to bones to provide movement is called a _____.

1. xiphoid process; 2. C; 3. brain; 4. voluntary, cardiac, cardiac, involuntary, voluntary; 5. joint

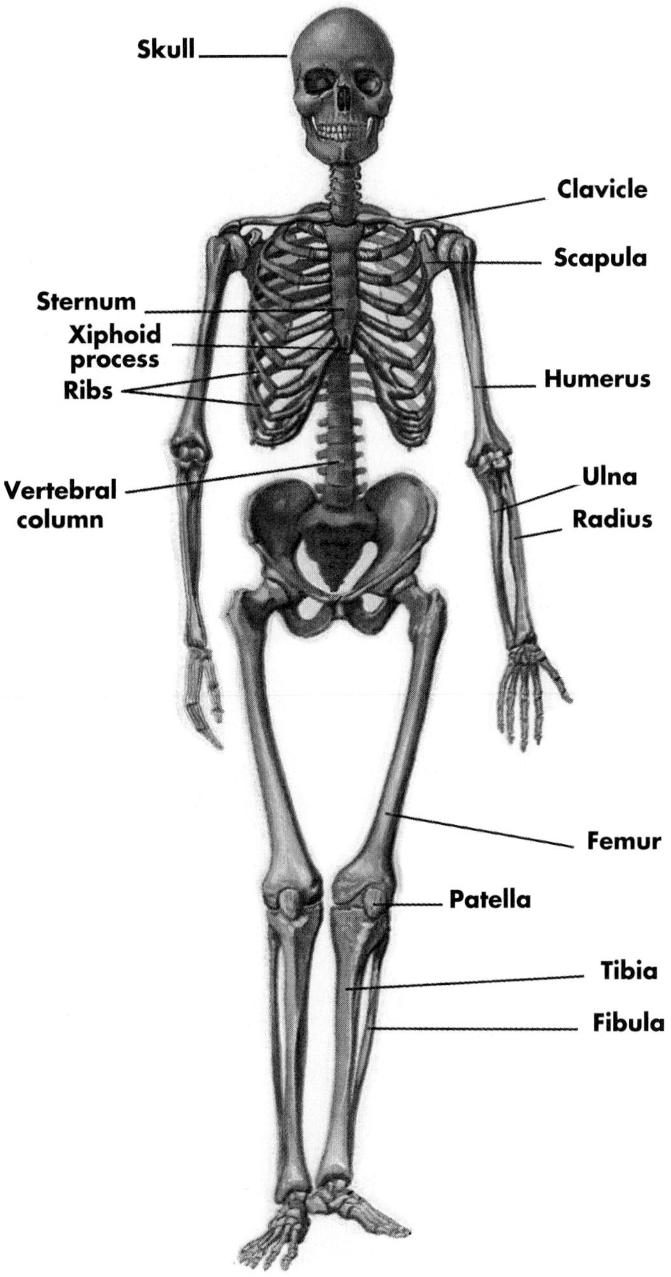

Skull
Clavicle
Scapula
Sternum
Xiphoid process
Ribs
Humerus
Vertebral column
Ulna
Radius
Femur
Patella
Tibia
Fibula

Fig. 11-1 The skeletal system.

INJURIES TO BONES AND JOINTS

Various injuries to bones and joints are described in the following sections. In order to properly care for patients with bone or joint injuries, you must understand the mechanism of injury. First Responders should maintain a high index of suspicion for patients who have sustained a serious mechanism of injury.

MECHANISM OF INJURY

The mechanism of injury can help you determine the potential severity of the injury. The mechanism of injury is the force that acts upon the body to produce an injury. Musculoskeletal injuries are the result of a force applied to an area of the body.

Some injuries result from a direct force (Fig. 11-3A). A **direct injury** is the result of a force applied to the body. An example of a direct

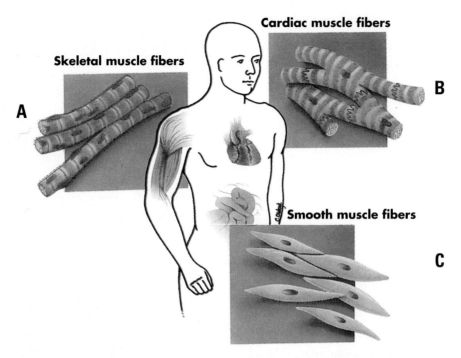

Skeletal muscle fibers

A

Cardiac muscle fibers

B

Smooth muscle fibers

C

Fig. 11-2 The three types of muscles are **A,** voluntary (skeletal), **B,** cardiac, and **C,** involuntary (smooth).

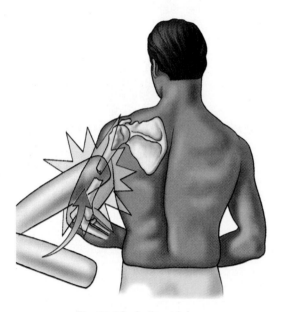

Fig. 11-3A A direct injury.

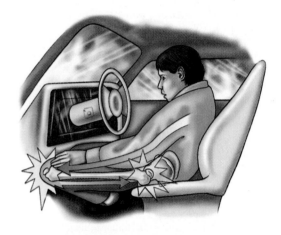

Fig. 11-3B An indirect injury.

injury is one caused by a baseball bat swung into a person's arm. The arm's injury results from direct contact with the baseball bat.

Other injuries are caused by indirect forces (Fig. 11-3B). An **indirect injury** is an injury caused by a force applied to another part of the body. An example of indirect injury is an auto collision in which a patient's knees are thrown forward into the dashboard. The knees are directly injured from contact with the dash. The hips and pelvis are indirectly

injured because the knees are pushed backward with a great force that reaches the hips and pelvis.

Some injuries are caused by twisting forces (Fig. 11-3C). If an extremity becomes pulled and twisted, a **twisting injury** may result from that force. For instance, a wrestler who becomes entangled in an opponent's hold may pull and twist his body. This force may produce an injury to the muscles and bones that are twisted.

Always consider the force that caused the injury. It takes a much greater force to injure the thigh, for example, than it takes to injure the forearm. This is because the bone is much larger, more dense, and protected by larger muscles.

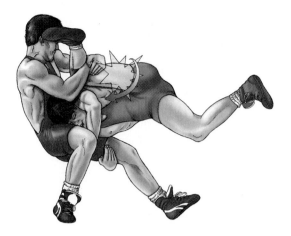

Fig. 11-3C A twisting injury.

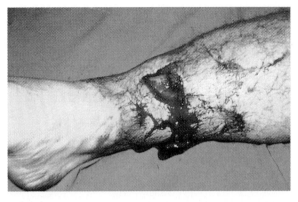

Fig. 11-4 An open injury of the lower leg with protruding bone ends.

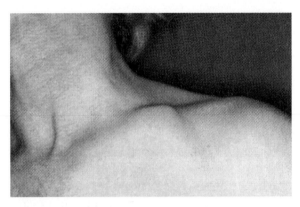

Fig. 11-5 A collarbone injury with obvious deformity.

Gather as much information as possible regarding the mechanism of injury, and include this in your report to EMS personnel. For more information on the mechanism of injury, refer to Chapter 7, "Patient Assessment."

BONE OR JOINT INJURIES

Musculoskeletal injuries are either open or closed. An **open injury** involves a break in the continuity of the skin and usually produces some external bleeding (Fig. 11-4). A **closed injury** does not involve a break in the skin or external bleeding, although it may produce internal bleeding (Fig. 11-5).

There are several signs and symptoms characteristic of bone or joint injuries. The area of injury may have some deformity or angulation and may be painful to move and tender to touch. If the bone ends are separated, you may hear or feel some grating during the examination, caused by the bone ends rubbing together. Do not purposefully seek this sign, and do not try to repeat it if you note it during the assessment. Grating bone ends together may produce further injury. The area of injury may be swollen, appearing larger than the same area on the other side of the body, and may be bruised and discolored. In an open bone injury, the ends of the bones that are injured may be protruding through the skin and exposed to the outside environment. With a joint injury, the joint may be locked in position and unmovable. Box 11-1 summarizes the signs and symptoms of a bone or joint injury.

ROLE OF THE FIRST RESPONDER

A First Responder's emergency medical care for patients with bone or joint injuries always includes taking appropriate body substance isolation

---

BOX 11-1 Signs and Symptoms of a Bone or Joint Injury

- Deformity or angulation
- Pain and tenderness
- Grating
- Swelling
- Bruising (discoloration)
- Exposed bone ends (open injury)
- Joint locked into position

---

precautions before examining the patient. Even a closed injury that is not bleeding may become an open injury because of movement or pressure. Perform a scene size-up, and make sure the scene is safe before you approach the patient.

Perform an initial assessment. Bone and joint injuries are often obvious and eye-catching, but control of the airway, breathing, and circulation always takes priority. Make sure the patient has a patent airway and is breathing adequately. Control any major bleeding or life-threatening situations using methods, such as direct pressure, described in Chapter 10, "Bleeding and Soft Tissue Injuries." If you suspect the patient may also have spinal injuries, stabilize their head in a neutral position and do not allow them to move until they can be immobilized.

If the injury is to an extremity, allow the patient to remain in a position of comfort after life threats have been controlled. Apply a cold pack to an extremity that is painful, swollen and deformed to reduce pain and swelling. Manually stabilize the extremity until additional EMS resources arrive with immobilization equipment. See Principle 11-1 for the steps of stabilizing.

Do not allow the patient to move the extremity until it can be immobilized with a splint. Splinting extremities is within the scope of practice for some First Responders. If you are responsible for splinting injuries in your system, refer to Appendix E, "Principles and Techniques of Splinting."

INJURIES TO THE SPINE

MECHANISM OF INJURY

The mechanism of injury can provide information about the cause and the severity of the patient's injuries. By considering the damage to a vehicle or the height of a fall, you can determine if the mechanism of injury involved a significant force to the patient's body. Figure 11-7 illustrates a scene in

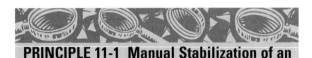

PRINCIPLE 11-1   Manual Stabilization of an Extremity

1. Support above and below an injury (Fig. 11-6A).
2. Cover open wounds with a sterile dressing (Fig. 11-6B).
3. Pad to prevent pressure and discomfort to the patient (Fig. 11-6C).
4. When in doubt, manually stabilize the injury (Fig. 11-6D).
5. Do not intentionally replace any protruding bones.

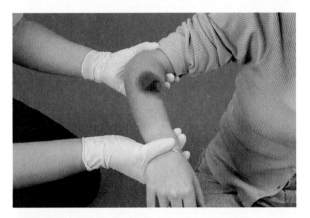

Fig. 11-6A Support above and below an injury.

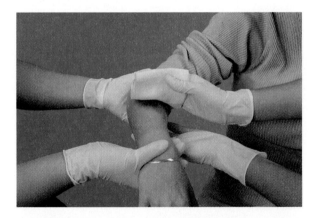

Fig. 11-6B Cover open wounds with a sterile dressing.

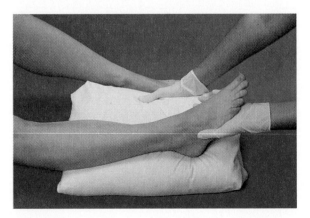

Fig. 11-6C Pad to prevent pressure and discomfort to the patient.

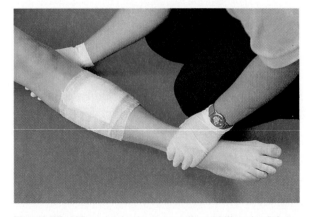

Fig. 11-6D When in doubt, manually stabilize the injury.

which the patient has sustained a significant mechanism of injury. In most situations, the mechanism of injury can be determined as part of the scene size-up. Many mechanisms of injury can cause trauma and injury to the spine. Box 11-2 lists some mechanisms of injury that should make you suspect that the patient may have a significant injury requiring spinal immobilization.

If you have any doubt about the mechanism of injury or if the patient is unresponsive, you should assume that the patient has significant life-threatening injuries.

SIGNS AND SYMPTOMS

Patients with spinal injuries may feel tenderness in the area of the injury or pain associated with movement of the area. However, do not ask the patient to move just to try to elicit a pain response, and do not move the patient just to test for a pain response. The patient may feel pain independent of movement or palpation along the spinal column or the extremities. The pain may be intermittent. Tell the patient not to move while you are asking questions. Stay within the patient's field of vision when talking or asking questions so that the patient does not move his/her head to look at you.

Soft tissue injuries may also be a sign of associated trauma to the spine. The head and neck may be injured along with the cervical spine. A shoulder,

---

REVIEW QUESTIONS

Injuries to Bones and Joints

1. A person hitting their head on the windshield of a car and receiving only a cut on their forehead would be an example of _____ force.

2. List three signs or symptoms of a bone/joint injury:

   _____

   _____

   _____

3. Of the two types of bone/joint injuries, which type involves a break in the continuity of the skin?

   _____

4. List the following steps for the care of bone/joint injury in order:
   A. Place a dressing on open wounds
   B. Support above and below the injury
   C. Pad the area to prevent discomfort to the patient

1. direct. 2. Deformity, angulation, pain, tenderness, swelling, discoloration, protruding bone ends, locked joints, grating; 3. Open; 4. B, A, C

BOX 11-2 Significant Mechanisms of Injury

- Motor vehicle crashes
- Pedestrian-vehicle collisions
- Falls
- Blunt trauma
- Penetrating trauma to head, neck, or torso
- Motorcycle crashes
- Hangings
- Springboard or platform diving accidents

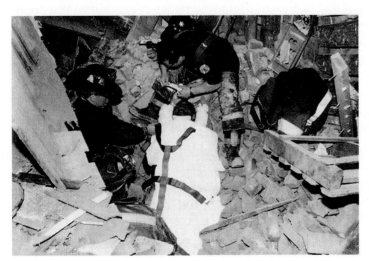

Fig. 11-7 The mechanism of injury may make you suspect that the patient has extensive injuries.

back, or abdominal injury could indicate an injury to the spinal column in the thorax or abdomen. Soft tissue damage to the lower extremities could indicate an injury to the lumbar or sacral spine.

Patients may feel numbness, weakness, or tingling in the extremities or may have complete loss of sensation or paralysis below the suspected level of injury. These patients may also have lost control of their bowels or bladder. The patient may have loss of sensation or paralysis in the upper or lower extremities and may have respiratory impairment.

The absence of pain does not rule out spinal column or cord damage along the spinal column. You also cannot rule out spinal column or cord damage if the patient can walk, move the extremities, or feel sensations.

During the assessment process, you need to gather important additional information about the condition of both responsive and unresponsive patients.

ASSESSING THE POTENTIALLY SPINE-INJURED PATIENT

The scene size-up and the initial assessment are the first critical areas of assessment. You should treat any life threats found during this time such as an airway problem or massive bleeding.

Responsive Patients

Assess the scene and notice the mechanism of injury. Once you are with the patient, tell the patient not to move while you ask questions. Important questions to ask the patient are listed in Box 11-3.

You should assess the patient's circulation, ability to move (motor function) and sensation in each of their extremities. You can assess circulation by feeling a pulse in the extremity. For the feet, assess the pulse on the top of the foot. For the arms, assess the radial pulses. Have the patient move both feet and both hands. Touch the patient on the foot and ask them if they can feel you touching them. Assess pulse, motor function, and sensation for each extremity.

Gather pertinent information, such as what happened, what hurts, and how the patient feels, from responsive patients in a timely fashion. A responsive patient could become unresponsive at any moment.

Unresponsive Patients

After assessing the scene and noticing the mechanism of injury, approach the patient and determine unresponsiveness. When caring for the unresponsive trauma patient, take precautions to minimize movement of the patient's neck and spine. Methods for stabilizing the patient's head and neck are discussed later in this chapter. Talk to others at the scene to determine more information about the mechanism of injury and the patient's mental status before you arrived.

COMPLICATIONS

Complications that can arise with a spinal injury include inadequate breathing effort and paralysis. To help prevent these complications, continually reassess the patient's airway and breathing and do not move the patient. Any patient movement might produce paralysis that was not previously present. Similarly, reassess a combative or uncooperative patient after any significant movement or attempted movement. Thoroughly document any changes in the patient's ability to move their extremities or changes in sensation.

A spinal cord injury that affects the nerves controlling the movement of the diaphragm and accessory muscles of breathing (a cervical or thoracic injury) may cause a patient to have difficulty breathing. Watch these patients closely and ventilate as needed.

ROLE OF THE FIRST RESPONDER

Before beginning patient care, perform a scene size-up and take appropriate body substance isolation precautions. Establish and maintain control of the airway and breathing. Stabilize the head and

BOX 11-3 Important Questions for Responsive Trauma Patients

- What happened?
- Where does it hurt?
- Does your neck or back hurt?
- Can you move your hands and feet?
- Where am I touching you now? (while touching fingers and toes)

neck manually using in-line cervical spinal stabilization, which is described in Technique 11-1. Do not release this stabilization until the patient is properly immobilized to the long backboard.

After the cervical spine is manually stabilized, complete the initial assessment. If needed, provide airway control and artificial ventilation while maintaining cervical in-line stabilization. Assess the pulse and motor and sensory function in all extremities.

If the patient vomits, you will need to roll them onto their side to prevent an airway obstruction. The First Responder stabilizing the head will direct the movement of all rescuers. One First Responder should support the patient's shoulders, one the patient's hips, and one the lower extremities. Roll the patient onto their side with the body in a straight line. Be careful to maintain the position of the head, neck, and spinal column in one straight line. Sweep any material out of the patient's mouth and roll him onto his back. Manage the airway using a head-tilt, jaw thrust as described in Chapter 6, "The Airway."

INJURIES TO THE BRAIN AND SKULL

Many injuries involving the spine also involve the brain and skull. Any patient with suspected brain and skull injuries should be suspected of having a spinal injury.

HEAD INJURIES

Injuries to the head may be closed or open. Closed and open injuries may present with discoloration, swelling, or a depression of the skull bones. Open injuries, in addition, may present with bleeding. Wounds to the scalp often look severe because many capillary beds are located there, and even a small cut can produce major bleeding. Control this bleeding with direct pressure.

An injury to the skull may damage brain tissue directly or may result in bleeding inside the

TECHNIQUE 11-1 Manual Cervical In-line Stabilization

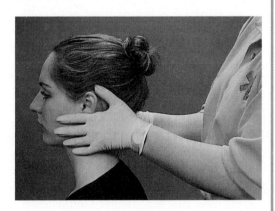

Fig. 11-8 Get into position at the top of the patient's head (with a patient lying down) or behind the patient (for a seated patient). Place your hands at the corner of the patient's jaws on both sides. Grasp the corner of the jaw and provide stabilization to the neck by wrapping your hands around the back of the neck. Place the patient's head in the neutral position in alignment with the spine. Do not attempt this positioning if the patient complains of pain, if the head is not easily moved into position, if muscle spasm occurs, or if the airway becomes compromised. Constant manual in-line stabilization may be released when additional EMS resources have properly secured the patient to a backboard with the head stabilized.

REVIEW QUESTIONS

Injuries to the Spine

1. Two complications that arise in patients with an injured spine are _____ and _____.

2. List the following steps for the care of the patient with an injured spine in order:
   A. Perform the initial assessment.
   B. Take body substance isolation precautions.
   C. Establish and maintain manual stabilization.
   D. Assess pulse, motor and sensation in all extremities.

3. Soft tissue injuries to the head and neck may indicate injury to the _____ spine.

4. If the patient can walk or move their extremities, they do not have a spinal injury. True or False?

1. Inadequate breathing effort, paralysis; 2. B, C, A, D; 3. cervical; 4. False

skull. Internal bleeding causes increased pressure inside the skull that can result in changes in mental status.

ROLE OF THE FIRST RESPONDER

Perform a scene size-up and take appropriate body substance isolation precautions. The first priority for patients with traumatic head injuries is to ensure a patent airway. Maintain the airway and provide artificial ventilation if appropriate. Do not use the head-tilt, chin-lift maneuver for the trauma patient, instead, use the jaw thrust without head-tilt. The initial assessment should be done and spinal stabilization performed. With any head injury, suspect a spinal injury and do not move the patient or allow them to move until they are completely immobilized. The patient's airway, breathing, pulse, and mental status must be continuously monitored for deterioration.

BOX 11-4 Emergency Medical Care for the Head Injured Patient

- Take body substance isolation precautions
- Perform initial assessment and provide manual stabilization of the head
- Maintain an open airway and provide artificial ventilation if needed
- Control bleeding
- Monitor mental status

REVIEW QUESTIONS

Injuries to the Brain and Skull

1. Control bleeding of the head with _____.

2. Place the following steps for managing a head injury in order:
   A. Control bleeding
   B. Body substance isolation
   C. Initial assessment with spinal stabilization
   D. Maintain airway and provide artificial ventilations

3. The two types of head injuries are _____ and _____.

1. direct pressure; 2. B, C, D, A; 3. open, closed

Control any bleeding. Apply enough pressure to control the bleeding, without disturbing the underlying tissue. Dress and bandage open wounds as described in Chapter 10, "Bleeding and Soft-Tissue Injuries." Be prepared for changes in the patient's condition and treat them appropriately. The patient with head injuries may experience nausea and vomiting. Be prepared to roll the patient to the side and clear the airway using suction. Box 11-4 summarizes the emergency medical care for the head-injured patient.

CHAPTER SUMMARY

REVIEW OF THE MUSCULOSKELETAL SYSTEM

The skeletal system helps provide body shape, protects internal organs, and assists in body movement. Muscles and bones, together with other connective tissue, allow for body movement. Muscles give the body shape, protect internal organs, and provide movement. Voluntary, or skeletal, muscles are attached to bones. They can be contracted and relaxed at will and are responsible for movement. Involuntary, or smooth, muscles are found in the walls of the hollow structures of the gastrointestinal tract and urinary system, as well as the blood vessels and bronchi. Cardiac muscle exists only in the heart.

INJURIES TO BONES AND JOINTS

The mechanism of injury can help you determine the potential severity of the injury. Injuries can result from a direct force onto an area of the body, an indirect force, or a twisting force. Always consider the force that was involved in the cause of the injury.

Musculoskeletal injuries are either open or closed. Signs and symptoms of a bone or joint injury include deformity or angulation, pain and tenderness, grating, swelling, bruising (discoloration), exposed bone ends (open injury), and joints locked into position.

Emergency medical care for bone or joint injuries for the First Responder always includes taking appropriate body substance isolation precautions. Establish a patent airway and control any major bleeding or life-threatening situations. Allow the patient to remain in the position of comfort. Any extremity that is painful, swollen, and deformed should have a cold pack applied to it to reduce pain and swelling. The extremity should be manually stabilized until additional EMS resources arrive.

INJURIES TO THE SPINE

By considering factors such as the damage to a vehicle or the height of a fall, you can determine if the mechanism of injury involved a significant force to the patient's body. In most situations, the mechanism of injury can be determined as part of the scene size-up.

Signs and symptoms of a spine injury include tenderness; pain with or without movement, soft tissue injuries with trauma, numbness, weakness or tingling; loss of sensation, paralysis, or respiratory impairment; or loss of bladder control.

To assess the responsive patient, the responder should ask questions to the patient to determine what happened, where he/she is injured, and to judge his/her mental status. For the unresponsive patient, the bystanders and family members may have the needed information. Complications in a spine-injured patient include inadequate breathing effort and paralysis.

Emergency care includes body substance isolation, establishing and maintaining manual spinal stabilization, establishing and maintaining airway/ventilation without moving the patient, and assessing the pulse, motor function, and sensation in the extremities.

INJURIES TO THE BRAIN AND SKULL

Head injuries may be open or closed. Open head injuries may bleed a lot and look worse than they actually are because of the large number of blood vessels on the scalp.

Emergency care includes body substance isolation, maintaining airway/ventilation, performing initial assessment, and manual spinal stabilization. Closely monitor the patient's mental status, control bleeding, and be prepared for changes in the patient's condition.

UNITED STATES DEPARTMENT OF TRANSPORTATION NATIONAL HIGHWAY TRAFFIC SAFETY ADMINISTRATION FIRST RESPONDER OBJECTIVES

Check your knowledge. The National Registry of EMTs and many state EMS agencies use the objectives below to develop First Responder certification examinations. Can you meet them?

COGNITIVE OBJECTIVES

1. Describe the function of the musculoskeletal system.
2. Differentiate between an open and a closed painful, swollen, deformed extremity.
3. List the emergency medical care for a patient with a painful, swollen, deformed extremity.
4. Relate mechanism of injury to potential injuries of the head and spine.
5. State the signs and symptoms of a potential spine injury.
6. Describe the method of determining if a responsive patient may have a spine injury.
7. List the signs and symptoms of injury to the head.
8. Describe the emergency medical care for injuries to the head.

AFFECTIVE OBJECTIVES

9. Explain the rationale for the feeling patients who have need for immobilization of the painful, swollen, deformed extremity.

10. Demonstrate a caring attitude towards patients with a musculoskeletal injury who request emergency medical services.
11. Place the interests of the patient with a musculoskeletal injury as the foremost consideration when making any and all patient care decisions.
12. Communicate with empathy to patients with a musculoskeletal injury, as well as with family members and friends of the patient.

PSYCHOMOTOR OBJECTIVES

13. Demonstrate the emergency medical care of a patient with a painful, swollen, deformed extremity.
14. Demonstrate opening the airway in a patient with suspected spinal cord injury.
15. Demonstrate evaluating a responsive patient with a suspected spinal cord injury.
16. Demonstrate stabilizing of the cervical spine.

Principles and Techniques of Splinting

I. Injuries to Bones and Joints
  A. Signs and Symptoms of Bone or Joint Injury
  B. Emergency Care for Patients with Bone or Joint Injuries

II. Splinting
  A. Reasons for Splinting
  B. Principles of Splinting
  C. Splinting Equipment and Techniques
  D. Risks of Splinting

KEY TERMS

Distal   A directional term meaning further away from the trunk.

Pneumatic splint   A device that uses air or vacuum to stabilize an injury.

Position of function   The relaxed position of the hand or foot in which there is minimal movement or stretching of muscle.

Rigid splint   A type of immobilization device that does not conform to the body.

Sling and swathe   Bandaging used to immobilize a shoulder or arm injury.

Splint   A device used to immobilize a musculoskeletal injury.

The specialized emergency medical care for a patient with a painful, swollen or deformed extremity includes applying a splint to immobilize the injury and prevent further damage. This appendix describes various types of splints, and discusses the principles and some techniques for splinting.

Musculoskeletal injuries are among the most common injuries you will encounter. Usually, these injuries are not life-threatening, although they are often painful. Prompt identification and treatment of musculoskeletal injuries is crucial to reduce pain, prevent further injury, and minimize permanent damage.

Splinting an extremity is within the scope of practice for some First Responders. If splinting is not within your scope of practice, you should care for injuries as described in Chapter 11, "Injuries to Muscles and Bones."

INJURIES TO BONES AND JOINTS

SIGNS AND SYMPTOMS OF BONE OR JOINT INJURY

Various signs and symptoms are characteristic of bone or joint injuries. The area of injury may have some deformity or angulation and may be painful to move and tender to touch. If the bone ends are separated, some crepitation or grating may be heard or felt during the examination. Crepitation is caused by bone ends rubbing together. Do not purposefully seek this sign, and do not try to repeat it if you note it during the assessment. Bone ends rubbing together may produce further injury.

The area of injury may be swollen, appearing larger than the same area on the other side of the body, and may be discolored. If the injury is open,

bone ends may be protruding through the skin and exposed to the outside environment. With a joint injury, the joint may be locked in position and unmovable. Box E-1 summarizes the signs and symptoms of a bone or joint injury.

EMERGENCY CARE FOR PATIENTS WITH BONE OR JOINT INJURIES

As described in Chapter 11, emergency medical care for bone or joint injuries consists of both basic techniques and specialized techniques. First, always take appropriate body substance isolation precautions before examining the patient. Even a closed injury that is not bleeding may become an open injury because of movement or pressure.

Establish a patent airway, and ensure the adequacy of breathing. Assess the patient's circulation and look for major bleeding. Any major bleeding or life-threatening situations should be controlled.

FIRST RESPONDER ALERT

Always care for life-threatening injuries before focusing on a painful, swollen, deformed extremity. Do not waste time caring for an extremity if the patient is not breathing adequately or has other threats to life!

BOX E-1 Signs and Symptoms of a Bone or Joint Injury

- Deformity or angulation
- Pain and tenderness
- Crepitation (grating)
- Swelling
- Bruising (discoloration)
- Exposed bone ends (open injury)
- Joints locked into position

REVIEW QUESTIONS

Injuries to Bones and Joints

1. Emergency medical care includes the application of a(n) _____ and _____ to reduce swelling and pain.

2. Injuries to the arm should always be splinted, even if the patient has more serious injuries. True or False?

3. List three signs and symptoms of a musculoskeletal injury:

   _____

   _____

   _____

1. Cold pack, splint; 2. False; 3. Deformity or angulation, pain and tenderness, crepitation, swelling, bruising, exposed bone ends, joints locked into position

Always care for life-threatening injuries before focusing on a painful, swollen, deformed extremity. Do not waste time caring for an extremity if the patient is not breathing adequately or has other threats to life!

Splint the injury appropriately to prevent movement of bone ends or fragments (described later in this appendix), and prepare the patient for transport. After splinting the injury, a cold pack may be applied to the injured area to reduce swelling and pain. An injured extremity should be elevated to reduce blood flow to that area, unless other injuries are present that would cause complications.

SPLINTING

The specialized emergency medical care provided for a painful, swollen, deformed extremity includes applying a splint to immobilize the injury and prevent further damage. A splint is a device used to immobilize a musculoskeletal injury. This appendix describes some types of splints and how they are used.

REASONS FOR SPLINTING

Splinting a painful, swollen, deformed extremity prevents movement of bone fragments, bone ends, or injured joints. The splint minimizes damage to muscles, nerves, and blood vessels caused by broken bones. Immobilization helps to prevent a closed injury from becoming an open injury. It also minimizes the restriction of blood flow resulting from bone ends compressing blood vessels and

---

BOX E-2 Reasons for Splinting

- Prevent movement of bone fragment, bone ends, or injured joints
- Minimize damage to muscle, nerves, and blood vessels
- Minimize the chance of converting a closed injury to an open injury
- Minimize the restriction of blood flow resulting from bone ends compressing blood vessels
- Minimize bleeding from damaged tissue caused by bone ends
- Minimize the pain associated with movement of bone ends
- Minimize chance of paralysis of extremities due to spinal damage

---

limits the bleeding caused by tissue damage from the bone ends. Splinting reduces pain by limiting the movement of bone ends. Paralysis resulting from spinal damage is also minimized. Box E-2 summarizes the reasons for splinting.

PRINCIPLES OF SPLINTING

Before splinting, always assess the patient as a whole first. After performing an initial assessment, a physical exam and treating any life threats, you should care for the injury. Evaluate the pulse (obtained at the end of the extremity), motor function (ability to move the extremity), and sensation (ability to feel) distal to the injury. Assessing distal to the injury means assessing further away from the trunk than the injury. For example, if the injury was to the knee, you should assess the pulse, motor function, and sensation in the lower leg or foot. If the injury is to the wrist, you should assess the fingers. Assess the pulse, motor function and sensation both before and after applying a splint, and record the findings. A splint that is placed improperly or secured too tightly may impede circulation. If there is a change in circulation, loosen the splint and reassess. If the circulation does not return, you may need to remove the splint and apply it again.

The bones and joints above and below an injury site must be immobilized with the splint to minimize muscle movement near the injury. Before splinting, cut clothing away to expose the area and make the splint more effective. Open injuries should be dressed and bandaged before application of the splint.

If there is a severe deformity or the extremity is cyanotic or lacks a pulse, the injury should be aligned with gentle traction before splinting in an attempt to regain circulation. If resistance is felt, splint the extremity in the position in which you find it. If no pulse returns in the injured extremity, rapid transport is indicated to prevent possible loss of the extremity. If any bones are protruding through the skin, do not try to replace them, although they may retract when the splint is applied. Splints should be padded to prevent pressure and discomfort to the patient.

When splinting a hand or foot, immobilize it in the position of function. This is the most comfortable position for the hand or foot and requires the least amount of muscle use or stretching. The position of function is a natural resting position. For the hand, place a roll of gauze in the palm to

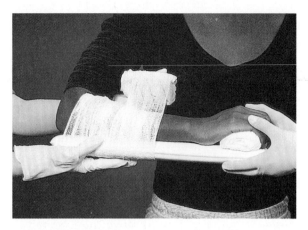

Fig. E-1 For a hand injury, place a roll of gauze in the palm to support and immobilize the hand in the position of function.

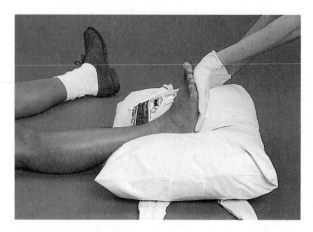

Fig. E-2 For a foot injury, support the sole and immobilize in the position of function.

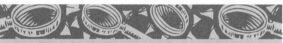

PRINCIPLE E-1 Principles of Splinting

1. Assess pulse, motor function, and sensation distal to the injury before and after splinting, and record your findings.
2. Immobilize the joint above and below the musculoskeletal injury. If the joint is injured, immobilize the bone above and below the injury.
3. Remove or cut away clothing before splinting.
4. Cover open wounds with sterile dressings before splinting.
5. Splint the injury in the position found, unless there is severe deformity or the extremity is cyanotic or lacks a pulse. If these conditions are found, attempt to align the extremity with gentle traction before splinting.
6. Do not intentionally replace protruding bones, but note them in your report.
7. Pad the splint to prevent pressure and discomfort to the patient.
8. Splint the injury before moving the patient unless there are life-threatening situations present.
9. If in doubt whether an injury is present, apply a splint.
10. If the patient has the signs and symptoms of shock, use full-body immobilization, align the patient in the normal anatomical position on a backboard and assist in the transport as soon as possible.

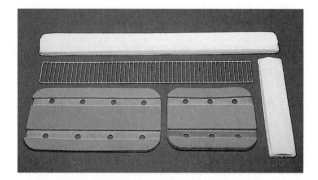

Fig. E-3 Common types of splints include padded-board splints (top and right), ladder splints (middle), and cardboard splints (bottom).

unacceptable to fail to treat an injury that does require splinting. Without an X-ray, it is impossible to differentiate between a broken ankle and a sprain or strain; therefore, you should assume the ankle is broken. Do not waste time trying to identify the actual injury. See Principle E-1 for the principles of splinting.

If the patient is showing the signs and symptoms of shock, align the patient in the normal anatomic position and transport using total body immobilization, including backboard and cervical collar. Do not waste time splinting each injury separately.

SPLINTING EQUIPMENT AND TECHNIQUES

Many types of splints are used to immobilize various musculoskeletal injuries. For all types of splints, remember the general principles previously described.

support the hand. For the foot, support the sole (Figs. E-1 and E-2).

If you are in doubt whether to splint an injury, splint it. Err on the side of caution. It is acceptable to splint an injury that did not need it, but it is

TECHNIQUE E-1 Splinting a Long Bone With a Rigid Splint

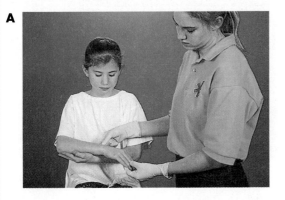
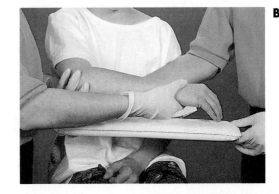
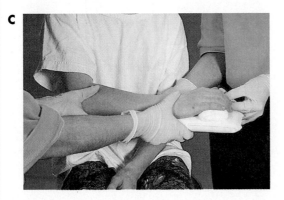
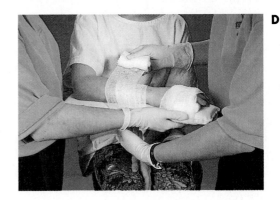

Fig. E-4 Use appropriate personal protective equipment for body substance isolation precautions. **A,** Check the patient's pulse, motor function, and sensation distal to the injury. **B,** Provide manual stabilization and support the injured extremity and maintain gentle traction if indicated while applying the rigid splint. Measure the rigid splint to the extremity. **C,** Pad the open spaces between the splint and the extremity to place pressure evenly over the entire area of the extremity. **D,** Secure the rigid splint to the extremity with cravats or roller gauze tied snugly. Tie the knots over the splint, not the skin, for comfort. Immobilize the joints above and below the injury site. Secure and immobilize the hand or foot in the position of function. Secure the entire injured extremity to the body. Repeat the assessment of pulse, motor function, and sensation distal to the injury.

Rigid splints are nonformable splints. They can be used to support a painful, swollen, and deformed extremity and immobilize the joints or bones above and below the injury. Common examples are padded-board splints, cardboard splints, and ladder splints (Fig. E-3). Technique E-1 describes one method for using rigid splints.

Pneumatic splints are flexible splints that use air to maintain rigidity. Air splints are an example of a pneumatic splint. Vacuum splints are also pneumatic splints that work by removing the air in the splint, so that it becomes rigid and immobilizes the injured extremity (Fig. E-5).

The air splint is applied to the injured area and then inflated with air until it is snug. The air splint

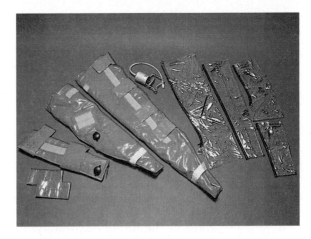

Fig. E-5 Vacuum splints (left) and air splints (right) are commonly used pneumatic splints.

usually has a zipper and is used primarily for injuries below the elbow and the knee. The advantages of the air splint include placing uniform pressure on bleeding areas, and it is comfortable for the patient. The disadvantages of the air splint are that air may leak from the splint or the pressure may change with changes in temperature or altitude. Air splints are difficult to clean, and the method of inflation may compromise body substance isolation precautions.

When using an air splint, cover all wounds with clean dressings before applying the splint. Place the injured extremity within the splint, and inflate the splint by blowing into the valve (Fig. E-6). The port for the air may be cleaned with an alcohol wipe prior to inflation. Some air splints may come with an adapter and a pump to inflate them with air. Using an air splint requires two rescuers, one to support the extremity and one to apply the splint. As when applying any splint, check the patient's pulse, motor function, and sensation distal to the injury before and after application.

Improvised splints, such as pillows, may be used to support joint injuries and are commonly used for ankle injuries. The pillow is wrapped completely around the ankle and secured. The toes are left visible so that assessment may be made of the pulse, motor function, and sensation (Fig. E-7). Cardboard splints are also useful for joint injuries, because they may be cut to form to an angle and then secured in place.

The sling and swathe is a common splinting technique used for a shoulder injury. The arm is placed into the sling and the swathe is wrapped around the arm and the body so that the arm and shoulder cannot move (Fig. E-8). The sling and swathe may be used along with other types of splints for arm injuries (Figs. E-9 and E-10).

Always use properly sized splints. Some devices come in infant and child sizes. Familiarize yourself with the equipment used by your local EMS agency.

RISKS OF SPLINTING

Using splints improperly can lead to complications. If splints are used incorrectly, they may cause more harm than benefit. A splint can compress nerves, tissues, and blood vessels; therefore, the pressure of the splint should be monitored continuously along with the pulse, motor function, and sensation of the injured extremity. A splint applied too tightly on an extremity can reduce distal circulation. An improperly applied

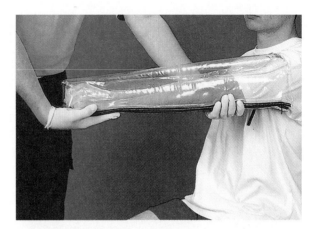

Fig. E-6 An injured arm immobilized by an air splint.

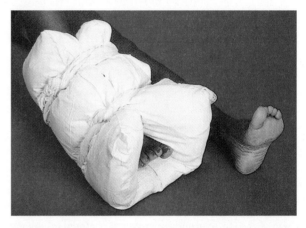

Fig. E-7 A pillow splint is an improvised splint that provides support for an injured ankle or foot.

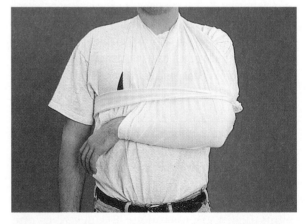

Fig. E-8 A sling and swathe is a common splinting technique for a shoulder injury to prevent movement of the arm and shoulder.

splint can increase bleeding and tissue damage associated with the injury, cause permanent nerve damage or disability, convert a closed injury to an open injury, or increase the pain caused by excessive movement.

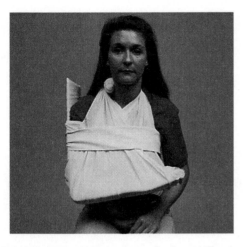

Fig. E-9 A deformed humerus can be immobilized using a sling and swathe.

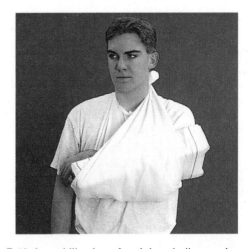

Fig. E-10 Immobilization of an injured elbow using a sling and swathe.

Splinting an injury takes time. If you are not able to complete splinting of a critically injured patient before the ambulance arrives, do not delay treating or transporting to complete splinting. Splinting may be done en route or not at all if the patient has life-threatening injuries. When moving the patient, take extreme care to keep the injury stable.

APPENDIX SUMMARY

INJURIES TO BONES AND JOINTS

Emergency medical care for musculoskeletal injuries includes body substance isolation precautions, airway assessment, control of major bleeding, and care for life-threatening situations. The injured area may be elevated to reduce blood flow to that area, and cold packs may be applied to reduce swelling. Splints can be used to restrict movement and prevent further damage to the injured tissue. Never delay transport of a critical patient to splint an extremity.

SPLINTING

Splinting a painful, swollen, deformed extremity minimizes movement and pain, and helps prevent further damage. Always follow appropriate splinting principles.

When splinting, assess the pulse, motor function, and sensation distal to the injury before and after splinting, and record your findings. Immobilize the joints or bones above and below the injury. Remove or cut away clothing before splinting, and cover any open wounds with sterile

dressings. Splint the injury in the position found unless there is impaired distal circulation or sensation, or the patient has a life-threatening condition. Types of splints include rigid or nonformable splints, pneumatic splints and improvised splints.

Because a splint might compress nerves, tissues, and blood vessels, the pressure of the splint should be checked continually along with the pulse, motor function, and sensation distal to the injury. Excessive movement may cause or aggravate tissue, nerve, vessel, or muscle damage. Do not delay treating or transporting a critical patient to splint.

UNITED STATES DEPARTMENT OF TRANSPORTATION NATIONAL HIGHWAY TRAFFIC SAFETY ADMINISTRATION EMT-BASIC OBJECTIVES

Check your knowledge. Many state EMS agencies use the objectives below to develop First Responder certification examinations. Can you meet them?

COGNITIVE OBJECTIVES

1. State the reasons for splinting.
2. List the general rules of splinting.
3. List the complications of splinting.
4. List the emergency medical care for a patient with a painful, swollen, deformed extremity.

AFFECTIVE OBJECTIVES

5. Explain the rationale for splinting at the scene versus load and go.

6. Explain the rationale for immobilization of the painful, swollen, deformed extremity.

PSYCHOMOTOR OBJECTIVES

7. Demonstrate the emergency medical care of a patient with a painful, swollen, deformed extremity.

Childbirth and Children

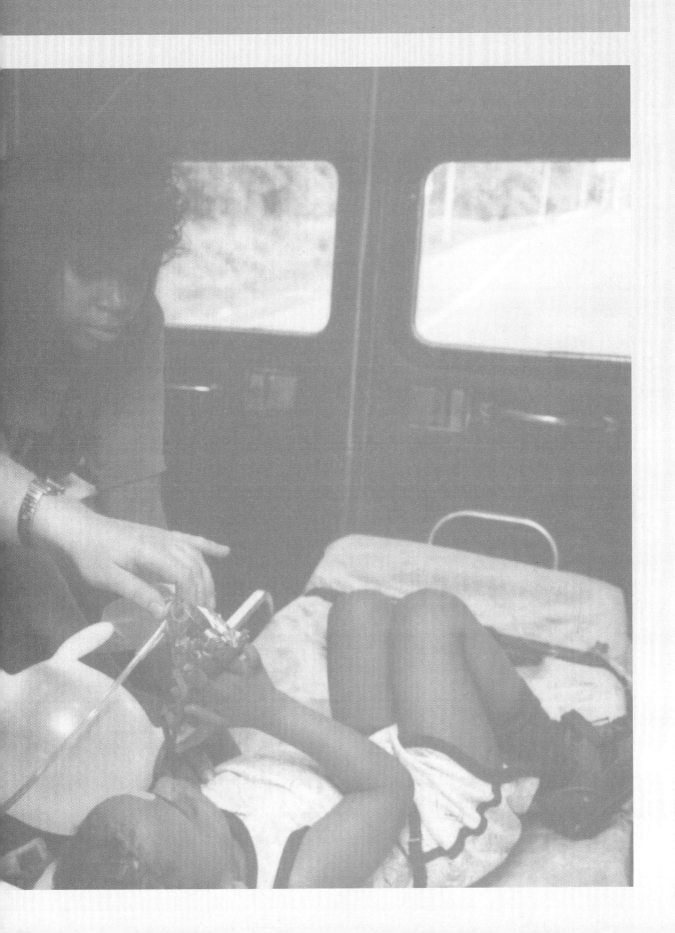

Childbirth

KEY TERMS

Abortion The medical term for any delivery or removal of a human fetus before it can live on its own.

Amniotic sac The membrane forming a closed, fluid-filled sac around a developing fetus.

Birth canal The lower part of the uterus and the vagina.

Bloody show The expulsion of the mucous plug as the cervix dilates, which is sometimes mixed with blood; it often occurs at the beginning of labor.

Cervix The neck of the uterus.

Crowning The stage in which the head of the baby (or other presenting part) is seen at the vaginal opening.

Fetus An unborn, developing baby.

Miscarriage Spontaneous delivery of a human fetus before it is able to live on its own.

Perineum The area of skin between the vagina and anus.

Placenta The fetal and maternal organ through which the fetus absorbs oxygen and nutrients and excretes wastes; it is attached to the fetus via the umbilical cord.

Presenting part The part of the fetus that appears at the vaginal opening first.

Umbilical cord The cord that connects the placenta to the fetus.

Uterus The female reproductive organ in which a baby grows and develops.

Vagina The canal that leads from the uterus to the external opening in females.

FIRST RESPONSE

First Responders Carlos and Sally were teaching an infant CPR class to expectant mothers and fathers at the local YMCA. Halfway through the practice session, one of the women, further along in her pregnancy than most in the class, said she had been experiencing some contractions during the day and that her water had just broken. She said her contractions were strong and regular now. Because she was expecting her third baby, Carlos and Sally knew the delivery might occur soon. Carlos went to call dispatch for an ambulance while Sally assessed the patient.

Although Sally had never assisted with a delivery, she was well educated and knew what questions to ask. When she confirmed that the patient's water had broken and that her contractions were about two minutes apart, Sally and Carlos prepared for delivery on the scene. The closest ambulance was about 45 minutes away, and the baby probably would not wait that long. Sally and Carlos, along with the patient and her husband, were a little nervous, but they knew childbirth is a natural process and is rarely an emergency for the mother or the newborn.

The delivery went well. After the baby was born, the mother, father, and healthy baby girl were all transported to the hospital for evaluation. Carlos and Sally had just participated in one of the most professionally rewarding calls a First Responder can experience.

Although most babies in the United States are born in the hospital, this is not true worldwide. Most babies in the world are not born in any type of medical facility. Birth is a natural process that usually does not require any medical intervention.

When an ambulance is called for a woman in labor, there is usually adequate time for the mother to be transported to the hospital. In some cases, however, First Responders may arrive on the scene to find a woman who is so far along into labor that there is not enough time to get to the hospital before delivery. In situations when prehospital delivery is likely to occur, First Responders must be ready to assist the mother with the delivery.

This chapter discusses what First Responders need to understand to assist with a prehospital delivery, beginning with a description of the anatomy of the woman and the developing baby. Emergency medical care for predelivery emergencies is discussed, as well as the procedure for assisting with a normal delivery. Resuscitation of the newborn and postdelivery care of the mother are included.

REPRODUCTIVE ANATOMY AND PHYSIOLOGY

The anatomy of the human female and the growing baby allow pregnancy and delivery to occur with few problems (Fig. 12-1). The mother's uterus, or womb, is the structure in which the baby grows and develops. The uterus is a muscular organ that eventually contracts and expels the fetus during childbirth. During pregnancy, the cervix, the neck of the uterus, contains a mucous plug. As the cervix dilates (widens) during labor to allow the fetus to pass through, the mucous plug becomes dislodged.

When the muscles of the uterus contract, the fetus is pushed into the birth canal, which consists of the lower part of the uterus and the vagina. The vagina is the canal that leads from the uterus to the external opening in females. The fetus is pushed through the birth canal into the outside world during childbirth. The perineum is the area of skin between the vagina and anus. This skin often tears as a result of the pressure exerted by the fetus during childbirth.

An unborn developing baby is called a fetus. The fetus is nourished through the placenta. The placenta attaches to the wall of the uterus and is composed of fetal and maternal tissue. It is attached to the baby via the umbilical cord. The placenta is an organ that develops during pregnancy. It is not present when a woman is not pregnant and is expelled from the body following childbirth. The placenta is also known as the afterbirth, because it is delivered after the baby is born. The placenta allows oxygen and nutrients to pass from the mother's bloodstream to the fetus. The placenta also allows carbon

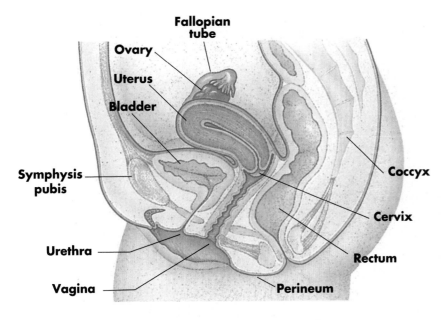

Fig. 12-1 The female reproductive system.

dioxide and waste products to pass from the fetus to the mother for elimination.

The transfer of material from the placenta to the fetus and back to the placenta is accomplished through the umbilical cord. The umbilical cord is an extension of the placenta and contains two arteries and one vein. Blood flows from the fetus to the placenta and back to the fetus. Maternal and fetal circulatory systems are independent of each other, and blood does not flow directly from mother to fetus.

The fetus is surrounded by a bag of fluid, which is called the amniotic sac. The amniotic sac contains 1 to 2 liters of liquid called amniotic fluid. The amniotic fluid cushions the baby and helps protect it from injury. The amniotic sac generally ruptures before childbirth (often described by the patient as "my water broke"). The amniotic fluid lubricates the birth canal during delivery. Figure 12-2 illustrates the anatomic structures of pregnancy.

The fetus grows and develops for approximately 9 months, or 40 weeks. During pregnancy, the mother's uterus expands for the growing fetus (Fig. 12-3, A through D). Her blood volume increases along with the amount of blood traveling through her heart each minute and her heart rate. Her blood pressure decreases slightly and her digestion slows.

LABOR

Labor is the process by which babies are born. Labor is generally divided into three stages, beginning with the first uterine contractions and ending when the placenta is delivered after childbirth (Fig. 12-4).

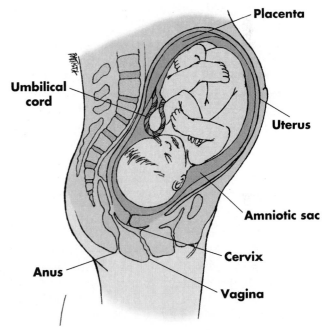

Fig. 12-2 The anatomical structures of pregnancy.

Labor consists of contractions of the walls of the uterus that push the fetus through the cervix and into the birth canal.

FIRST STAGE OF LABOR

The first stage of labor begins with regular contractions of the uterus and continues until the fetus enters the birth canal. During this stage of labor, the cervix must dilate to allow the baby to pass through into the birth canal. As the cervix dilates, mucous and blood may pass through the vagina. This mucous and blood, called the bloody show, is normal. Each contraction thins and shortens the cervix to

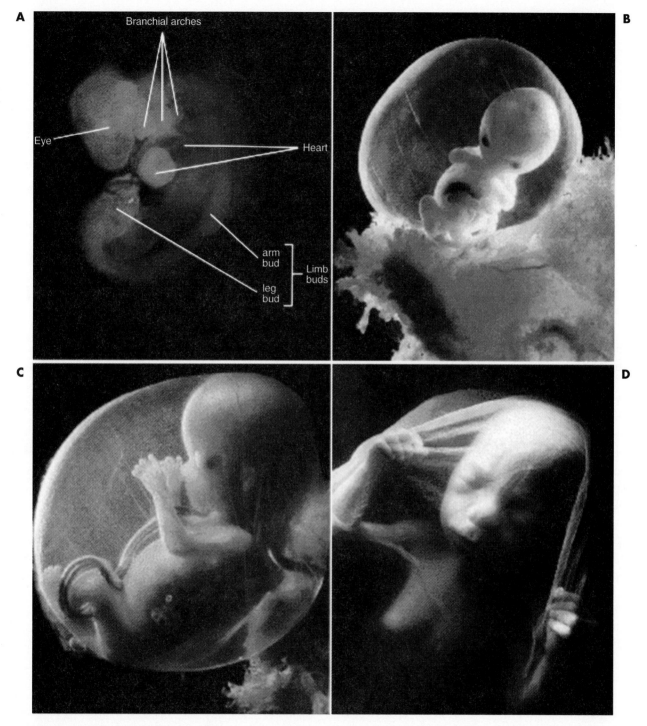

Fig. 12-3 The uterus enlarges and expands to encompass the growing infant. **A,** At 35 days. **B,** At 49 days. **C,** After the first trimester. **D,** At 4 months.

allow the head of the fetus to pass. Once the cervix dilates to approximately 10 cm (4 in.), the head can pass through and the second stage of labor begins.

SECOND STAGE OF LABOR

The second stage of labor begins when the fetus enters the birth canal and ends when the baby is born. Rhythmic contractions of the uterus push the fetus through the birth canal into the vaginal opening. Most babies are born with their head as the presenting part. The **presenting part** is the part that appears at the vaginal opening first. **Crowning** occurs when the head (or other presenting part) bulges against the vaginal opening. When you see

REVIEW QUESTIONS

Reproductive Anatomy and Physiology

Match the terms in the left column with their definitions in the right column.

1. Uterus
2. Cervix
3. Birth canal
4. Perineum
5. Fetus
6. Placenta
7. Amniotic sac
8. Umbilical cord

A. The passageway from the uterus through which the baby is born.
B. The organ where the baby develops.
C. The skin between the vagina and the anus.
D. The neck of the uterus.
E. The organ that allows nutrients to pass from mother to fetus and waste from fetus to mother.
F. The fluid filled sac that cushions the fetus.
G. The connection from the placenta to the fetus.
H. The unborn developing baby.

1.B; 2.D; 3.A; 4.C; 5.H; 6.E; 7.F; 8.G

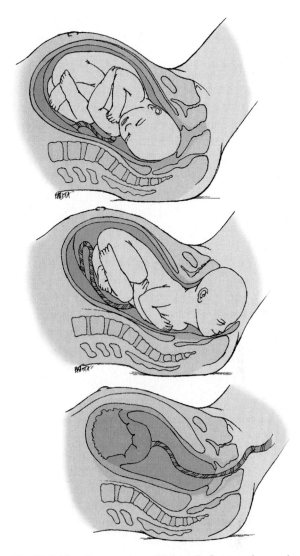

Fig. 12-4 The three stages of labor. **A,** Contraction and dilation. **B,** Baby moves through birth canal and is born. **C,** Delivery of placenta.

crowning, delivery is imminent and you should be prepared for immediate delivery (Fig.12-5).

THIRD STAGE OF LABOR

In the third stage of labor, which starts after the baby is born, the placenta, umbilical cord, and other tissues are delivered. The placenta detaches from the uterine wall and passes through the birth canal. This tissue is still connected to the fetus by the umbilical cord unless the cord has already been cut.

Labor pains occurring with each contraction are normal. Women generally experience pain when the uterus contracts and experience relief from pain as the contraction ends. A support person should be available to help the mother. The father, a friend, or another First Responder should encourage her, help her to breathe regularly through the contractions, and make her as comfortable as possible. The length of normal labor varies greatly among women, depending on the woman's age, previous deliveries, and other individual factors and circumstances. The

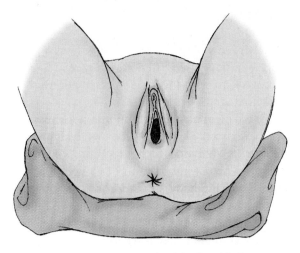

Fig. 12-5 Crowning occurs when the head bulges against the vaginal opening.

length of time a woman spends in labor generally decreases with each delivery.

PREDELIVERY EMERGENCIES

A miscarriage is the delivery of the fetus before it can live independently of the mother. The medical term for this early delivery is abortion, but it is generally referred to as a miscarriage when it occurs spontaneously. A miscarriage usually occurs within the first 3 months of pregnancy. A woman experiencing a miscarriage generally has abdominal cramping that may be severe. She may be bleeding and there may be noticeable vaginal discharge of clots and tissue. Any pads or towels that contain clots or tissue should be transported to the hospital with the patient. Be prepared to treat for shock if the mother exhibits signs and symptoms of hypoperfusion. Along with medical care, emotional support is very important for the mother. Grief is normal and should be expected from both parents.

DELIVERY

Childbirth is not an emergency unless complicating factors are involved. In a normal delivery, your role as a First Responder is to provide support and assistance to the mother as she delivers her child and to provide care and, if necessary, resuscitation to the newborn.

In general, it is best to transport the expectant mother to the hospital unless delivery is anticipated within five minutes. When deciding whether to transport or to assist in delivery on the scene, the following questions will help in making that decision.

1. What is your due date?
2. Is there any bleeding or discharge?
3. Do you have the sensation of having a bowel movement with increasing pressure in the vaginal area?

If the patient answers yes to questions two and three, examine for crowning. If crowning is present, prepare for delivery. If the decision is made to deliver on the scene, take the following precautions. Practicing body substance isolation precautions is a must when you assist in childbirth. Blood and amniotic fluid should be expected and may splash. The mother may feel the need to go to the bathroom, but should not be allowed to use the toilet. The feeling of a bowel movement is common

and is caused by the baby's head pressing against the walls of the rectum. The baby may deliver while she is trying to have a bowel movement.

Do not try to delay the delivery by measures such as holding the mother's legs together. These measures are ineffective and can harm the baby.

Once the decision has been made to assist in delivery on the scene, you must prepare for the delivery. While making these preparations, ask the mother if there is any chance of multiple births. Request more assistance if there is a possibility of two or more babies.

Follow these steps for delivery:

1. Follow body substance isolation precautions.
2. Position the mother by having her lie with her knees flexed, drawn up, and widely separated.
3. Elevate the buttocks with blankets or a pillow (Fig.12-6).
4. Place absorbent, clean material such as towels or pads under the patient's buttocks. Place towels over her legs.
5. When the infant's head appears, place the palm of your hand on top of the delivering baby's head and exert very gentle pressure to prevent explosive delivery.
6. If the amniotic sac does not break or has not broken, tear it with your fingers and push it away from the infant's head and mouth.
7. As the infant's head is being delivered, determine whether the umbilical cord is around

the infant's neck. If it is, attempt to slip the cord over the baby's head. If you are unable to do that, attempt to lessen pressure on the cord.

8. Once the head delivers, support the head as it rotates and suction the baby's mouth and then nostrils two or three times, using a bulb syringe. The bulb syringe should be compressed before placing it in the baby's mouth. Once the bulb syringe is in the mouth, release the bulb and allow the fluids to fill the syringe. Withdraw the syringe and release the contents of the syringe onto a towel. Suction the mouth two or three times and then suction each nostril once or twice. Do not place the bulb syringe in so far that it touches the back of the mouth and gags the baby (Fig. 12-7). If a bulb syringe is not available, wipe the baby's mouth and then the nose with gauze.

9. As the torso and full body are delivered, support the infant with both hands. As the feet are delivered, grasp the feet. Do not pull on the infant.

10. Keep the infant level with the vagina.

11. When the umbilical cord stops pulsating, it should be tied with gauze between the mother and the newborn and the infant may be placed on the mother's abdomen.

12. Wipe blood and mucus from the baby's mouth and nose with sterile gauze; suction the mouth and nose again.

13. Dry the infant, wrap him in a warm blanket, and place the infant on its side with the head slightly lower than the trunk to aid the draining of fluid from the mouth and nose (Fig. 12-8).

14. Rub the baby's back or flick the soles of his feet to stimulate breathing.

15. Record the time of delivery.

16. If there is a chance for multiple births, prepare for the second delivery.

17. Observe for delivery of the placenta. This may take up to thirty minutes.

18. If the placenta is delivered, wrap it in a towel with $3/4$ of the umbilical cord and place in a plastic bag. Keep the bag at the level of the infant.

19. Place a sterile pad over the vaginal opening, lower the mother's legs, and help her hold them together.

There is no need to cut the cord in a normal delivery. Keep the infant warm and wait for additional EMS resources who will have the proper equipment to clamp and cut the cord. Figure 12-9 shows a delivery from crowning through delivery of the shoulder.

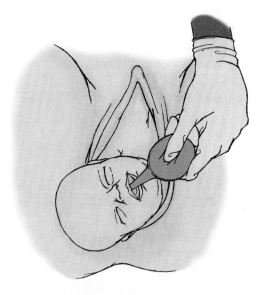

Fig. 12-7 After the infant's head is born, support the head and wipe the mouth and nose. Suction the baby's mouth and nose with a bulb syringe.

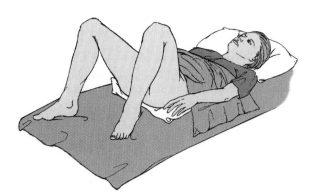

Fig. 12-6 Position the mother for delivery.

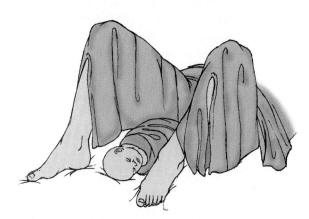

Fig. 12-8 Positioning for newborn infants.

Following delivery, vaginal bleeding of 300 to 500 ml of blood can be expected. This is usually well tolerated by the mother. It is important for the First Responder to be aware of this so as not to cause undue psychological stress on him/herself or the mother. If the mother continues to bleed well beyond the expected amount, it will be necessary to massage the uterus. With the fingers of one hand fully extended, place the palm of the hand on the lower abdomen above the pubic bone and continue to massage this area until the bleeding stops (Fig. 12-10).

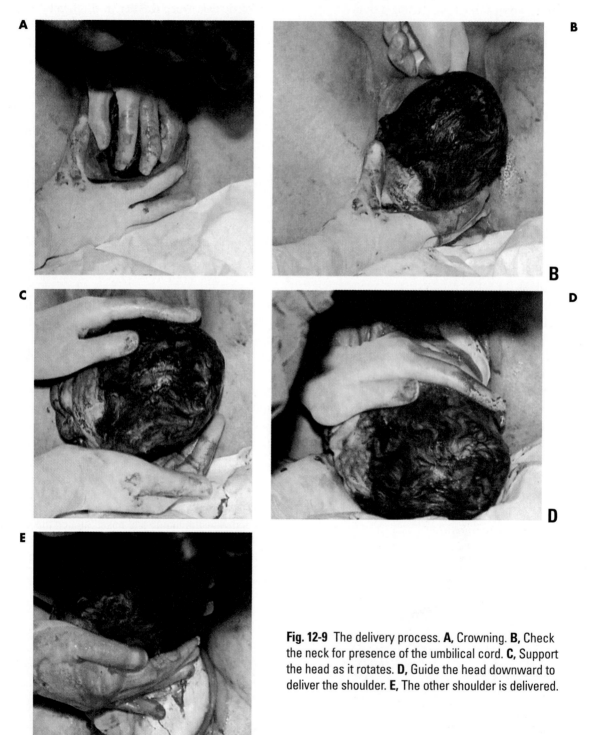

Fig. 12-9 The delivery process. **A,** Crowning. **B,** Check the neck for presence of the umbilical cord. **C,** Support the head as it rotates. **D,** Guide the head downward to deliver the shoulder. **E,** The other shoulder is delivered.

If during delivery, the presenting part is not the head, the delivery may be complicated. The First Responder should tell the mother not to push, and update responding EMS personnel about the situation. Calm and reassure the mother until additional EMS personnel arrive on scene.

ROLE OF THE FIRST RESPONDER

INITIAL CARE OF THE NEWBORN

Immediately after birth, dry the baby and wrap him in a warm blanket with the head covered to preserve body heat. Position the infant on its side with the head slightly lower than the feet to aid

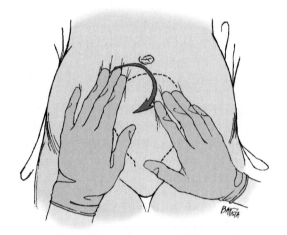

Fig. 12-10 Uterine massage to help control bleeding after delivery.

fluid drainage from the mouth and nose; repeat suctioning as necessary.

Count the infant's respiratory rate. A normal respiratory rate for a newborn is greater than 40 breaths per minute with crying. Next, determine the pulse rate, either at the umbilical cord or the brachial artery. Normal pulse rates for a newborn are greater than 100 beats per minute. If the baby is not breathing flick the soles of the feet or rub the infant's back to stimulate. If the baby does not begin breathing or continues to have difficulty after one minute, you will need to assist the infant's respiratory efforts. This would include ensuring an open and patent airway, and ventilating at a rate of 40 breaths per minute. Reassess the infant's respiratory efforts after one minute. Refer to Chapter 6, "The Airway," for a review of techniques of ventilation.

If the heart rate is less than 80 beats per minute, initiate chest compressions following infant CPR guidelines. Chapter 8, "Circulation," lists the steps of infant CPR.

POST DELIVERY CARE OF THE MOTHER

After initial care for the newborn baby, do not forget to address the mother's needs as a patient. It is important to keep contact with the mother throughout the process. Monitor the mother's respirations and pulse. Replace any blood-soaked sheets and blankets while awaiting transport to the hospital. Remember that delivery is an exhausting process for the mother also. Be attentive to her needs, both physical and psychological.

REVIEW QUESTIONS

Delivery

1. A _____ is the spontaneous delivery of the fetus before it is able to live outside of the womb.

2. After the head delivers, you should check to see if the _____ is wrapped around the baby's neck.

3. The _____ usually delivers within 30 minutes of the baby and should be taken to the hospital to be checked for completeness.

1. Miscarriage; 2. Umbilical Cord; 3. Placenta

REVIEW QUESTIONS

Role of the First Responder

1. Infants who have poor respiratory effort or slow heart beats may require _____ or _____.

2. If the newborn's heart rate is less than _____ beats per minute, begin CPR.

3. List two ways to stimulate a baby who is not breathing:

_____

_____

1. Ventilations, chest compressions; 2. 80; 3. Flick the soles of the feet, rub the back

CHAPTER SUMMARY

REPRODUCTIVE ANATOMY AND PHYSIOLOGY

The fetus grows and develops in the mother's uterus. The fetus is attached to the placenta by the umbilical cord. The fetus is surrounded by a bag of fluid called the amniotic sac.

LABOR

There are three stages of labor. During the first stage, contractions of the uterus cause the cervix to dilate. The baby enters the birth canal and is born during the second stage. The placenta delivers in the third stage of labor. A miscarriage is the spontaneous delivery of a fetus before it is able to survive on its own.

DELIVERY

If the mother feels the need to push, or if she has had any bleeding or discharge, you should evaluate her for crowning. If the baby is crowning, delivery will occur soon, and you should prepare to assist. Take body substance isolation precautions including gloves, eyewear, gown and mask. Prepare the mother for delivery and assist her.

ROLE OF THE FIRST RESPONDER

Dry the infant and wrap him to keep him warm. Position the infant on his side with the head lower than the feet. If the infant is not breathing on its own, you should stimulate it by rubbing the back or flicking the soles of the feet. Ventilate the infant if necessary. If the heartbeat is less than 80 beats per minute, initiate chest compressions. Keep in contact with the mother while caring for the infant.

UNITED STATES DEPARTMENT OF TRANSPORTATION NATIONAL HIGHWAY TRAFFIC SAFETY ADMINISTRATION FIRST RESPONDER OBJECTIVES

Check your knowledge. The National Registry of EMTs and many state EMS agencies use the objectives below to develop First Responder certification examinations. Can you meet them?

COGNITIVE OBJECTIVES

1. Identify the following structures: birth canal, placenta, umbilical cord, amniotic sac.
2. Define the following terms: crowning, bloody show, labor, abortion.
3. State the indications of an imminent delivery.
4. State the steps in the pre-delivery preparation of the mother.
5. Establish the relationship between body substance isolation and childbirth.
6. State the steps to assist in delivery.
7. Describe care of the baby as the head appears.
8. Discuss the steps in delivery of the placenta.
9. List the steps in the emergency medical care of the mother post-delivery.
10. Discuss the steps in caring for a newborn.

AFFECTIVE OBJECTIVES

11. Explain the rationale for attending to the feelings of a patient in need of emergency medical care during childbirth.

12. Demonstrate a caring attitude towards patients during childbirth who request emergency medical services.
13. Place the interests of the patient during childbirth as the foremost consideration when making any and all patient care decisions.
14. Communicate with empathy to patients during childbirth, as well as with family members and friends of the patient.

PSYCHOMOTOR OBJECTIVES

15. Demonstrate the steps to assist in the normal delivery.
16. Demonstrate necessary care procedures of the fetus as the head appears.
17. Attend to the steps in the delivery of the placenta.
18. Demonstrate the post-delivery care of the mother.
19. Demonstrate the care of the newborn.

Infants and Children

KEY TERMS

Child abuse Improper or excessive action by parents, guardians, or caretakers that injures or causes harm to children.

Crowing A harsh noise heard on inspiration.

Grunting A sound made when the patient in respiratory distress attempts to trap air to keep the alveoli open.

Nasal flaring An attempt by the infant in respiratory distress to increase the size of the airway by expanding the nostrils.

Neglect The act of not giving attention to a child's essential needs.

Respiratory distress A clinical condition in which the infant or child begins to increase the work of breathing.

Respiratory failure Clinical condition in which the patient is continuing to work hard to breathe, the effort of breathing is increased, and the patient's condition begins to deteriorate.

Retractions The use of accessory muscles to increase the work of breathing, which appears as the sucking in of the muscles between the ribs and at the neck.

Stridor An abnormal high-pitched inspiratory sound, often indicating airway obstruction.

Sudden infant death syndrome (SIDS) The sudden, unexplained death of an infant, generally between the ages of 1 month and 1 year, for which there is no discernable cause on autopsy.

FIRST RESPONSE

Denise and Sandra were watching the kindergarten children play on the swings during recess. All of the teachers in the elementary school had recently been trained as First Responders. As they watched, a 5-year-old boy fell approximately 5 feet from a swing, landing on his left arm and side. Immediately, both Denise and Sandra felt the adrenaline starting to pump. They heard the little boy cry and ran towards him. The thought of caring for an injured child caused anxiety for both of them, but they knew that they had been well educated for this. They knew to start with the basics of airway, breathing, and circulation. Denise told another teacher to call 9-1-1.

When they reached the child's side, they were both ready to take on the challenge of dealing with the injured child. The ambulance arrived shortly after, and care was transferred to the ambulance crew. Both Denise and Sandra felt comfortable with their skills and were glad they could provide early care for the injured child.

Emergency medical care providers have long been challenged by the unique aspects of caring for ill or injured infants and children. Understanding the anatomical and physiological differences is essential to providing good patient care. It is important that First Responders understand that these patients are not little adults. They are patients with unique anatomy and functional differences that must be considered. Since the percentage of responses involving infants and children is relatively small, First Responders should practice these skills to ensure they are prepared when confronted with an ill or injured infant or child.

Special attention should be given to pediatric patients in areas such as airway management, oxygenation and ventilation, assessment, trauma, and near drowning. Unfortunately, some children are also the victims of abuse and neglect. In these instances, the First Responder must know the necessary steps to deal with these situations.

Finally, First Responders need to deal with parents who are having strong emotional responses because their child is ill or injured. In addition to the parents' emotional response, First Responders must deal with their own feelings associated with caring for an ill or injured child.

THE AIRWAY

ANATOMICAL AND PHYSIOLOGICAL CONCERNS

The most important anatomical and physiological differences in an infant or child relate to the airway. In general, the airway is smaller and more easily blocked by secretions and swelling than an adult's airway. Methods of positioning the airway are different for an infant or child than an adult. Do not hyperextend the neck because the airway is so flexible it may actually become occluded because of kinking.

The infant or child's tongue is relatively large compared to their small mandible and oropharynx. The tongue can easily cause an airway obstruction in unresponsive infants and children when they are lying on their back. A proper head-tilt, chin-lift or jaw thrust maneuver without head-tilt can overcome this problem. Take special care not to place pressure on the soft tissues under the jaw, as this may occlude the airway.

Infants are obligate nose breathers: they do not open their mouth to breathe when their nose is occluded. Suctioning a secretion-filled nasopharynx can improve breathing problems in an infant.

Infants and children can compensate for a breathing problem for a short period of time by increasing the rate and effort of breathing. This increased work of breathing uses a tremendous amount of energy. After a short period of compensating, the child may experience rapid decompensation. This decompensation is characterized by general and muscular fatigue and is a sign of respiratory failure. Because of this, a normal respiratory rate following a fast rate may be a bad sign, especially if the child looks tired or is otherwise doing poorly. Watch for signs of mental status changes, including drowsiness, and unusual tolerance of assessment procedures and treatment.

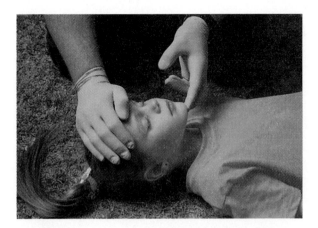

Fig. 13-1 When performing a head tilt on an infant or child, be careful not to hyperextend the neck, but to use the sniffing position. Placing a folded towel under the shoulders may assist in mainainting an open airway.

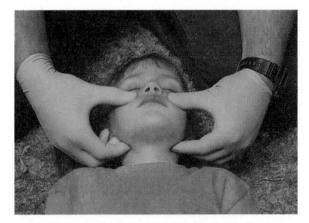

Fig. 13-2 A jaw thrust without head-tilt is performed using the same technique for children and adults.

OPENING THE AIRWAY

Chapter 6, "The Airway," describes the techniques for opening an airway using the head-tilt, chin-lift and the jaw thrust without head-tilt. Because most problems leading to the death of infants and children are related to airway difficulties, you must be knowledgeable and skilled in these techniques.

When a patient loses consciousness, the muscles relax and the tongue may fall back and occlude the airway. Because these structures are attached to the lower jaw, the airway can be opened by lifting up on the lower jaw. This can be accomplished with the head-tilt, chin-lift, or, when trauma is suspected, the jaw thrust without head-tilt. When performing a head-tilt, be careful not to hyperextend the neck. Hyperextension may occlude the small flexible airway of infants and young children. Extend the head or the neck only until the bottom of the nose points straight up. This is referred to as the "sniffing position" for infants and children (Fig. 13-1). Placing a folded towel placed under the shoulder may assist in maintaining an open airway.

When you suspect trauma, use the jaw-thrust without head tilt. With the jaw thrust maneuver, maintain the head in a neutral position, and lift the chin up and out by applying pressure to the angle of the posterior jaw (Fig. 13-2). Be sure to maintain stabilization of the spine while using this technique.

SUCTIONING

Suction may be required to clear the airway of secretions, blood, or vomit. In infants, take care not to stimulate the back of the patient's throat with the suction catheter. This stimulation can dramatically slow the infant's heart rate, cause a gag reflex or vomiting.

Suction the infant or child's airway only as deeply as you can see. In general, use a soft flexible catheter for infants and children. Measure the distance from the corner of the patient's mouth to the angle of the jaw. Place your finger on the catheter at this measurement, and do not insert the catheter any further than this. To ensure that the patient does not become hypoxic, limit the suctioning to 10 to 15 seconds. Rinse the catheter and suction tubing as necessary. When using a suction device on an infant or child, the vacuum should be limited to 80 to 120 mm Hg.

It is important to consider the need for nasal suctioning. In infants, nasal secretions can cause significant upper airway obstruction. The mechanical suction may be used; however, a bulb syringe is simple and effective at removing nasal secretions. When using the bulb syringe, remember to evacuate the air prior to inserting the tip into a nostril.

If the infant or child has an airway obstruction, follow the American Heart Association guidelines for foreign body airway obstruction as outlined in Chapter 6, "The Airway."

USING AIRWAY ADJUNCTS

Oropharyngeal airways are useful in maintaining an open airway in infants and children when the head-tilt, chin-lift or jaw thrust maneuvers are ineffective. Airway adjuncts are not used for initial ventilation efforts.

Oropharyngeal airway

An oral airway should be used following the head-tilt, chin-lift only if the patient is unresponsive and has no gag reflex. If the oral airway is used in a patient who has a gag reflex, the patient may gag and vomit. This can seriously threaten the airway. The preferred method of inserting an oral airway in an infant or child is to use a tongue depressor to insert the airway without rotating. This will reduce the potential for damage to the soft palate. Technique 13-1 demonstrates the steps for inserting an oral airway.

Nasal airways are not recommended for use by First Responders in infants or children.

ASSESSMENT

Once you have sized up the scene and are prepared to assess the patient, perform an initial assessment. Be sure to include the parents in your assessment and management of infants and children. If the parents are agitated, the child may become agitated. If the parents are calm, this may help calm the child. In many cases, you can begin your assessment from a distance. Mental status, respiratory distress, and many signs of shock can be assessed long before you touch the patient. Use your experience and clinical judgment to determine the assessment order that is most appropriate. Always try to assess painful areas last.

In general, begin the assessment from a distance. Observe the child's surroundings and, if the patient is injured, note the mechanism of injury. Form a general impression of the child being well or sick based on overall appearance. Look at the patient as you enter the room. Is he or she interacting appropriately with the people or items in the environment? Does he or she recognize the parents? Infants begin to recognize their parents at about two months of age. Failure to recognize parents is an ominous sign. Is the infant or child quiet and disinterested, or is the infant or child playing with a favorite toy? Is the patient appropriately distressed or scared, or is he or she unusually quiet?

Assess mental status. Mental status changes should be recognized. For example, a child who is uninterested in any activity or person may be experiencing a mental status change. In some cases mental status changes may be indicated simply in the parent's statement that "There is something wrong." Mental status is characterized

TECHNIQUE 13-1 Inserting the Oral Airway in Infants and Children

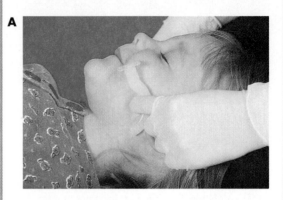

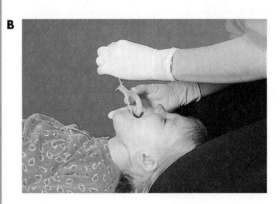

1. Observe body substance isolation precautions.
2. **A,** Select the proper size airway by measuring from the corner of the patient's mouth to the tip of the jaw
3. Position yourself at the top of the patient's head.
4. Open the patient's mouth and use a tongue depressor to move the tongue forward by pushing down against the base of the tongue while lifting upwards.
5. **B,** Insert the airway right side up (with the tip facing toward the floor of the of the patient's mouth).
6. Advance the airway gently until the flange comes to rest on the patient's lips. Be sure not to push the tongue into the back of the throat.
7. Ventilate the patient as needed.

and documented as A = Alert, V = responds to voice, P = responds to pain, and U = unresponsive. For newborns and infants, "responds to voice" can be interpreted as turns to parent's voice, as young children may not obey commands under normal

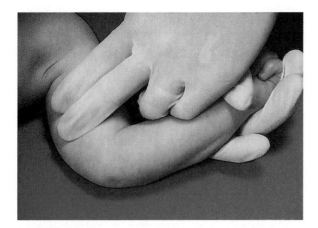

Fig. 13-4 Assessing the brachial pulse in the infant.

circumstances. Try to make eye contact with the child. Observe the child's general response to you, as well as their body tone and position.

If necessary, open the airway. Look, listen, and feel for the presence of breathing. Assess the rate and effort of breathing. Increased effort may be seen as nasal flaring, the use of accessory muscles, retractions, and airway noises. Airway noises include stridor, crowing, and grunting, and they will be explained later in this chapter. Any noise made when breathing indicates a respiratory problem. Evaluate the quality of the cry or speech. If necessary, provide artificial ventilation. Look for equal expansion of both sides of the chest. As part of your respiratory assessment, assess skin color. Look for skin that is pale, blue, or mottled.

Assess circulation using the brachial and femoral pulses in infants (Fig.13-4). In addition to heart rate, assess for quality and equality. The quality of the two pulses should be compared. Any differences may be an indicator of inadequate perfusion. Assess the patient's skin color, temperature, and condition.

Based on the findings from the initial assessment, you can determine a patient priority. Infants and children with altered mental status, respiratory distress, or poor perfusion should be considered priority patients.

How you perform the First Responder physical exam depends on the situation and the patient's age. In general, this examination is often best done in a trunk-to-head approach. The components remain the same as for an adult. Even though you start with the trunk you should still assess for deformities, open wounds, tenderness, and swelling. This approach provides valuable

REVIEW QUESTIONS

The Airway and Assessment

1. Compared to adults, the airways of infants and children are _____ and more easily _____ by secretions and swelling.

2. To open the airway of an injured child, the First Responder should perform the

   _____.

3. When assessing infants and younger children, the First Responder should start with the _____ of the body and finish with the _____.

4. Suctioning in the infant and child should be limited to:

   a. 5-10 seconds

   b. 10-15 seconds

   c. 15-20 seconds

5. The oral airway must be inserted by using a _____ without _____.

1. smaller, obstructed; 2. jaw thrust; 3. trunk, head; 4.B; 5. tongue depressor, rotation

information about the patient while building the infant or child's trust and confidence.

COMMON MEDICAL PROBLEMS IN INFANTS AND CHILDREN

This section reviews common medical emergencies. A solid understanding of the nature of illness and the signs and symptoms related to various illnesses will help prepare you to deal with pediatric medical emergencies in the field.

AIRWAY OBSTRUCTION

Airway obstructions in infants or children are often caused by foreign bodies such as toys or food (Fig. 13-5). It is important to recognize the difference between partial and complete airway obstruction. If you interfere with a child's attempt to clear a partial airway obstruction you could cause a complete obstruction.

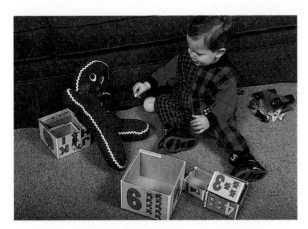

Fig. 13-5 Small removable parts that toddlers can place in their mouths, such as this button from a stuffed toy, can cause airway obstruction.

Partial Obstruction

Partial airway obstructions are characterized by noisy respirations, sometimes with stridor, an abnormal high-pitched inspiratory sound, or crowing, a harsh noise heard on inspiration. The child may be coughing.

Retractions may be seen on inhalation. In general, if the nailbeds and the mucous membranes are pink, that signals good peripheral perfusion. This is because even though there is a partial obstruction, there is adequate air exchange. During your assessment of mental status, these infants and children will often be awake and agitated. If there is cyanosis or altered mental status, there may be a complete obstruction.

Emergency care

To assist an infant or child with a partial airway obstruction, first pay attention to positioning. Allow the child to maintain a position of comfort: assist a younger child to sit up, but do not allow the patient to lie supine, as this may worsen the obstruction. Many children will be more comfortable sitting in their parent's lap. The patient should be transported to a hospital for further evaluation. Be aware that transporting a child sitting in a parent's lap may compromise your ability to assure them safety through proper restraints. Never buckle a lap belt over both parent and child. For safety you may need to separate the parent and child; if so, keep the parent restrained close and within the child's field of vision.

Make every effort to keep the child comfortable; do not agitate the child. Agitation will increase the work of breathing and further complicate the situation. Perform only a limited examination. Avoid assessing blood pressure because this may upset the child. If there is a deterioration in color or mental status, it is most likely that a complete obstruction has probably occurred.

Complete obstruction

Complete airway obstruction is a life-threatening emergency. Any partial airway obstruction with altered mental status or cyanosis should be treated as a complete obstruction. These obstructions require immediate intervention.

Patients with complete airway obstruction have no effective crying and cannot speak. Cyanosis is often present. When complete obstruction follows partial airway obstruction, the infant's or child's efforts to clear the airway by coughing become ineffective. Increased respiratory effort is seen. The patient may lose responsiveness or have an altered mental status.

Clear the airway using the foreign body airway procedures described in Chapter 6, "The Airway." Attempt artificial ventilation using the mouth-to-mask technique.

RESPIRATORY EMERGENCIES

The rapid recognition and treatment of respiratory emergencies in infants and children is the priority equivalent to recognition of shockable rhythms, early CPR, and early defibrillation in adults. More than 80% of all cases of cardiac arrest in infants and children start as respiratory arrest. The two best ways to prevent unexpected death in children are to prevent injuries and to recognize and intervene early in respiratory emergencies.

Respiratory distress

Respiratory distress is a clinical condition in which the infant or child begins to experience an increase in the work of breathing. Infants and children increase the work of breathing at the expense of other physiological functions. Signs and symptoms of respiratory distress include a rapid respiratory rate (greater than 60 breaths per minute in infants, 30 or 40 breaths per minute in children), nasal flaring, retractions, stridor, use of accessory muscles, lethargy, apathy, and grunting. Often see-saw respirations may be present. This is the pronounced use of the abdomen to assist in breathing. The chest is pulled in and the abdomen is thrust out.

Nasal flaring occurs as the infant tries to get more air by increasing the size of the airway by expanding the nostrils. Retractions are contractions of muscles to increase the ability to expand and contract the chest cavity. Retractions appear as the sucking

BOX 13-1   Signs and Symptoms of Respiratory Distress

Respiratory distress is indicated by any of the following:

- Increased rate of breathing
- Nasal flaring
- Intercostal, supraclavicular and subcostal retractions
- Mottled skin color or cyanosis
- Stridor
- Grunting
- Altered mental status (combative, decreased mental status, unresponsive)

BOX 13-2   Signs and Symptoms of Respiratory Failure

Respiratory failure/arrest is the presence of any of the findings of respiratory distress along with any of the following:

- Breathing rate less than 10 per minute in a child
- Breathing rate of less than 20 per minute in an infant
- Limp muscle tone
- Unresponsive
- Slow or absent heart rate
- Weak or absent distal pulses
- Cyanosis

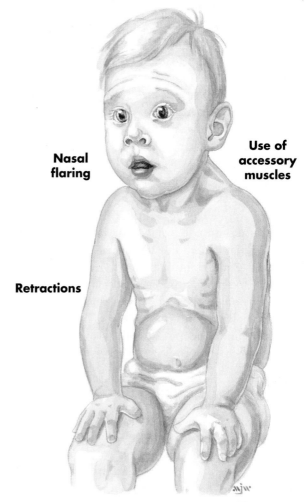

Fig. 13-6 Nasal flaring, retractions, accessory muscle use and positioning are signs of respiratory distress in infants and children.

in of the muscles between the ribs (intercostal muscles), at the neck (supraclavicular muscles) and below the margin of the rib (subcostal muscles). Retractions occur as the effort of breathing increases (Fig. 13-6). Grunting is an expiratory sound made when the patient attempts to trap air to keep the alveoli open. Box 13-1 lists the signs and symptoms of respiratory distress.

Respiratory Failure

If uncorrected, respiratory distress can progress to respiratory failure. In this clinical condition, the patient is continuing to work hard to breathe, and the patient's condition begins to deteriorate. As the work of breathing increases, the infant or child will become tired and no longer able to compensate for respiratory distress. Respiratory failure is seen in the combination of the signs and symptoms of respiratory distress with decreased peripheral perfusion, cyanosis, and mental status

changes. Box 13-2 lists the signs and symptoms of respiratory failure.

If respiratory failure is not treated, the patient will become too tired to breathe. A complete failure of the respiratory system will occur. As the infant or child fatigues or shows signs of decompensation, the First Responder must begin more aggressive interventions.

Role of the First Responder

Begin with a scene size-up and initial assessment. Complete a physical exam as needed.

Regardless of the origin of the clinical condition presented, the goal is to restore effective respiratory function. The easiest way to correct this problem is first to recognize the seriousness of the condition. Act quickly and calmly to avoid upsetting the child or the parents.

In cases of respiratory failure, the patient is focused on breathing. When the patient focuses on breathing they will not resist your interventions. The child should be allowed to remain in a position of comfort. Make sure an ambulance is en route and notify the crew of the patient's condition.

If the respiratory failure progresses, you will need to ventilate the child. This will be done with the child in a supine position. If the child is able to struggle against being placed in this position and your assistance with ventilation, the child does not need to be ventilated. In all cases of respiratory arrest, your goal is to prevent cardiac arrest. Immediately begin to ventilate the child at one breath every three seconds. Airway management and ventilation are the highest priority for these patients. Patients in respiratory arrest should be transported rapidly to a facility capable of dealing with this emergency. Perform an ongoing assessment if the ambulance has not yet arrived. Carefully monitor the patient's respiratory efforts and heart rate.

CIRCULATORY FAILURE

Shock is the failure of the cardiovascular system to supply adequate oxygenated blood to the vital organs. If uncorrected, it can rapidly lead to death. Attention to assessment findings helps you identify this condition. Shock in infants and children rarely results from a cardiac problem. Common causes include dehydration from vomiting and/or diarrhea, trauma, blood loss, and infection.

When assessing the infant or child, be alert for the following circulatory signs and symptoms. As the body attempts to compensate, respirations become rapid, and the skin becomes pale, mottled, cool, and clammy. The pulse becomes rapid and distal pulses may be weak or absent compared to central pulses. You may see mental status changes ranging from agitation and disorientation to unresponsiveness.

Role of the First Responder

The goal in the management of shock is to transport the patient to a facility capable of establishing vascular access and rapidly administering fluid. In some EMS systems this may be accomplished by ALS providers; for others this requires transport to a hospital by EMS personnel. Your actions at the scene must be rapid and organized. After completing the scene size-up, perform an initial assessment. During the initial assessment, ensure a patent airway. Be prepared to artificially ventilate. Manage bleeding if pre-

sent. Keep the patient warm. Carefully monitor the patient's pulse, and begin chest compressions if necessary.

SEIZURES

Seizures represent a nervous system malfunction and are among the most common complaints seen by EMS providers in infants and children. Some infants and children have chronic seizures; others have seizures because of acute illness or injury. There are many types and causes of seizures including chronic medical conditions, rapid rise of fever, infections, poisoning, low blood sugar, head injury or other trauma, decreased levels of oxygen, and unknown causes. Inadequate breathing and/or altered mental status may occur following a seizure.

The role of the First Responder is to support the patient's vital functions and prevent the patient from injuring themselves. Do not worry about determining the cause of the seizure. Be alert for violent muscle contractions called convulsions. Keep in mind that not all seizures have this violent muscle contraction. Seizures may be brief or prolonged. Seizures must be considered a serious emergency, however, seizures themselves are rarely life-threatening.

When gathering a history concerning seizures be sure to include the following questions: Has the child had previous seizures? Does the child take anti-seizure medications? Is it possible that the child ingested any other medications? If the answer to either of the last two questions is yes, the First Responder should determine whether the medication was taken as prescribed and also whether or not this seizure is similar to previous seizures.

Role of the First Responder

Following the completion of scene size-up, the initial assessment and physical exam (as needed), protect the patient from the environment. Move any objects that the patient might come in contact with during the seizure. Ask bystanders, with the exception of the parents, to leave the area. Ensure a patent airway. Never restrain a seizing patient or put anything in their mouth. Patients who are seizing will often have significant oral secretions, so have suction available. If the patient is bluish, assure an adequate airway and begin ventilation if possible. Observe and describe the seizure activity to EMS personnel who will be transporting the patient to the hospital.

Following the seizure, place the patient in the recovery position if there is no possibility of spinal trauma. If there is a partial airway obstruction, correct head positioning, check for a foreign body, and consider insertion of an airway. Although brief seizures are usually not harmful, there may be a dangerous underlying condition. If a seizure lasts for more than 5 to 10 minutes, a specific anti-seizure medication may be required. Comfort, calm, and reassure the patient and family that an ambulance is on the way.

ALTERED MENTAL STATUS

Another common medical condition that First Responders may encounter in an infant or child is altered mental status. There are many common causes of altered mental status; no one cause predominates in infants or children. Altered mental status may be caused by low blood sugar, poisoning, seizure, infection, head trauma, decreased oxygen levels, and shock (hypoperfusion).

Altered mental status in infants and young children may be characterized by a lack of an appropriate response to the environment or persons, lack of interest in items in the environment, and failure to recognize parents. As with adults, the AVPU acronym can be used to assess and communicate the level of responsiveness in infants and children.

Role of the First Responder

Support the patient. Do not worry about trying to determine a specific cause of the altered mental status, except by obtaining a patient history. Maintain an open airway. Place the patient in the recovery position if there is no possibility of spinal trauma. Have suction available. If the patient is cyanotic, ensure a patent airway and artificially ventilate. Comfort and reassure the child's parents that an ambulance is on the way. Complete ongoing assessments as needed.

SUDDEN INFANT DEATH SYNDROME (SIDS)

Sudden infant death syndrome (SIDS) is the sudden death of an infant who is generally less than 1 year old. Infants who have died from SIDS are often discoverd early in the morning. This is a death not apparently related to anything in the infant's history and remains unexplained by a thorough autopsy. SIDS is the leading cause of death in infants less than 1 year of age.

Role of the First Responder

Unless the baby is stiff, try to resuscitate the infant. Follow good basic life support procedures and alert the responding EMS personnel of the

REVIEW QUESTIONS

Common Medical Problems in Infants and Children

1. Define respiratory distress, and list possible signs and symptoms.

_____

_____

_____

2. Define respiratory arrest, and list possible signs and symptoms.

_____

_____

_____

3. Management of the seizure patient includes which of the following?
   1. Maintaining airway
   2. Assuring adequate ventilation
   3. Maintaining circulation
   4. Protecting the patient from his environment

   A. 1 and 3
   B. 2 and 4
   C. 1, 2, and 3
   D. 1, 2, 3, and 4

4. Management efforts of sudden infant death syndrome include:
   1. Attempting to resuscitate the infant
   2. Transport of the infant to an appropriate facility
   3. Supporting the parents
   4. Telling the parents that they performed CPR incorrectly

   A. 1 and 3
   B. 2 and 4
   C. 1, 2, and 3
   D. 1, 2, 3, and 4

1. Respiratory distress is a clinical condition in which the infant or child begins to increase the work of breathing. Signs and symptoms: Nasal flaring, intercostal retraction (chest muscles), supraclavicular, subcostal retractions, stridor, use of abdominal muscles, audible wheezing, grunting, increased respiratory rate.; 2. Respiratory arrest is the result of respiratory failure. Signs and symptoms: Breathing rate less than 10 per minute, limp muscle tone, unconscious, slow or absent heart rate, weak or absent distal pulses.; 3. D; 4. C

infant's condition. Be especially observant of scene details and document well. Unfortunately, some infants who seem to be victims of SIDS are actually victims of abuse. Your documentation may be critical to any investigation that is conducted.

The death of a child is very difficult for parents and health professionals. Parents experience intense feelings of guilt, anger, denial, and disbelief. The initial reaction may range from hysteria to complete silence. It is essential to allow the family to express their grief. Be careful to avoid comments that might suggest blame to the parents. Be prepared to provide emotional support to the parents. Some EMS and law enforcement agencies provide bereavement teams to help families deal with their emotional trauma. Check to see if any agencies in your area provide this service.

This is an extremely emotional event for the First Responder. Do not hesitate to consider the need for and request critical incident stress debriefings for you and others involved (see Chapter 2, "Well-Being of the First Responder"). Communicating these feelings with one another can greatly reduce the stress.

For additional information about SIDS, contact the National Sudden Infant Death Syndrome Foundation (1-301-459-3388), or your local SIDS chapter.

TRAUMA

Trauma is a leading cause of death in children and adolescents. Blunt trauma is most common, although unfortunately, in our society, penetrating trauma is on the rise. In infants and children, the injury patterns are different than those in adults. Because the child is smaller, the traumatic forces are more generalized and may spread throughout the body rather than dissipating over a small area. Often more than one body system is involved. With the small size and the closeness of internal organs, more energy is transmitted to more organs. The bones of a child are less calcified and are more resilient. This makes the musculoskeletal system less likely to absorb the impact of trauma. In addition, there may be more significant internal damage without serious outward signs (Fig. 13-7).

Children are often injured in motor vehicle crashes. If the infant or child is not restrained in an infant or child car safety seat, or if the seat is

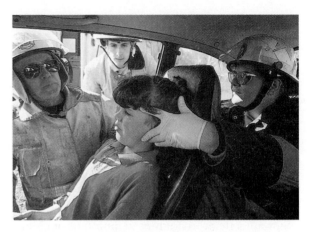

Fig. 13-7 Children who have been injured will often initially appear to be fine, but they deteriorate more rapidly than adults. Your treatment should therefore be based on the mechanism of injury and suspicion of internal injuries.

secured improperly, they often have head and neck injuries. When improperly restrained they often have abdominal and lower spine injuries. Air bag deployment may cause facial trauma. Children may be injured as pedestrians or bicycle riders who are struck by vehicles, resulting in head, spinal, and abdominal trauma. Children may also be injured in falls from a height, as a result of burns, from sports injuries and as a result of child abuse. The following sections describe certain common injuries and their appropriate emergency medical care.

HEAD INJURY
The head is proportionally larger in infants and children than adults. Head injury is the most common cause of death in pediatric trauma patients. Unfortunately, many severe injuries result in death regardless of the treatment given.

Vomiting is common in head injuries, and, therefore, the airway must be protected. The most common cause of decreased oxygen in unresponsive head injury patients is the tongue obstructing the airway. For this reason, the jaw-thrust technique is critically important. Respiratory arrest is common secondary to severe head injuries and may occur during transport.

CHEST INJURY
Suspect chest injury based on the mechanism of injury. Children have soft, pliable ribs. When the child is injured in the chest, the resiliency of the

chest wall allows the forces to be transferred to the heart, lungs, and blood vessels. There may be significant internal injuries without obvious external signs. If abrasions or contusions are present on the chest, they signal an increased risk of internal chest injury.

ABDOMINAL INJURY

The abdomen is a common site of injury to infants and children. Often the injury is not obvious. Always suspect internal injuries when evaluating trauma patients. Always consider abdominal injury in a deteriorating trauma patient without external signs of trauma or blood loss. The abdomen may collect a lot of blood that cannot be seen. Distension may be present.

EXTREMITY INJURY

Infants and children are not exempt from extremity injuries. In cases of extremity injury, provide manual stabilization as in injuries to adult patients.

For all trauma patients, begin with a scene size-up and initial assessment. Note the mechanism of injury. Complete a physical exam, looking for specific injuries. Have your partner hold the child's head in a neutral position and do not move the patient. Make sure the patient has an open airway and is breathing adequately. If you need to open the airway, use the jaw thrust without head-tilt. Have suction ready. If there are injuries to the extremities, stabilize them in the position you find them until they can be splinted. Complete ongoing assessments until transporting EMS personnel arrive.

CHILD ABUSE AND NEGLECT

Child abuse is an improper or excessive action by parents, guardians, or caretakers that injures or causes harm to an infant or child. This includes direct physical abuse, sexual abuse, and emotional battery. Some children may also be neglected. Neglect is giving insufficient attention or respect to the infant or child, which may result in problems such as poor nutrition, inappropriate exposure to environmental conditions, or inadequate health care. You must be aware of these conditions to recognize the problem. It is estimated that 2.5% of all American children are abused or neglected, and the number is growing.

REVIEW QUESTIONS

Trauma

1. Which of the following areas is most often injured in infants and children?
   A. Head
   B. Chest
   C. Abdomen
   D. Extremities
2. When assessing an injured infant or child with deteriorating perfusion, the First Responder should suspect hidden injuries in the _____?
   A. Head
   B. Chest
   C. Abdomen
   D. Extremities

1.A; 2.C

SIGNS AND SYMPTOMS OF ABUSE AND NEGLECT

You should be able to recognize the signs and symptoms of abuse so that you can report situations as necessary and give appropriate treatments. Boxes 13-3 and 13-4 list signs and symptoms of abuse and neglect. Central nervous system injuries are most lethal, such as those caused by vigorous shaking of a baby. In this type of injury, there are rarely external signs of injury. The term "shaken baby syndrome" has been applied to this type of injury.

ROLE OF THE FIRST RESPONDER

Remember that the care of the infant or child is most important. Do not accuse parents or caretakers on the scene. Accusation and confrontation delay transportation and patient care. Provide appropriate medical care based on the signs and symptoms present and provide objective information to the transporting EMS personnel.

Every state has reporting requirements for child abuse and neglect. Your report will set into motion the local agency responsible for investigating the problem. Keep in mind that your report should be objective. Include pertinent environmental findings from the scene. Document potential significant remarks from

BOX 13-3 Signs and Symptoms of Abuse

- Multiple bruises in various stages of healing.
- Injury inconsistent with the mechanism described by parent or caretaker.
- Mechanism of injury inconsistent with child's developmental characteristics. Examples: 2-week-old rolling off of a bed, 7-month-old pulling a pot off of the stove.
- Repeated calls to the same address.
- Patterns of injury
    Whip marks
    Hand prints
- Fresh burns
    Untreated burns
    Scalding burns
    Dip pattern burns (consistent with an extremity dipped into hot water)
- Parents or caretakers who seem inappropriately unconcerned.
- Conflicting histories given by parents or caretakers.
- The child being afraid to discuss how the injury occurred.
- Central nervous system (CNS) injuries.
    Unresponsive or seizure patients
    Severe internal injuries
    No evidence of external injuries

BOX 13-4 Signs and Symptoms of Neglect

- Lack of adult supervision.
- Malnourished appearing child.
- Unsafe living environment.
- Untreated chronic illness; e.g., asthmatic patient not taking medication.
- Untreated soft tissue injuries.

caregivers in quotes. Report only what you see and what you hear — not what you think. Take a helpful rather than vindictive approach to the parent.

REACTIONS TO ILL AND INJURED INFANTS AND CHILDREN

Many First Responders feel anxiety when dispatched to a call involving an ill or injured child. This anxiety often comes from a lack of experience

REVIEW QUESTIONS

Child Abuse, Neglect and Reactions to Ill and Injured Infants and Children

1. Define the term child abuse:

   _____

   _____

   _____

2. The most lethal injuries from child abuse are:
   A. Burns
   B. Extremity trauma
   C. Brain injuries
   D. Spinal injuries

3. It is important to be aware of child abuse so that the First Responder can:

   _____

4. A First Responder is having nightmares following a serious injury to an infant. The First Responder should:
   A. Quit, because these situations occur all the time.
   B. Try to take every call involving children to make the nightmares go away.
   C. Openly discuss these feelings and fears.
   D. Ignore the nightmares, they will go away.

1. Child abuse is improper or excessive action so as to injure or cause harm by parents, guardians or caretakers.; 2. C.; 3. Recognize the signs and symptoms and report suspicious cases.; 4. C

treating children or a fear of failure. First Responders who have children of their own often experience stress from identifying the patient with their own child. Cases of child abuse or neglect or dealing with a child who is seriously injured or dies is especially difficult. Chapter 2, "Well-Being of the First Responder," describes measures you can take to manage the stress resulting from these situations. A debriefing after the event can help you think about your emotions.

Remember that you have skills that you can apply to children. Much of what you have learned about adults applies to children, but you need to remember the differences.

If you rarely see infants and children in your EMS practice, staying prepared is important. Often a local pediatrician can assist you in refining these skills. Observe normal children of all ages. Finally, consider every patient encounter with an infant or child as a learning experience. Remember that most of the children using EMS are not gravely ill or injured and you will be able to help them. Allow yourself to enjoy the time you spend with your smallest patients.

CHAPTER SUMMARY

AIRWAY

Anatomical and physiological concerns related to airway are the most important. In general, airways are smaller and more easily obstructed. Positioning the airway is different; take caution not to hyperextend the neck as this may occlude the airway. The tongue is relatively large in infants and young children. It occupies a proportionally larger amount of space. Proper positioning is important in these patients.

Airway adjuncts may be used to assist in maintaining an open airway. Insert an oral airway using a tongue depressor.

ASSESSMENT

Assessment of the infant or child begins from a distance. Use your general impression to decide if the child is sick or well. In general, use a trunk-to-toe-to-head approach in infants and young children. Assess the airway, breathing, and circulation of the child.

COMMON PROBLEMS IN INFANTS AND CHILDREN

The first priority when dealing with ill infants and children is airway and breathing. The leading cause of death in infants and children is an uncorrected respiratory problem. Follow the proper sequence for relieving a foreign body airway obstruction.

Respiratory failure is the next step in the progression of respiratory distress. Respiratory failure/arrest is characterized by an increased or decreased respiratory rate, cyanosis, decreased muscle tone, and mental status changes. These patients should have airway positioning as a top priority. Ventilation may be absent or just inadequate. Ensure airway patency and provide ventilation.

Other medical emergencies in infants and children include altered mental status, shock, and seizures. In general, the First Responder will provide care that supports the vital functions. Ensure an open airway, have suction available, and support ventilation. Make sure an ambulance is en route and notify the crew of the patient's condition.

TRAUMA

Trauma is a leading cause of death for children and adolescents. The pattern of injury will be different than in adults. Because of the smaller size, multiple body systems may be involved. Management of injuries is similar to that for adults, however, it is important to have appropriately sized equipment. Vehicular trauma, burns, and falls are the most common causes of childhood trauma. Head injuries are common. Chest injury should be suspected based on mechanism of injury. It is possible to have a significant chest injury without obvious external signs. Abdominal injuries are common and are often hidden. The First Responder must suspect abdominal injury in any trauma patient who is deteriorating without obvious external injury.

CHILD ABUSE AND NEGLECT

The First Responder must be aware that child abuse and neglect do occur. The First Responder must be able to recognize the signs and symptoms to be able to identify abuse or neglect. The First Responder must remain objective and provide appropriate medical care. It is important to understand and follow your local reporting procedures and requirements.

REACTIONS TO ILLNESS AND INJURED CHILDREN

Realize that most of your First Responder skills for adults also apply to infants and children. Take time to gain additional experience and knowledge related to infants and children. Use every opportunity to provide care to an infant or child as a learning experience.

UNITED STATES DEPARTMENT OF TRANSPORTATION NATIONAL HIGHWAY TRAFFIC SAFETY ADMINISTRATION FIRST RESPONDER OBJECTIVES

Check your knowledge. The National Registry of EMTs and many state EMS agencies use the objectives below to develop First Responder certification examinations. Can you meet them?

COGNITIVE OBJECTIVES

1. Describe differences in anatomy and physiology of the infant, child, and adult patient.
2. Describe assessment of the infant or child.
3. Indicate various causes of respiratory emergencies in infants and children.
4. Summarize emergency medical care strategies for respiratory distress and respiratory failure/arrest in infants and children.
5. List common causes of seizures in infants and children.
6. Describe management of seizures in infants and children.
7. Discuss emergency medical care of the infant and child trauma patient.
8. Summarize the signs and symptoms of possible child abuse and neglect.
9. Describe the medical/legal responsibilities in suspected child abuse.
10. Recognize need for First Responder debriefing following a difficult infant or child transport.

AFFECTIVE OBJECTIVES

11. Attend to the feelings of the family when dealing with an ill or injured infant or child.
12. Understand the provider's own emotional response to caring for infants or children.
13. Demonstrate a caring attitude towards infants and children with illness or injury who require emergency medical services.
14. Place the interests of the infant or child with an illness or injury as the foremost consideration when making any and all patient care decisions.
15. Communicate with empathy to infants and children with an illness or injury, as well as with family members and friends of the patient.

PSYCHOMOTOR OBJECTIVES

16. Demonstrate assessment of the infant and child.

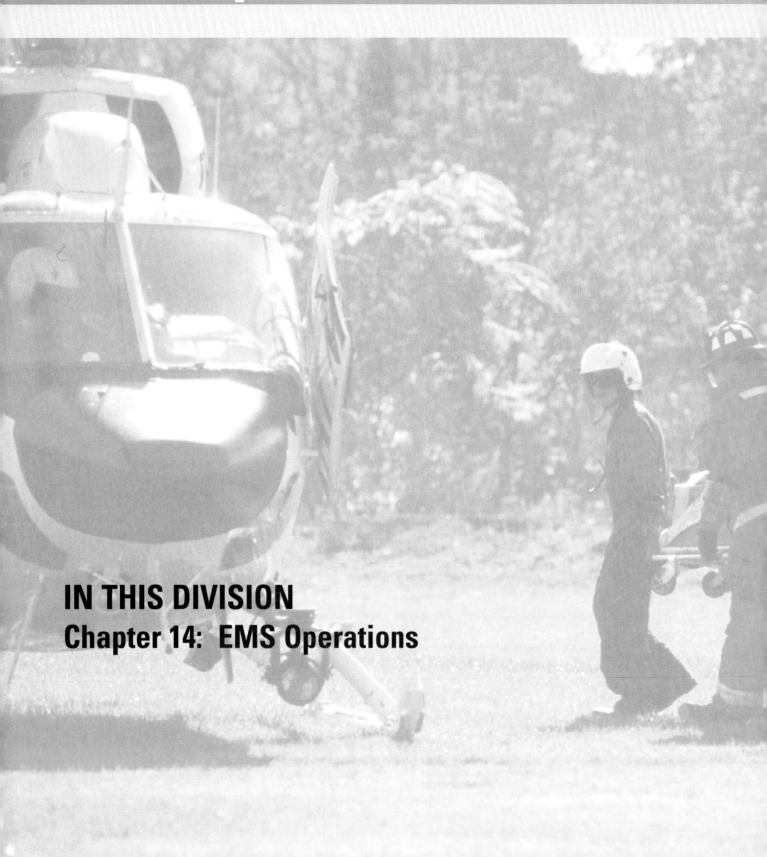

EMS Operations

IN THIS DIVISION
Chapter 14: EMS Operations

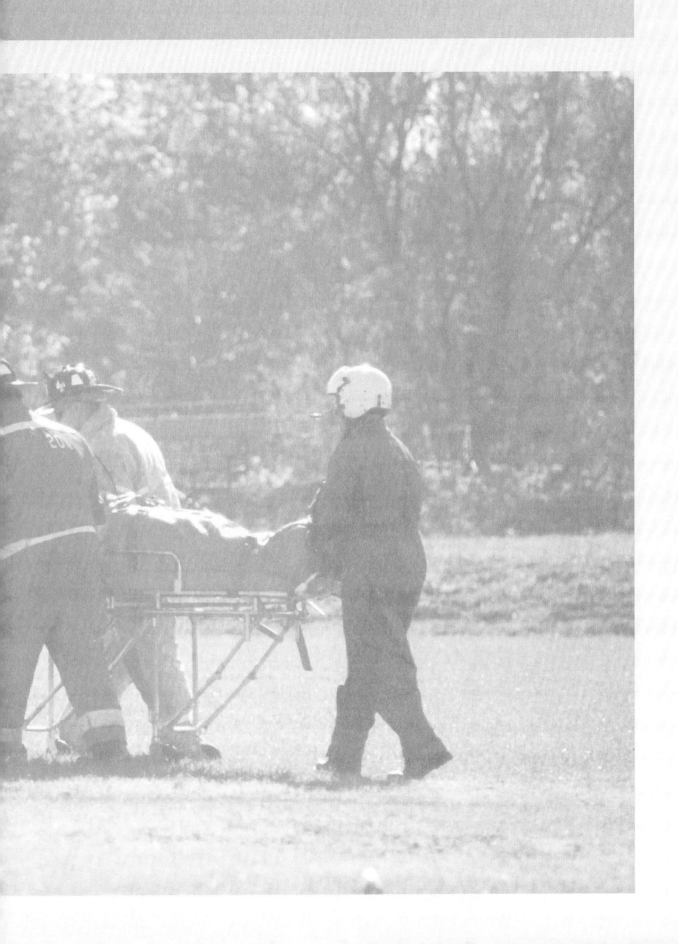

EMS Operations

KEY TERMS

Extrication The process of removing a patient from entanglement in a motor vehicle or other situation in a safe and appropriate manner.

Hazardous material Any substance or material that can pose an unreasonable risk to safety, health, or property.

Incident management system A system for coordinating procedures to assist in the control, direction, and coordination of emergency response resources.

Placard An information sign with symbols and numbers to assist in identifying the hazardous material or class of material.

Triage A method of categorizing patients into treatment or transport priorities.

FOURTEEN

FIRST RESPONSE

The shift was about to begin for Firefighter/First Responders Jane and Roy. They arrived at the station a few minutes early to prepare for their workday. In the past, they sometimes began a shift without adequate time to check the equipment, but this time they planned ahead. Roy began to inventory the medical supplies, checking that there were adequate supplies for an emergency call and that the battery-operated equipment was functioning properly. At the same time, Jane was inspecting the mechanics of the vehicle. She completed the daily checklist, recording fluid levels, checking tire pressure, and assuring that all lights and warning devices were functioning properly.

With the vehicle check complete, Jane and Roy stored their personal protective equipment and checked to see that the street maps were available. They reported to dispatch that they were in service and available. As they headed to the kitchen for a glass of orange juice, the radio interrupted: "Truck 37, respond to 1818 Elm Street... First Responder Assignment with Medic 5104, unknown problem; patient is unresponsive, unknown if breathing. Call-back in progress." As they returned to the unit, they were confident they were prepared for the call.

Just as competent patient care skills are critical, nonmedical operational skills are equally important. As a First Responder, you need a solid understanding of the skills required for all phases of an EMS response, as well as an understanding of your roles and responsibilities in each phase. As you read this chapter, please remember that it is intended only as an overview of ambulance operations. You should seek additional educational programs in emergency vehicle operations and assistance from your EMS service.

PHASES OF AN EMS RESPONSE

A typical EMS response consists of nine stages or phases: 1) preparation for the call; 2) dispatch; 3) en route to the scene; 4) arrival at the scene; 5) transferring the patient to the ambulance; 6) en route to the receiving facility; 7) arrival at the receiving facility; 8) en route to the station; and 9) the post-run phase. First Responders are generally not involved in the "en route to the receiving facility" phase or the "arrival at the receiving facility" phase. Each phase blends into the next, but you have a clear role in each.

PREPARATION FOR THE CALL

Preparation for the call refers to the phase before an EMS response, during which you prepare to respond. This is the phase that allows you to check that all equipment is completely stocked in the emergency vehicle (Fig. 14-1), that the unit is mechanically sound (Fig. 14-2), and that you are mentally and physically prepared to respond to an emergency call.

As a First Responder, you have a responsibility to yourself, your family, your partner, and your patient to be mentally and physically fit to respond to any emergency call. This includes a proper diet and exercise as described in Chapter 2, "The Well-Being of the First Responder." In addition to your physical and mental status, you must remain prepared to respond through skills and knowledge learned and maintained in your initial First Responder program and continuing education programs.

Continuing education is extremely important in emergency medical services, and you should attend as many additional classes as possible. Discussing operations and patient care experiences with other EMS personnel is also beneficial. Prehospital emergency care is a dynamic field that continually evolves along with trends and advances in medicine. You must remain flexible and open to new ideas and procedures while progressing in your EMS career.

The emergency vehicle must also be prepared to respond to any call, and must always be stocked with medical and nonmedical supplies. Your EMS system, along with state and local regulations, dictates what specific equipment is required in the vehicle (Fig. 14-3). Most EMS services stock the typical emergency vehicle with a wide range of basic medical supplies (Box 14-1).

Besides medical supplies, certain nonmedical supplies are required for the safe and efficient operation of a First Responder unit. Many states and local governments mandate specific safety equipment and personal protective equipment that First Responder services should have on the unit. This equipment includes gloves, gowns, masks, and protective eye wear. First Responders should also have the appropriate gear to respond to a rescue situation.

Other beneficial nonmedical supplies and equipment include local street maps, preplanned routes, DOT Emergency Response Guidebooks, binoculars, and patient care reports. As a First Responder, you should be familiar with your response area, including a basic knowledge of traffic patterns, one-way streets, and alternate routes to receiving facilities.

EMS personnel should be available to respond to an emergency call at any time. The recommended minimum staffing for an ambulance is one EMT in the patient compartment and one qualified to drive the emergency vehicle. Some services require two EMTs in the patient compartment. Review the local policies and requirements in your area to determine your role in the EMS system.

DISPATCH

Dispatch is a critical phase of an emergency response. Many dispatch centers have a central access number, often "9-1-1." If this access number is not available in your area, a specific number is usually available for the public to reach the EMS

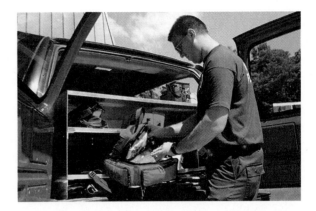

Fig. 14-1 Check all medical supplies and equipment in the emergency vehicle to make sure it is completely stocked.

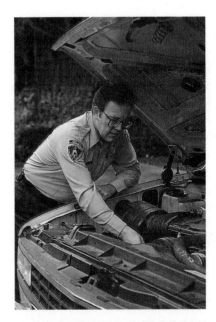

Fig. 14-2 Check all of the unit's mechanical systems.

BOX 14-1 Emergency Vehicle Equipment

- Basic supplies
- Airways
- Suction equipment
- Artificial ventilation devices
- Basic wound care supplies

Note - Box 14-1 is only a suggested minimum list for a typical emergency vehicle. State and local policy may require additional specific supplies.

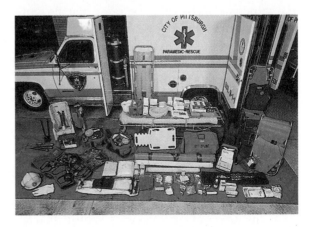

Fig. 14-3 The emergency vehicle should be well stocked with a variety of equipment and supplies for all emergencies.

system. The communication center is staffed 24 hours a day with personnel who may be able to provide medical instructions to the caller before the EMS response arrives. This system allows the family, friend, or bystander to begin emergency medical care while help is en route. In addition, many dispatch centers have preplanned response policies that allow the dispatcher to use a computer-assisted dispatch program or cardex system to determine what units to dispatch and to give the units a mode of response based on patient information.

Once the dispatcher notifies you of a response, you must have specific information. This information depends on your particular communications center and the caller providing the information. Usually you are informed of the location and the nature of illness or the mechanism of injury. In some systems, the dispatcher provides the caller's name, location, and call-back number. Additional information may be available at the time of dispatch or become available while you are en route, including the exact location of the patient (e.g., third-floor apartment), the number of patients, the severity of injuries or illness, the patient's age, the patient's level of responsiveness and respiratory status, and any other special problems or complications at the scene, including hazards and safety issues.

Dispatch information should also alert you to the possible need for additional public safety personnel such as firefighters or law enforcement officials.

EN ROUTE TO THE SCENE
To respond to the request for help, you must reach the scene safely. Use common sense, but also consciously remind yourself not to run to the vehicle (or later at the scene) because of the risk of injury. You should notify the dispatch center that you are responding to the call. Record the essential information from dispatch and keep this information available for review as you respond.

As an added safety measure to keep you, the crew, and other passengers safe, everyone in the vehicle, should always wear safety belts. This protection may save your life and is often a state law (Fig. 14-4).

As the driver of an emergency vehicle, you are responsible for knowing and following all state and local regulations regarding the use of emergency warning devices.

While traveling to the scene, a First Responder not operating the vehicle should obtain additional information from the dispatcher to help in your scene size-up. This is also a good time to assign personnel to specific duties and consider any special equipment needs. Preplanning now may save time at the scene. This time may also be used to decide what equipment to take with you initially and to prepare it.

Before beginning patient care, you must consider your arrival at the scene carefully. The first step is to position the unit. Position the unit primarily for safety and secondly for departure from the scene. Safety considerations include parking uphill or upwind from any hazardous substance, and at least 30 m (100 ft) from any wreckage. Local policy dictates whether to park the unit in front of or beyond the wreckage.

Position the vehicle to allow safe loading of the patient and easy departure from the scene. Use the parking brake and turn on the warning lights to alert other vehicles of your presence. At night, avoid blinding other drivers approaching the scene by turning off the headlights unless they are needed to illuminate the scene.

ARRIVAL AT THE SCENE
Notify dispatch of your arrival at the scene. Remember to size up the scene before approaching; this is an opportunity to protect yourself from harm. If there is a potential for violence or if the

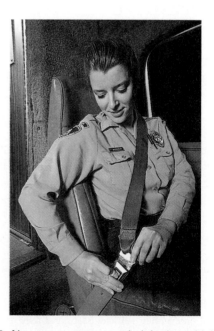

Fig. 14-4 Always wear your seatbelt in the vehicle.

scene is unsafe, wait for law enforcement assistance before approaching. Consider the need for body substance isolation precautions, and assess the scene for hazards. Is the vehicle parked in a safe location? Is it safe to approach the patient? Does the patient need to be moved immediately because of any hazards?

Next, note the mechanism of injury or the nature of illness. If there are more patients than you and your crew can handle, request additional help and begin triage. The principles of triage are discussed later in this chapter. If there is only one patient, begin your initial assessment with the general impression. If the patient has sustained trauma, provide in-line spinal immobilization.

All actions at the scene should be rapid, organized, and efficient.

TRANSFERRING THE PATIENT TO THE AMBULANCE

Using the principles you learned in Chapter 5, "Lifting and Moving Patients," assist the EMS personnel when they transfer the patient to the vehicle for transport. After performing all critical interventions, assure that all dressings and bandages or splints, if used, are secure. Cover the patient to provide protection from the weather, and secure the patient to the appropriate lifting and moving device.

REVIEW QUESTIONS

Phases of an EMS Response

Match the activity in the second column with the phase in the first column:

1. Predispatch
2. Dispatch
3. En route to the scene
4. Arrival at the scene
5. Transferring the patient to the ambulance
6. Post-run

A. Crew assignments
B. Scene size-up
C. Lifting and moving
D. Checking equipment
E. Filing paperwork
F. Location of the incident

1.D; 2.F; 3.A; 4.B; 5.C; 6.E

POST-RUN

If the vehicle needs fueling or other mechanical work, this should be handled at this phase. All paperwork from the call should be filed as required by your service. Restock any supplies that were used, and clean and disinfect equipment. Follow your service procedure for disinfecting equipment. When you are finished with these tasks, notify dispatch that you are clear of the call.

AIR MEDICAL TRANSPORT

Air medical transportation should be considered when the patient's condition warrants and significant time can be saved, or when patients must be transported to specialty care facilities (e.g., trauma centers, burn centers, neonatal centers, and other tertiary care facilities). Helicopters fly in a direct route from the scene to the hospital at speeds averaging 120 mph, bypassing traffic congestion and barriers on the ground. The important issues involve when to use air medical transport, how to set up and use landing zones, and maintaining safety.

USE OF AIR MEDICAL TRANSPORT

Helicopter transport has become a standard of care for certain medical emergencies and traumatic injuries in many areas. The decision to request air medical transport should be made in consultation with the medical director. You may have guidelines that determine when to request a helicopter, or this decision may be made at the time of the individual situation. Remember that aircraft do have some limitations: they cannot fly in certain weather conditions, and they require maintenance, both scheduled and unscheduled, that may preclude their use at a time when you need them.

In general, consider using air medical transport for patients experiencing a serious mechanism of injury, or when the hospital is far away and flying the patient would save a considerable amount of time. Become familiar with the policies of your local air medical care provider.

LANDING ZONES

Once you have determined the need for air medical transport, you should follow certain guidelines. Identify one communications person. This person should have a good sense of direction, be

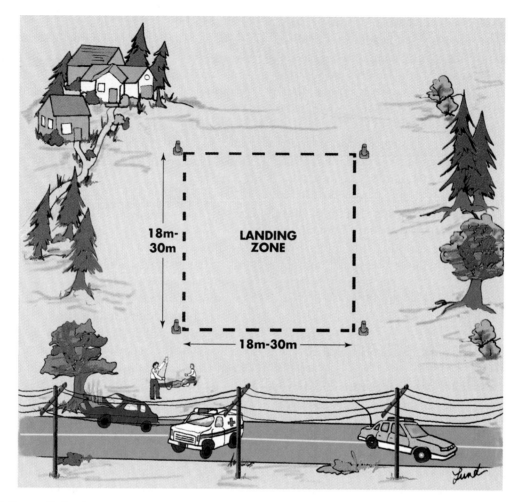

Fig. 14-5 Set up the landing zone in an area clear of obstructions such as overhead wires, trees, and fences.

familiar with the area around the landing zone, and not be directly involved in patient care. The communications officer should then contact the air medical dispatch center. Be sure to give the following essential information to the communications center: unit calling and call sign, radio frequency, number of aircraft needed, location of the incident, and prominent landmarks in the area.

A landing zone should be set up. Ideally, the landing zone should be 30 m by 30 m (100 ft by 100 ft), and minimally, 18 m by 18 m (60 ft by 60 ft). It should be free from debris, obstruction, and hazards such as overhead wires, fences, trees, or loose objects. Ideally the ground should not slope (Fig. 14-5). The person setting up the landing zone should mark each corner with an independent lighting system. Flares, light sticks, or cones that are adequately secured, or emergency vehicles with headlights pointing to the center of the landing zone all make good markers. If vehicles are used, remember to turn headlights off at

night as the helicopter descends into the landing zone, to avoid blinding or distracting the pilot.

The communications officer should notify the pilot when the aircraft is heard or seen. Before the aircraft arrives, provide descriptive landmark information. Good landmarks include water or radio towers, schools, tennis courts, swimming pools, high power lines, and major road intersections. You can direct the pilot to the landing zone using the clockface method. The pilot is always facing the twelve o'clock position (Fig. 14-6). If you are facing the aircraft and it is heading toward you, and you see the aircraft to the right of the landing zone, you would report that the landing zone is at the three o'clock position. Provide the pilot with a brief but detailed description of the landing zone, such as a field, road, or construction site, and the type of surface, such as grass, concrete, gravel, or dirt. Also, give boundary information such as trees, buildings, wires, fences, and towers. Information

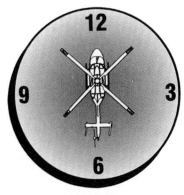

Fig. 14-6 In the clockface method of providing direction to EMS helicopters, the pilot faces the twelve o'clock position.

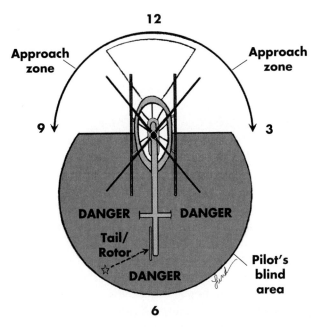

Fig. 14-7 All movement around the helicopter should be within the nine o'clock to three o'clock position.

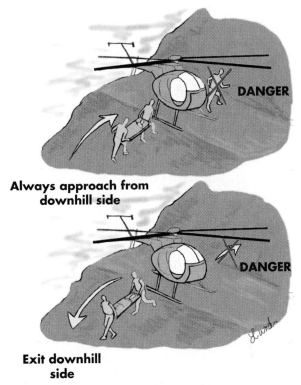

Fig. 14-8 If the pilot lands on a slope, approach the aircraft from the downhill side. It is very dangerous to approach from the uphill side.

regarding the location of power lines is extremely important. Make attempts to illuminate any potential hazards.

SAFETY

Safety around an aircraft is everyone's responsibility. If the flight crews in your area provide a continuing education course regarding aircraft operations and safety, try to attend this course.

Most safety considerations around helicopters are based on common sense. Cover your eyes to protect yourself from flying particles such as dust and gravel. Always stay a safe distance from the helicopter when the blades are turning. Even when the blades have stopped turning, keep vehicles 9 m (30 ft) from the landing zone, and keep crowds 30 m (100 ft) away. Avoid running or smoking in or around the landing zone.

No one should approach the aircraft unless directed by the pilot or medical crew. If directed, you should approach only from the front of the aircraft in the view of the pilot. The tail rotor of a helicopter is often low to the ground and spinning so fast that it is nearly impossible to see. Whether or not the helicopter engine is running, all personnel should avoid the tail section. Movement in the landing zone and around the aircraft should occur only within the nine o'clock to three o'clock positions (Fig. 14-7), which is the pilot's area of vision. Never take a short cut under the body, the rear section, or the tail boom. If you are helping the flight crew, do not operate any of the aircraft doors. The flight crew is responsible for opening and closing all doors and latches.

When approaching the helicopter, stay low. Unexpected wind gusts may change the height of the blade unexpectedly. Use caution when carrying equipment to the aircraft. Approaching the helicopter carrying any equipment over your head, even if you duck low, is extremely dangerous and must be avoided. Loose equipment and hats may be blown off by the wind from the rotor blades and should be secured or not worn. If the pilot parks the aircraft on a slope, always approach from the downhill side since the main rotor blade will be lower to the ground on the uphill side (Fig. 14-8). Always follow the directions of the flight crew regarding approach to and departure from the aircraft.

If you assist the EMS crew and air medical crew load the patient into the aircraft, be sure that all straps are secured and there is no loose material. The patient should be informed about the noise and wind around the aircraft. Follow the direction of the air medical crew when operating around the aircraft.

Remember that the pilot may choose a different route of departure based on winds and obstacles. The departure may require that the helicopter be turned when still close to the ground. As the aircraft prepares for departure, all personnel and equipment should be clear of the landing zone.

Many organizations and agencies can provide additional information regarding EMS helicopters, including the Association of Air Medical Services, the National Association of EMS Pilots, and your local EMS air medical provider.

FUNDAMENTALS OF EXTRICATION

First Responders are called to many situations involving motor vehicle collisions or other situations in which a patient may be trapped (Fig. 14-9). Personal safety is very important in these situations. A First Responder who is injured not only is unable to help the patient but requires additional EMS or rescue resources. In some EMS systems, First Responders are required to have special knowledge and education in rescue techniques. In other systems, rescue is handled by fire service, special rescue, or law enforcement personnel (Fig. 14-10). Therefore, you must become familiar with the system used in your area and seek additional education as necessary. This chapter provides an overview of the safety equipment First Responders use at rescue scenes and the medical aspects of extrication.

Extrication is the process of removing a patient from entanglement in a motor vehicle or other situation in a safe and appropriate manner. In some situations extrication must be preceded by removing objects from around the patient to access the patient and provide a path from the vehicle or other structure. This process, often called disentanglement, usually involves the use of special equipment. In many EMS systems, such rescues are the responsibility of specially educated EMS providers. In other areas, rescue services are provided by specially educated firefighters or law enforcement personnel. In all systems, however, First Responders respond to situations that require extrication. Therefore, it is important to understand the role of EMS personnel at crash scenes, industrial accidents, structure collapses, and other settings of entrapment.

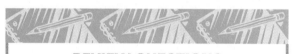

REVIEW QUESTIONS

Air Medical Transport

1. Which of the following is not an essential element of information to provide the communications center?
   A. Patient name
   B. Ground contact name and call sign
   C. Frequency
   D. Location of incident

2. Which of the following is not a consideration for calling for air medical transport?
   A. Distance
   B. Cost
   C. Time
   D. Mechanism of injury

3. Who has the responsibility for safety around an aircraft?
   A. The pilot
   B. The flight crew
   C. The First Responders on the ground
   D. All of the above

4. What is the minimum size for a landing zone?
   A. 7.5 m by 7.5 m (25 ft by 25 ft)
   B. 15 m by 15 m (50 ft by 50 ft)
   C. 18 m by 18 m (60 ft by 60 ft)
   D. 30 m by 30 m (100 ft by 100 ft)

1.A; 2.B; 3.D; 4.C

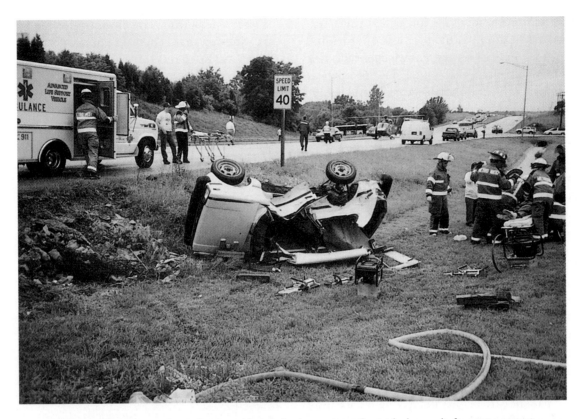

Fig. 14-9 First Responders often provide medical care to patients during and after entrapment.

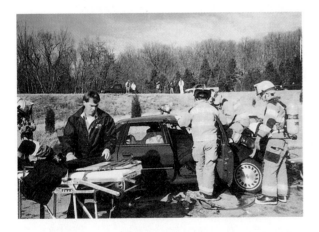

Fig. 14-10 In some areas, First Responders work with specially educated teams to rescue patients from entrapment.

ROLE OF THE FIRST RESPONDER

Depending on your system, you may be responsible for rescue. Regardless of your rescue responsibilities, however, everyone's actions at a rescue scene must follow a chain of command. In some systems, an incident management system coordinates the emergency efforts involving extrication.

The incident commander coordinates the efforts of both medical and rescue personnel (Fig. 14-11),

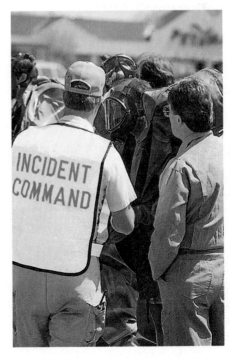

Fig. 14-11 The incident commander coordinates rescue efforts by medical and rescue personnel.

as well as those responsible for patient transport. Teamwork is important in these operations. Extrication depends on the knowledge, skill, and equipment of rescue personnel, just as medical care depends on your knowledge, skill, and equipment. You cooperate with the rescuers, but rescue activities should not interfere with your patient care activities.

All critical emergency care should be provided before and during the extrication. If a rescue crew is performing the extrication, work with them to ensure that the patient is removed in a way that minimizes the risk of further injury. In all cases of entrapment, critical patient care precedes extrication unless delay would endanger the life of the patient or rescuers, in which case extrication is done immediately. While the rescue crew works, prepare the equipment necessary to remove the patient and begin to initiate care such as assessment and bleeding control.

This same principle applies for First Responders who also perform as rescue personnel. Provide all critical patient care before and during the extrication. Patient care precedes extrication unless an emergency move is necessary. Rescue First Responders must cooperate with medical First Responders to ensure that the patient is removed in a way that minimizes the risk of further injury.

SAFETY AND EQUIPMENT

When a patient must be extricated, your safety is the first priority, followed by the safety of the patient and bystanders.

Personal safety is always your number one priority. This rule applies to all workers involved in rescue activities or medical care. Wear protective clothing that is appropriate for the situation (Fig 14-12). The National Fire Protection Administration (NFPA) and the Occupational Safety and Health Administration (OSHA) have guidelines for personal safety equipment that many EMS services follow when purchasing equipment. Box 14-2 lists the minimum personal protective equipment for First Responders working around vehicle collisions.

BOX 14-2 Personal Protective Equipment

- Impact-resistant protective helmet with ear protection and chin strap.

- Protective eyewear. Ideally the protective eye wear has an elastic strap and vents to prevent fogging. The shield on a helmet is not considered protective eyewear.

- Light-weight, puncture-resistant ``turn-out'' coat.

- Leather gloves.

- Boots with steel insoles and steel toes.

- Most rescuers also use light-weight, puncture-resistant turn-out pants.

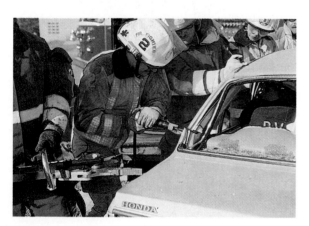

Fig. 14-12 In rescue situations, First Responders should use protective equipment.

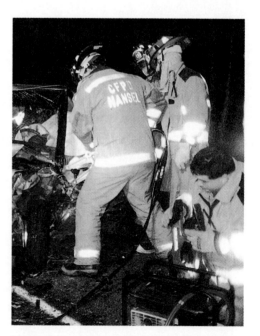

Fig. 14-13 Protect the patient from glass, metal, and other hazards during the disentanglement process.

In addition to using personal protective equipment, take body substance isolation precautions. As described in Chapter 2, "The Well-Being of the First Responder," body substance isolation precautions are required any time you may come in contact with blood or other body fluids.

Once the safety needs of both medical and rescue personnel are met, consider the safety of the patient and bystanders. Explain the extrication process to patients, including the sounds they will hear. Cover patients with blankets or tarps to protect against broken glass, sharp metal, and other hazards (Fig. 14-13), as well as to keep them warm.

Bystanders and uninvolved people should be kept clear of the scene. The presence of curious onlookers at the scene increases the risk of additional injuries (Fig. 14-14).

Motor vehicle crashes and other cases of entrapment may involve hazardous materials, which could prevent you from gaining access to the patient. Also be alert for the possibility of fire at a crash scene. To reduce this risk, turn off the ignition of the vehicle and prevent smoking at the scene (Fig. 14-15). Unless you have had special education in vehicle firefighting, do not attempt to extinguish a fire. With a small fire, you may be able to use a fire extinguisher to stop the fire from spreading. Again, attempt this only if you have the proper knowledge, skills, and equipment.

In addition to the risk of fire, there is a risk of electric shock from downed power lines. Only utility or rescue workers who are educated in the handling of live power lines should approach downed power lines to secure them. If victims are inside a vehicle, advise them to remain inside the vehicle. If you cannot approach the vehicle because of downed power lines, try to talk to the patient through a loud speaker system, such as the vehicle radio's public address system. Remember, if the scene is unsafe, either make it safe or do not enter. If you cannot make it safe yourself, request the appropriate agency to respond.

Unstable vehicles also pose a problem for rescuers and First Responders. As you are caring for an injured patient, the balance of the vehicle may change, causing the unstable vehicle to shift and roll or fall and potentially injure you or other personnel.

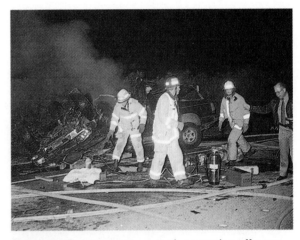

Fig. 14-15 Safety measures such as turning off a car ignition can prevent a car fire.

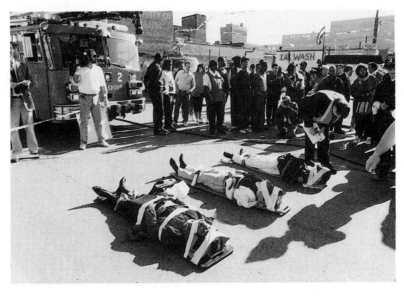

Fig. 14-14 Establish a safe zone at the rescue scene, and only those persons responsible for patient care or extrication should be in the inner circle.

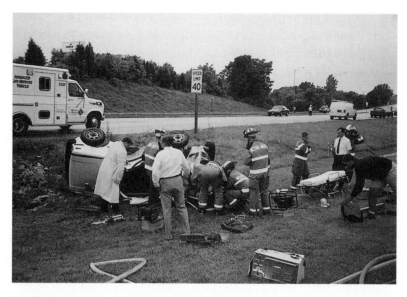

Fig. 14-16 Be sure every effort has been made to secure vehicle stability before entering. Continue to assess the vehicle's stability throughout the extrication process.

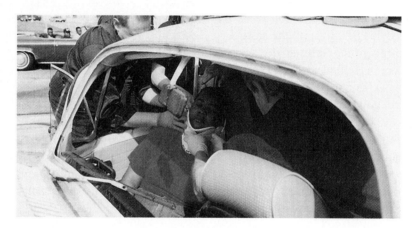

Fig. 14-17 Simple access does not require mechanical tools.

Before entering a crashed vehicle, assess its stability (Fig. 14-16). Assist the rescue workers to ensure that the vehicle is stabilized before caring for the patient.

A rescue scene always must be managed. In addition to an incident commander, if enough personnel are present, a safety officer should be appointed. A person who is not directly involved in the rescue or patient care should have this responsibility. This person should be an objective observer and should watch for safety issues and additional hazards that the rescue workers may not be able to see, such as development of fires, movement of the vehicle, or unsafe acts by the rescuers or First Responders. This person can also cycle in new rescuers when others become fatigued.

ACCESSING THE PATIENT

Accessing, or getting to the patient, may be simple or complex. Simple access does not require the use of rescue equipment and can be performed by all First Responders. Opening the door, rolling down a window, and having the patient unlock the doors are all simple access (Fig. 14-17). Complex extrication requires additional education, skills, and equipment.

If you are interested or required to become a rescue technician, you should investigate the variety of available programs that provide this additional education, skills, and equipment. Different basic rescue courses deal with vehicle rescue and the use of ropes and self-contained breathing apparatus. In addition, special rescue programs

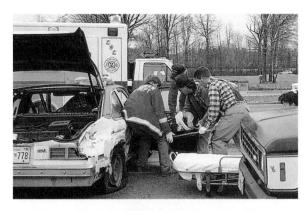

Fig. 14-18 Except in cases of emergency moves, immobilize the patient's spine before removal.

REVIEW QUESTIONS

Fundamentals of Extrication

1. Define extrication. _____

2. What is the difference between simple and complex extrication?

   _____

   _____

3. Unless there is danger to the patient or rescuers, all patients involved in motor vehicle crashes should have _____.

1. The removal of a patient from entanglement in a safe and appropriate manner.; 2. Complex extrication requires special education, skills, and equipment; simple extrication does not.; 3. Spinal immobilization.

include water rescue, trench rescue, and high-angle rescue. Check with your instructor or service about the availability of these courses.

REMOVING THE PATIENT

Once you have gained access to the patient, you should extricate or remove the patient. When removing the patient, work with the additional EMS response to maintain spinal immobilization at all times. Move a patient without spinal immobilization only in situations when the patient or rescuers are in danger if the patient is not moved immediately.

Complete the initial assessment and provide critical interventions before removing the patient. Except in a situation that requires rapid extrication,

work with the additional EMS response to ensure that the spine is immobilized using a short spine board or other immobilization device (Fig. 14-18).

Before removing the patient from the vehicle, ensure sufficient personnel are present to move the patient. Remember to pick up the patient rather than the immobilization device, unless the device is designed to be lifted. Choose the path of least resistance, protect the patient from hazards, ensure an open airway, and maintain spinal immobilization.

HAZARDOUS MATERIALS

A **hazardous material** is any substance or material that can pose an unreasonable risk to health, safety, or property. Because there is a great chance that you will be involved in a hazardous materials incident during your emergency services career, you should, at a minimum, attend a First Responder Awareness Level education program. This education involves approaching hazardous materials in a manner safest for everyone involved. Check with your instructor to learn more about hazardous materials courses in your area.

SAFETY

The issue of hazardous materials is an everyday concern and problem. Although some may think of hazardous materials only in terms of transportation incidents such as vehicle crashes, in reality many household chemicals, pesticides, and other compounds found in the home and industrial sites may cause a hazardous materials situation. A patient's home may have carbon monoxide leaking from the heating system, a patient may use an oven cleaner in a poorly ventilated room, or chlorine gas may leak at a local municipal swimming pool. Any time there is a spill or leak of chemicals, there is a potential for a hazardous materials incident (Fig. 14-19). Any time First Responders, the public, or the environment is at risk, there is a hazardous materials situation.

In all hazardous materials situations, your primary concern should be safety. Safety concerns include your own well-being and that of other crew members, patients, bystanders, and the community.

Knowledge of what is involved and what to do is necessary for successful and safe management of hazardous materials situations. While traveling to the scene of a hazardous materials incident, obtain as much additional information as you can from

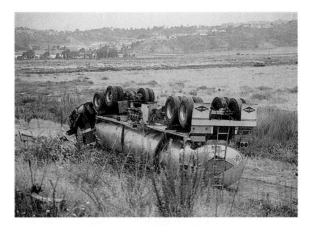

Fig. 14-19 Any spill of chemicals can become a hazardous materials incident.

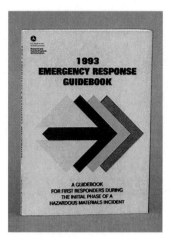

Fig. 14-20 The Emergencey Response Guidebook.

dispatch. This gathering of information is the start of your investigation into the scope of the problem. The United States Department of Transportation (USDOT) publishes a reference to assist in identifying and managing hazardous materials, the Emergency Response Guidebook (Fig. 14-20), which lists hazardous materials and the appropriate emergency procedures. This book should be in every response vehicle to help you identify potential hazards. It can be a great resource for you until more highly educated help arrives. Always remember the scene size-up rule: If the scene is not safe, make it safe, otherwise do not enter. In a hazardous materials scene, the expertise of a highly educated hazardous materials team is usually required to make the scene safe. Do not enter the scene unless you are educated to handle hazardous materials and have skills for use of the necessary equipment.

PROCEDURES

Once you suspect the scene may involve hazardous materials, because of either dispatch information or physical clues, follow these important safety guidelines as you approach the scene:
- Approach the scene from an uphill and upwind direction
- Isolate the area
- Avoid contact with the material
- Be alert for unusual odors, clouds, and leakage
- Remember that some chemicals are odorless
- Do not drive the response vehicle through leakage or vapor clouds
- Keep all personnel and bystanders a safe distance from the scene
- Remove patients to a safe zone if there is no risk to the First Responder

Approach the scene with extreme caution. Do not rush into a situation that may harm you. You cannot help others if you become a patient yourself. Until you know what the material or situation is, you cannot help.

Once the scene has been recognized as a hazardous materials incident, if you are educated and required to deal with decontamination issues, you should work at identifying the extent of the problem. At the site of a vehicle crash, try to determine if the vehicle is occupied and the size and shape of the container of hazardous materials. If the hazardous materials scene does not involve a vehicle, identifying the container by shape and size is also important. This information may allow the hazardous materials team to make an early identification of the materials involved. Often hazardous materials are identified by a placard (Fig. 14-21). The placard may also have a four-digit identification number to help you identify the material or class of material. Check the Emergency Response Guidebook for any placard numbers. Shipping papers, if you can safely locate and retrieve them without personal risk, are also a valuable resource. Shipping papers are typically located in the passenger compartment of the vehicle, with the driver. Some vehicles have a special compartment for the shipping papers. Shipping papers are not usually retrievable without the use of protective equipment.

Check the Emergency Response Guidebook for suggested interventions you may be able to perform before the specially educated team arrives.

An additional available resource is the Chemical Transportation Emergency Center (CHEMTREC), which is a service of the Chemical

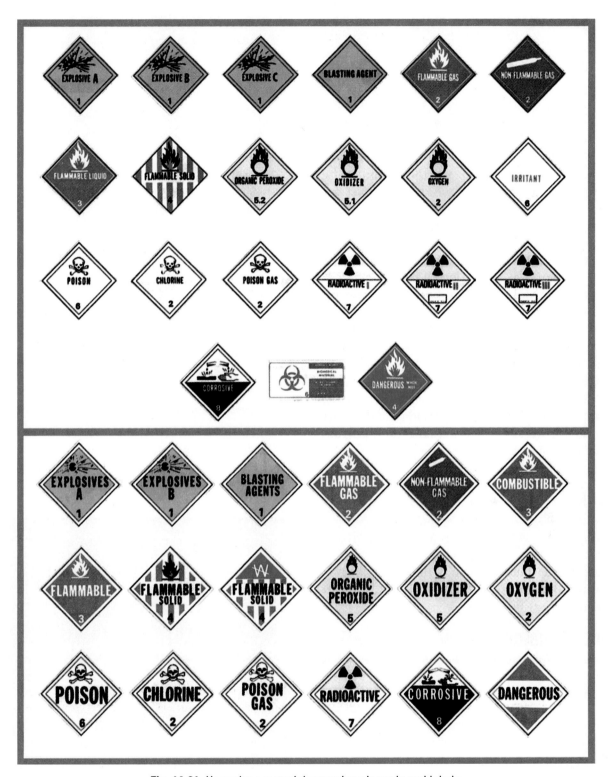

Fig. 14-21 Hazardous materials warning placards and labels.

Manufacturers Association. This public service agency can provide immediate on-line advice to emergency personnel at the scene of hazardous materials incidents. CHEMTREC operates 24 hours per day, 7 days a week, and can be reached through an emergency phone number (1-800-424-9300). It is recommended that you contact CHEMTREC as soon as possible during the incident. When you call, be prepared to provide as much information as possible regarding the incident, including the name of the substance, its identification number, and a description of the incident.

These are only some of the available resources. In general, do not rely on only one source of information when dealing with a hazardous materials incident. Other resources include poison centers and medical direction.

The Occupational Safety and Health Administration (OSHA) and the National Fire Protection Administration have guidelines for public safety personnel, including EMS, related to hazardous materials. Part 1910.120, 29 Code of Federal Regulations, regulates the safety and health of employees in any emergency response to incidents involving hazardous substances. NFPA 473, Professional Competence for EMS Personnel Responding to Hazardous Materials Incidents, identifies the competencies required of EMS personnel who respond to hazardous materials incidents. Note that your initial education program may not include the necessary components to meet these competencies. Therefore, if you are assigned to a unit responsible for hazardous materials responses, seek out and gain additional education in this area.

MASS CASUALTY SITUATIONS

A mass casualty situation is an incident involving more patients than the responding unit can safely and efficiently handle. In general, these situations require activation of the incident management system.

BASIC TRIAGE

In a multiple casualty situation, patient triage is a priority. Triage is a method of categorizing patients into treatment and transport priorities. There are generally three priority levels. A tagging system is typically used to assist in designating the category of each of the patients. Through the use of color-coded or numbered tags, patients are placed into one of the triage categories (Fig. 14-22). Box 14-3 lists the conditions that fall into each of these categories.

PROCEDURES

In general, the EMS provider most knowledgeable of patient assessment and intervention who arrives on the scene first becomes the triage officer.

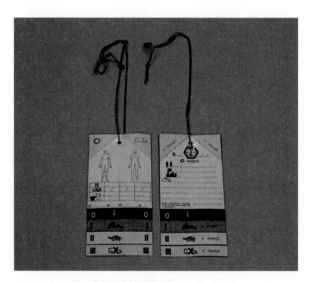

Fig. 14-22 METTAG Triage Cards

Immediately during the scene size-up, additional help should be requested. The triage officer rapidly performs an initial assessment of all patients. Care is not provided during triage, except for correction of immediate life threats,

BOX 14-3 Triage Priorities

Highest priority
- Airway and breathing difficulties
- Uncontrolled or severe bleeding
- Decreased mental status

Second priority
- Burns without airway problems
- Major or multiple extremity injuries
- Back injuries

Lowest priority
- Minor extremity injuries
- Minor soft tissue injuries
- Death

such as opening the airway or managing major bleeding.

The triage officer rapidly moves through the patients, doing an initial assessment and using triage tags to assign patients in treatment categories. As patients are assessed and tagged, they are moved to a treatment area for further evaluation and intervention. From the treatment area the patient is moved to a transportation area for transport. Transport decisions are based on patient priority, the receiving hospital's capabilities and capacity, and transportation resources.

Once all patients have been triaged, the triage officer reports to the incident commander. Often the triage officer remains in that position and continues to triage and update patient priorities based on available resources, or the triage officer may receive a new assignment.

The triage process forces First Responders to make difficult decisions. You may wish to practice using triage tags to be prepared when a true multiple casualty situation arises. For example, you could simply select one day a month and use triage tags on all patients in all calls just to practice. The important skill in triage is to be able to quickly prioritize patients to give the greatest amount of care, keeping in mind available resources, to allow the greatest amount of treatment to be provided to the greatest number of patients.

When you report to the scene of a mass casualty incident, report to the command post and identify yourself and your level of training. Follow the directions of the incident commander.

REVIEW QUESTIONS

Mass Casualty Situations

Match the patient to the appropriate priority.

A = Highest priority; B = Second priority;
C = Lowest priority

1. Respiratory difficulty _____

2. Signs and symptoms of shock (hypoperfusion) _____

3. Burns to the legs and abdomen _____

4. Pain, swelling, and deformity to both lower legs _____

5. Altered mental status _____

6. Death _____

7. The term triage means _____.

1. A; 2. A; 3. B; 4. B; 5. A; 6. C; 7. To sort or prioritize

CHAPTER SUMMARY

PHASES OF AN EMS RESPONSE

The nine phases of a typical EMS response are: 1) preparation for the call; 2) dispatch; 3) en route to the scene; 4) arrival at scene; 5) transferring patient to the ambulance; 6) en route to the receiving facility; 7) at the receiving facility; 8) en route to the station; and 9) post-run. First Responders are typically not involved in transporting the patient to the receiving facility.

Your roles and responsibilities depend on the phase of the call. The first phase allows you to prepare for the call and check the vehicle for medical equipment and mechanical readiness. Dispatch is an opportunity to gain information regarding the call. En route to the scene is the travel time to the scene and preplanning for the actions at the scene. Upon arrival, you size-up the scene to ensure the well-being and safety of the crew. Remember that your actions at the scene should be organized with the goal of transport in mind. Assist the EMS personnel with lifting and moving the patient to the ambulance. Finally, the post-run phase is a time to disinfect equipment, restock the vehicle, and prepare for the next response.

AIR MEDICAL TRANSPORT

Air medical transport is becoming the standard of care for some critically ill and injured patients. Considerations for the use of air medical transport include the mechanism of injury and the time and distance to the receiving facility. The set-up of a landing zone and communication should be delegated to persons not directly involved in patient care. The landing zone should be clear of debris and wires. Give the pilot as much information as possible.

Safety around the aircraft is the responsibility of everyone. Avoid running and do not smoke in or around the landing zone. The main rotor blades may dip as low as 4 feet from the ground. The tail rotor is spinning at a speed that makes it nearly invisible. Always approach the aircraft from the nine to three o'clock positions and only when directed by the flight crew. Never walk near the tail rotor or under the tailboom. Follow the instructions of the flight crew regarding safety around the aircraft.

FUNDAMENTALS OF EXTRICATION

Extrication is the process of freeing a patient from entanglement. This process may require disentanglement by specially educated rescue EMS providers or rescue technicians. An incident commander should coordinate the efforts of everyone responsible for extrication and the EMS providers responsible for medical care. Teamwork is important. Assess the patient and provide critical care before and during the extrication. Work with the rescue crew to ensure that the patient is removed in a way that minimizes further injury to the patient.

Personal safety is the number one priority for both rescue and non-rescue EMS providers. Wear protective clothing appropriate for the situation, and take the appropriate body substance isolation precautions. Perform a scene size-up. Situations requiring extrication may involve hazardous materials. Also be alert for the potential of fire at a crash scene and the risk of electrical shock from downed power lines. Unstable vehicles also pose a problem. If the scene is unsafe, make it safe or do not enter.

Simple access to the patient does not require the use of equipment. Try all the vehicle doors, or have the patient unlock a locked door or roll down a window. Complex access requires the use of rescue tools. Once extrication procedures have been completed, remove the patient. Complete the initial assessment. Provide only critical interventions before moving the patient. Before moving the patient from the vehicle, ensure that there are sufficient personnel to move the patient safely.

HAZARDOUS MATERIALS

Hazardous materials are a common problem today. Your primary responsibility in hazardous materials incidents is your own safety and well-being and that of the crew, patients, bystanders, and the environment. Unless you are specifically educated to deal with hazardous materials situations, you must protect the scene and wait for additional help to arrive. A number of resources are available to identify and provide guidance when dealing with hazardous materials. These resources include placards, shipping papers, the USDOT Emergency Response Guidebook, and CHEMTREC. You should become familiar with all of these resources. First Responders are recommended to be educated at least to the OSHA First Responder Hazardous Materials Awareness Level.

In a hazardous materials situation, approach the scene with extreme caution, identify the hazard, assure safety around the scene, do whatever is possible to isolate the area, and ensure the safety of the people and the environment, and move and keep all bystanders and crew away from the scene. Obtain additional help, do not walk through leakage, and do not touch spilled material. Avoid inhaling fumes, smoke, or vapors.

MASS CASUALTY SITUATIONS

Another incident requiring activation of the incident management system is a multiple casualty situation. These situations can occur when there are more patients than the responding unit can safely and effectively deal with. The first and most knowledgeable EMS provider on the scene begins triage, categorizing patients according to their injury into one of three categories. This is accomplished by rapidly performing an initial assessment of each patient and indicating the priority of each with a triage tag. This decision-making process allows the most patients to be treated and transported using available resources.

This chapter does not educate First Responders to deal with every situation but is an overview only. You should seek additional knowledge and skills through continuing education programs, practice drills, and experience.

UNITED STATES DEPARTMENT OF TRANSPORTATION NATIONAL HIGHWAY TRAFFIC SAFETY ADMINISTRATION FIRST RESPONDER OBJECTIVES

Check your knowledge. The National Registry of EMTs and many state EMS agencies use the objectives below to develop First Responder certification examinations. Can you meet them?

COGNITIVE OBJECTIVES

1. Discuss the medical and non-medical equipment needed to respond to a call.
2. List the phases of an out-of-hospital call.
3. Discuss the role of the First responder in extrication.
4. List various methods of gaining access to the patient.
5. Distinguish between simple and complex access.
6. Describe what the First Responder should do if there is reason to believe that there is a hazard at the scene.
7. State the role the First Responder should perform until appropriately trained personnel arrive at the scene of a hazardous materials situation.
8. Describe the criteria for a multiple-casualty situation.
9. Discuss the role of the First Responder in the multiple-casualty situation.
10. Summarize the components of basic triage.

AFFECTIVE OBJECTIVES

11. Explain the rationale for having the unit prepared to respond.

PSYCHOMOTOR OBJECTIVES

12. Given the scenario of a mass casualty incident, perform triage.

APPENDIX F: Functional Job Analysis

The attached Functional Job Analysis was developed at the request of the Board of Directors of the National Registry of EMTs. This job analysis should be used to assist in meeting the requirements of the Americans with Disabilities Act. Readers and persons interested in utilizing this functional job analysis should refer questions related to specific indicators to occupational health rehabilitation specialists for interpretation.

First Responder Characteristics

The First Responder must be a person who can remain calm while working in difficult and stressful circumstances, as well as one who is capable of combining technical skills, theoretical knowledge, and good judgment to insure optimal level of fundamental emergency care to sick or injured patients while adhering to specific guidelines within the given scope of practice.

The First Responder is expected to be able to work alone, but must also be a team player. Personal qualities such as the ability to "take charge" and control the situation are essential, as are the maintaining of caring and professional attitude, controlling one's own fears, presenting a professional appearance, staying physically fit, and keeping one's skills and abilities up to date. The First Responder must be willing to adhere to the established ongoing medical control and evaluation required for the maintenance of quality medical care.

Self-confidence, a desire to work with people, emotional stability, tolerance for high stress, honesty, a pleasant demeanor, and the ability to meet the physical and intellectual requirements demanded by this position are characteristics of the competent First Responder. The First Responder also must be able to deal with adverse social situations which include responding to calls in districts known to have high crime rates. The First Responder ideally possesses an interest in working for the good of society and has a commitment to doing so.

Physical Demands

Aptitudes required for work of this nature are good physical stamina, endurance, and body condition that would not be adversely affected by having to walk, stand, lift, carry, and balance at times, in excess of 125 pounds. Motor coordination is necessary because over uneven terrain, the patient's and the First Responder's well being, as well as other workers' well being must not be jeopardized.

Comments

Use of the telephone or radio dispatch for coordination of prompt emergency services is essential. Accurately discerning street names through map reading, and correctly distinguishing house numbers or business addresses are essential to task completion in the most expedient manner. Concisely and accurately describing orally to dispatcher and other concerned staff, one's impression of patient's condition, is critical as the First Responder works in emergency conditions where there may not be time for deliberation. The First Responder must also be able to accurately report all relevant patient data, which is generally, but not always, outlined on a prescribed form. Verbal and reasoning skills are used extensively. The ability to perform mathematical tasks is minimal, however, it does play a part in activities such as taking vital signs, making estimates of time, calculating the number of persons at a scene, and counting the number of persons requiring specific care.

Job Analysis Schedule

1. **ESTABLISH JOB TITLE:** First Responder
2. **CODE 079026 WTA GROUP:** Occupations in medicine and health
3. **JOB SUMMARY:** Activates the EMS system, surveys the scene for hazards, contains those hazards, gains access to the injured or sick, gathers relevant patient data, provides immediate emergency medical care using a limited amount of equipment, controls the scene, and prepares for the arrival of the ambulance.

4. WORK PERFORMED ESTIMATES:

Worker Functions	Data	People	Things
	3	7	4

3. Compiling
7. Serving
4. Manipulating
Work Field: 294 Health, Caring, and Medical
M.P.S.M.S. 920 (**M**aterials, **P**roducts, **S**ubject **M**atter, and **S**ervices) Medical and other health services.

5. WORKER TRAITS RATINGS:

GENERAL EDUCATION DEVELOPMENT (GED) encompasses three broad areas which are rated independently in relation to the occupation being assessed: Reasoning development, Mathematical development, and Language development.

General Educational Development (GED) embraces those aspects of education (formal and informal) which contribute to the worker's reasoning development, and ability to follow instructions, and to acquisition of "tool" knowledge such as language and mathematical skills. This is education of a general nature which does not have a recognized, fairly specific occupational objective. Ordinarily, such education is obtained in elementary school, high school, or college. However, it may be obtained from experience and self study.

Description of rating on the GED Scale: Level 1—lowest level; Level 6—highest level.

Lowest						Highest
GED	1	M1, L2	3	R4	5	6

Reasoning development (R)
Level 4—Apply principles of rational systems to solve practical problems and deal with a variety of concrete variables in situations where only limited standardization exists. Interpret a variety of instructions furnished in written, oral, diagrammatic, or schedule form.

Mathematical development (M)
Level 2—Add, subtract, multiply and divide all units of measure. Complete ratio, rate, and percent. Perform the four operations with like on common decimals, fractions. Perform arithmetic operations involving all American monetary units.

NOTE: In the analyst's opinion, the degree of math skills required for this position is minimal, however, reducing the mathematical component to a level 1, the lowest level, appears slightly too low. For example, in Level 1, a person would only be required to add and subtract up to two digit numbers. There could be instances where higher level skills are required, such as the total number of persons with slight injuries compared to those with more serious injuries.

Language development (L)
Level 2—Reading: Passive vocabulary of 5000–6000 words; read at a rate of 190–215 words per minute; read adventure stories and comic books; looking up unfamiliar words in dictionary for meaning, spelling and pronunciation; and read instructions for assembling model cars and airplanes.

Writing: Write compound and complex sentences using cursive style, proper end punctuation, and employing adjectives and adverbs.

Speaking: Speak clearly and distinctly with appropriate pauses and emphasis, correct pronunciation, variation in word order, using present, perfect, and future tenses.

SPECIAL VOCATIONAL PREPARATION (SVP) (Time requirement of 40 classroom hours)

SVP	1	2	3	4	5	6	7	8	9

Explanation of scale:

Level	Time[1]
1	Short demonstration only
2	Anything beyond short demonstration up to and including one month
3	Over one month up to and including three months
4	Over three months up to and including six months
5	Over six months up to and including one year
6	Over one year up to and including two years
7	Over two years up to and including four years
8	Over four years up to and including ten years
9	Over ten years

NOTE: The levels of this scale are mutually exclusive and do not overlap

[1]Time that applies to General Educational Development is not considered in estimating SVP.

Level 2.

NOTE: In the analyst's opinion, the requirement of 40 hours of formal classroom study, and competency based on formal written and practical examination, when judged only by a time perspective, appear to qualify the preparation time as less than 30 days. While this may be true in some instances, preparation time may vary and span a longer period of calendar time, depending upon the student, the instructor, and the locality of training. First Responder applicants typically make application in writing at least thirty days before the start of the training program. This requirement will vary depending upon locality. Because First Responder program guidelines can permit a student up to six months for course completion, the SVP could, in essence, be as high as a Level 4.

APTITUDE LEVELS: G 3 V 3 N 4 S 3 P 2 Q 3 K 2 F 2 M 2 E 2 C 1

Scale: Level 1 indicates the highest degree of particular aptitude;
         Level 5 indicates the lowest degree of an aptitude.

Lowest				Highest
5	4	3	2	1

G– Intelligence
Level 3
Level G-3:1 Renders general care to patients.

Intelligence is required to learn and apply principles of anatomy, physiology, and patient care used in emergency medical care; to make independent judgments in absence of doctor; to determine methods and treatments to use when caring for patients with varying illnesses or injuries; and to exercise judgment concerning ethical and legal considerations within scope of practice.

V– Verbal Aptitude
 Level 3
 Level V-3:9 Questions patients to obtain their medical history, personal data, and to determine if they
   are allergic to medications or have any complicating illnesses.

N– Numerical Aptitude (Perform arithmetic operations quickly and accurately)
 Level 4 Lower degree of aptitude required. No illustrations in medical area. Closely related skills
   appear comparable to 4:7. Records business transactions in journals, ledgers, on special forms,
   and transfers entries from one accounting record to another. Adds totals of entries and original
   record and compares to check for posting errors.

S– Spatial Aptitude (Comprehend forms in space and understand relationships to plane and solid objects)
 Level 3
 Level S-3:1 Spatial aptitude is required to visualize anatomic and the relationship between the point
   of application of forces and the area affected (as in traction); and to place treatment
   devices or administer manual treatment in relationship to the affected body part.

P– Form Perception (Ability to make visual comparisons and discriminations and see slight differences in shapes and shadings of figures and widths and lengths of lines)
 Level 2
 Level P-2:6 High degree of aptitude required. Form perception is required to perceive pertinent
   details of size, shape, and form in skeletal structure, organs, tissue, and specimens of
   various animals.

Q– Clerical Perception (Ability to perceive pertinent detail in verbal or tabular material-proof read)
 Level 3
 Level Q-3:13 Assists in care of hospital patients under direction of medical staff. Clerical perception is
   required to read and report such data as temperatures, pulse rate and respiration rate, to
   report patient's food and fluid intake and output, and to read charts and instructions accurately. Generally completes documentation of relevant data on pre-printed form. Must be
   able to read form accurately and report patient information in appropriate allocated space.
   Occasionally, may be required to submit short narrative report.

K– Motor Coordination (Ability to make a movement response quickly and accurately and coordinate eye-hand)
 Level 2
 Level K-2:5 Renders general care to patients. Aptitude and ability are required to coordinate vision,
   finger and hand movements, to take vital signs, to assist with freeing airway, and to balance self when lifting/moving or stabilizing patients.

F– Finger Dexterity (Ability to move fingers and manipulate small objects rapidly and quickly)
 Level 2 No illustrations in medical field. Recommended due to necessity of ability to open and maintain airway, ventilate patient, control hemorrhage, bandage wounds, and manually stabilize
   painful swollen and deformed extremities.

M– Manual Dexterity (Ability to move the hands easily and skillfully)
 Level 2 No illustrations given. Manual dexterity is required during emergency situations to control
   and extinguish fires, protect life and property, and maintain equipment as volunteer or em-
   ployee of city, township, or industrial plant. Manual dexterity is also required in positioning

ladders and nets, clasping rungs to climb ladders, giving artificial respiration, and in lifting of patient.

E– Eye-Hand-Foot Coordination (Ability to coordinate these)

Level 2 No illustrations given. Recommended as job may require balancing on ladders, stairs, or walking on uneven terrain while assisting in carrying patients. In the interest of time and safety, may be required to move quickly.

C– Color Discrimination (Ability to perceive difference in colors, shades, or harmonious combinations, or to match colors)

Level 1 High degree of aptitude and ability required.

C-1:4 Uses color discrimination and color memory in making diagnosis of patients' affliction or condition, by recognizing any deviations in color of diseased tissue from healthy tissue; evaluating color characteristics such as hue and saturation of affected body parts; and making determination as to extent or origin of condition

TEMPERAMENT

Temperament	A	D	F	I	J	M	P	R	S	V

Explanation of terms:

A– Working alone or apart in physical isolation from others.

D– Directing, controlling, or planning the activities of others.

I– Influencing adaptability to influencing people in their opinions, attitudes, or judgments about ideas or things.

J– Adaptability to making generalizations, evaluations or decisions based on sensory or judgmental criteria.

M– Adaptability to making generalizations, judgments, or decisions based on measurable or verifiable criteria.

P– Adaptability to dealing with people beyond giving and receiving instructions.

S– Adaptability to performing under stress when confronted with emergency, critical, unusual, or dangerous situations; or in situations in which working where speed and sustained attention are make or break aspects of the job.

V– Adaptability to performing a variety of duties, often changing from one task to another of a different nature without loss of efficiency or composure.

INTERESTS

Interests	1a	1b	2a	2b	3a	3b	4a	4b	5a	5b

4a– A preference for working for the presumed good of the people.

PHYSICAL DEMANDS

Physical Demands	S	L	M	H	V	2	3	4	5	6

Explanation of terms:

1. Strengths

   S– Sedentary (10 pounds maximum)

   L– Light work (10 pounds frequently, 20 pounds maximum)

   M– Medium work (25 pounds frequently, 50 pounds maximum)

   H– Heavy work (50 pounds frequently, 100 pounds maximum)

   V– Very heavy work (50 pounds frequently, no maximum)

2. Climbing and/or balancing
3. Stooping, kneeling, crouching, and crawling
4. Reaching, handling, fingering, and/or feeling
5. Talking and hearing
6. Seeing

ENVIRONMENTAL CONDITIONS

Environmental Conditions	I	O	B	2	3	4	5	6	7

Explanation of terms:
1. Work location (I = Indoors, O = Outdoors, B = Both)
2. Extreme cold, with or without temperature changes
3. Extreme heat, with or without temperature changes
4. Wet and/or humid
5. Noise and/or vibration
6. Hazards
7. Atmospheric conditions

NOTE: In the analyst's opinion, the general environmental conditions in which the First Responder works cannot be adequately assessed in an indoor evaluative environment. First Responders in actual situations are exposed to a variety of hot and cold temperatures and may be, at times, exposed to hazardous fumes and areas which are unsafe. Because of the variance in climate in the United States and because of the infinite possibilities to which a First Responder may be expected to respond, it must be assumed that some environments may be extremely hazardous, i.e., mine shafts, high exposed places, explosives, radiation, toxic chemicals, close proximity to moving vehicles or mechanical parts. First Responders may be required to walk, climb, crawl, bend, pull, push, or lift and balance over less than ideal terrain, and are also exposed to a variety of noise levels, which at times can be quite high, particularly when multiple sirens are sounding, and crowds/bystanders are upset and may be screaming or crying hysterically.

U. S. Department of Labor
Manpower Administration

Analyst: Cathy Cain, Ph.D.   **Date:** 1/27/95

Physical Demands and Environmental Conditions

ESTAB. JOB TITLE First Responder   **ESTAB. & SCHED. NO.**
DOT TITLE & CODE 079.010
GOE CODE & TITLE 100302 Medical services; SOC 3690
                    Code: F = Frequently
                             O = Occasionally
                             NP = Not Present
                             C = Constantly

Job Summary: Activates the EMS system, surveys the scene for hazards, contains those hazards, gains access to the injured or sick, gathers relevant patient data, provides immediate emergency medical care using a limited amount of equipment, controls the scene, and prepares for the arrival of the ambulance.

Physical Demands			Comments
1. Strength			
a. **Standing** 47%		1a	Walking and standing are major components of this job. Sitting is necessary for transportation to and from scene of emergency.
Walking 50%			
Sitting 3%			
b. **Lifting**	F	1b	First Responders are required to assist in lifting and carrying injured or sick persons to ambulance. May be required to engage in pushing and/or pulling to assist other EMS providers to extricate patient from scenes to include but not limited to closed upright vehicles, patient in closed overturned vehicle, patient pinned beneath vehicle, pinned inside vehicle, in vehicles with electrical hazards.
Carrying	F		
Pushing	O		
Pulling	O		
2. Climbing	F	2	Climbing and balancing may be required for First Responder to gain access to site of emergency, i.e., stairs, hillside, ladders, and in safely assisting in transporting patient.
Balancing	F		
3. Stooping	F	3	Patients are often found injured or sick in locations where assessment of patient is possible only through the First Responder's stooping, kneeling, crouching, or crawling.
Kneeling	F		
Crouching	F		
Crawling	F		
4. Reaching	F	4	Required for assessing pulse, assessing breathing, blocking nose and cheek for ventilation, lifting chin, head, or jaw for opening ventilation, lifting chin, head, or jaw for airway, following angle of ribs to determine correct position for hands after each ventilation, compressing sternum, and assisting in lifting of patient. Extension of arms to use hands and fingers to assess vital signs, feeling and touching of patient's skin to assess body warmth, handling limited equipment, and transporting of patient are important aspects of this position.
Handling	F		
Fingering	F		
Feeling	F		
5. Talking		5	Responding to patients, physicians, and co-workers through hearing is necessary in transmitting patient information and following directions.
Ordinary	F		
Other			
			May be required to shout for help and additional assistance.
Hearing		5	Verbally responding to dispatcher's messages on phone or radio is necessary for quick efficient service that can be vital to life in emergency situations. Communication on scene is critical for interviewing patient and in some instances, significant others, and in relaying this information in most expedient manner. Sounds of vehicles may alert First Responder that additional help is on the way. Other sounds can alert First Responder that other persons may be hurt or injured, i.e., someone thrown behind a bush in a vehicle accident who cannot be seen and whose voice may be barely audible.
Ord. Conv.	F		
Other	F		

6. **Seeing**   6   Sight is used to drive self, or in some cases, ambulance to scene
   Acuity, Near   F   of injury or illness, to visually inspect patient and area, and to
   Acuity, Far   F   administer treatment using limited equipment.
   Depth Perception F
   Accomodat   F
   Color Vision   F
   Field of Vision F

7. **General Education:** High school graduation or equivalency is not required.

8. **Vocational Preparation:**
   a. **College:**   None
   b. **Vocational Education Courses:**   Forty hours of specialized training at the First Responder
                                            level
   c. **Apprenticeship:**   None
   d. **In-plant Training:**   None
   e. **On-the-Job-Training:**   None
   f. **Performance on Other Jobs:**   None

9. **Experience:**   None

10. **Orientation:** Must be affiliated with public safety personnel such as a law enforcement agency, fire
    department (either as an employee or as a non-paid volunteer), and/or as industrial
    safety personnel, athletic trainers, ski patrol members, emergency management person-
    nel, disaster team personnel, first aid section attendants, lifeguards, teachers, hotel employ-
    ees, and others responsible for the safety of others where there are gatherings of people. As
    such, the First Responder will receive orientation relevant to tasks and scope of practice.

11. **Licenses, Etc.:** Certification or licensure.

12. **Relation to Other Jobs and Workers:**

    Promotion: In some locations, First Responders may take bridge courses which will permit them,
    upon successful completion of written and practical examination, to progress to higher
    level EMS providers. First Responders may also take additional course hours which will
    permit them to become trainers of First Responders.

    Transfers: None

    Supervision Received: Physicians

    Supervision Given: None

13. **Machines, Tools, Equipment, and Work Aids:**
    Radio/telephone, oral airway device, suction equipment, and resuscitation mask.

14. **Materials and Products:** Disposable latex gloves, bandages, universal dressings such as gauze pads,
    tape, blankets, and pillows.

Description of Tasks

Answers verbally to telephone or radio emergency calls from dispatcher to provide efficient and immediate care to critically ill and injured persons using a limited amount of equipment. Responds safely to the

address or location as directed by radio dispatcher. Visually inspects and assesses or "sizes up" the scene upon arrival to determine if scene is safe, to determine the mechanism of illness or injury, and the total number of patients involved. Directly reports verbally to the responding EMS unit or communications center as to the nature and extent of injuries, the number of patients, and the condition of each patient, and identifies assessment findings that may require communication with medical direction for advice.

Assesses patient constantly while awaiting additional EMS resources, administers care as indicated. Requests additional help if necessary. Creates a safe traffic environment in the absence of law enforcement. Renders emergency care to adults, children and infants based on assessment findings, using a limited amount of equipment. Opens and maintains patient airway, ventilates patient, performs cardiopulmonary resuscitation. Provides prehospital emergency care of simple and multiple system trauma such as controlling hemorrhage, bandaging wounds, manually stabilizing painful, swollen, and deformed extremities. Provides emergency medical care to include assisting in childbirth, management of respiratory problems, altered mental status, and environmental emergencies.

Searches for medical identification as clue in providing emergency care. Reassures patients and bystanders while working in a confident and efficient manner, avoids misunderstandings and undue haste while working expeditiously to accomplish the task. Extricates patients from entrapment, assesses extent of injury, assists other EMS providers in rendering emergency care and protection to the entrapped patient. Performs emergency moves, assists other EMS providers in the use of prescribed techniques and appliances for safe removal of the patient.

Assists other EMS providers in lifting patient onto stretcher, placing patient in ambulance, and insuring that patient and stretcher are secured. Radios dispatcher for additional help or special rescue and/or utility services. Reports verbally all observations and medical care of the patient to the transporting EMS unit, provides assistance to transporting staff. Performs basic triage where multiple patient needs exist. Restocks and replaces used supplies, uses appropriate disinfecting procedures to clean equipment, checks all equipment to ensure adequate working condition for next response. Attends continuing education and refresher courses as required by employers, medical direction, and licensing or certifying agencies. Meets qualifications within the functional job analysis.

Qualifications

Ability to communicate verbally, via telephone and radio equipment; ability to lift, carry, and balance up to 125 pounds (250 with assistance); ability to interpret and respond to written, oral, and diagnostic form instructions; ability to use good judgment and remain calm in high-stress situations; ability to work as the most basic fundamental unit of a team with personal recognition of limitations within the scope of practice of the First Responder.

Must have the ability to read road maps; drive vehicle; accurately discern street signs and address numbers; ability to communicate verbally to interview patient, family members, and bystanders; ability to document, in writing, all relevant information in prescribed format in light of legal ramifications of such; ability to converse with dispatcher and EMS providers via phone or radio as to status of patient. Proof of driver's license. Good manual dexterity with ability to perform all tasks related to level of care being provided. Ability to bend, stoop, balance, and crawl on uneven terrain; and the ability to withstand varied environmental conditions such as extreme heat, cold, and moisture. Ability to perform basic arithmetic.

Must have successful completion of approved curriculum, with achievement of passing scores on written and practical certification examinations as defined by programmatic guidelines, and be certified in cardiopulmonary resuscitation (CPR) by the American Heart Association or its equivalent. Reauthorization for certification is dependent upon an individual's currently being active as a prehospital emergency care provider, successful completion of an interagency-approved First Responder refresher course, or successful completion of all requirements of a higher level training course such as EMT-B, EMT-I, or EMT-P. Conditional reciprocity may be granted to individuals who have completed a First Responder program in another state. Documentation of course completion of a DOT First Responder course, current recognition as a First Responder in the state in which the individual was originally trained, a resident of the state to which the individual is applying, and successful completion of an interagency-approved written and practical examination.

Activates EMS system and provides immediate emergency medical care to sick and injured persons using a limited amount of equipment. Controls the scene, and prepares for the arrival of the ambulance. Receives call from dispatcher, responds verbally to emergency calls, reads maps, uses most expeditious route, and observes traffic ordinances and regulations. Uses own vehicle to arrive at site of emergency or designated public safety facility, drives ambulance to emergency site when called upon to do so. Works alone as well as member of team. Determines nature and extent of illness or injury, takes pulse, blood pressure, visually observes changes in skin color, establishes priority for emergency care, renders appropriate emergency care (based on the competency level required of a First Responder). Uses limited equipment to open airways and ventilate patient, and improve patient's blood circulation until higher skilled EMS providers arrive on scene. Assists in lifting, carrying, and transporting patient to ambulance. Reassures patients and bystanders, avoids mishandling patient and undue haste, searches for medical identification emblem to aid in care. Extricates patient from entrapment, assesses extent of injury, uses prescribed techniques and appliances, radios dispatcher for additional assistance or services, provides light rescue service if required, provides additional emergency care. Complies with regulations in handling deceased. Reports verbally and in writing observations about and care of patient at the scene, provides assistance to emergency staff as required. Checks and sanitizes all equipment for future readiness.

APPENDIX G: Continuing Education and Its Importance in Lifelong Learning

This curriculum is designed to provide the student with the essentials to serve as a First Responder. After completing this course, the First Responder will be able to care for a patient who is ill or injured with minimal equipment until other EMS personnel arrive. This textbook will not provide the First Responder with all of the information necessary to deal with every possible type of situation.

First Responders should actively seek continuing education in fields applicable to their field of service. For example, this text covers only the very basics of how to avoid becoming injured in a hazardous materials incident. If the First Responder will routinely be working around hazardous materials, he or she should take a course that will educate them to deal with the materials appropriately. First Responders will also need to continue their education to stay up to date on current medical practices and body substance isolation requirements.

We strongly urge employers and service chiefs to integrate new graduates into specific orientation training programs.

APPENDIX H

Cardiopulmonary Resuscitation (CPR) Review for Adults, Children, and Infants

	OBJECTIVES	ACTIONS		
		Adult (over 8 yrs)	**Child (1 to 8 yrs)**	**Infant (under 1 yr)**
A—Airway	1. Assessment: Determine unresponsiveness	Tap or gently shake shoulder.		
		Ask "Are you okay?"		Observe
	2. Position patient	Turn on back as unit, supporting head and neck.		
	3. Open airway	Open airway with head-tilt/chin-lift.		
B—Breathing	4. Assessment: Determine breathlessness	Maintain open airway. Place ear over mouth, observing chest. Look, listen, feel for breathing (3–5 sec).		
	5. Give two rescue breaths	Seal mouth-to-mouth with barrier device or bag-valve device.		Seal mouth-to-mouth/nose with barrier device.
		Give two rescue breaths 1.5–2 sec each	Give two rescue breaths 1–1.5 sec each.	
		Observe chest rise. Allow lung deflation between breaths.		
C—Circulation	6. Assessment: Determine pulselessness	Feel for carotid pulse (5–10 sec); maintain head-tilt/chin-lift.		Feel for brachial pulse; maintain head-tilt/chin-lift
	7. If pulseless, begin chest compressions. a. Landmark check b. Hand placement	Place two hands on lower third of sternum. Depress 1.5 to 2 inches.	Place heel of one hand on lower third of sternum. Depress 1 to 1.5 inches.	Place 2–3 fingers on sternum, 1 finger's width below nipple line. Depress 0.5–1 inch.
	c. Compression rate	Give 80–100 compressions per minute.	Give at least 100 compressions per minute	
CPR Cycles	8. Compressions to breaths	Give 2 breaths every 15 compressions.	Give 1 breath every 5 compressions	
	9. Number of cycles	4	20	
	10. Reassessment	Feel for carotid pulse		Feel for brachial pulse
		If there is no pulse, resume CPR.		
Entrance of second rescuer		Compression rate for two-rescuer CPR is 80–100 per min; the compression ratio is 5 chest compressions to 1 breath.		
Option for pulse return		If no breathing, give rescue breaths	Give 1 breath every 5 sec (12/minute).	Give 1 breath every 3 sec (20/minute).

GLOSSARY

Abandonment: Termination of care without the patient's consent and without making any provisions for continuing care at the same or a higher level.

Abortion: The medical term for any delivery or removal of a human fetus before it can live on its own.

Abrasion: An open injury involving the outermost layer of skin.

Accessory muscles: Muscles in the neck, chest, and abdomen used to assist breathing. The use of accessory muscles indicates difficulty in breathing.

Advance directive: Order from a patient and their physician regarding what care should be provided or withheld in certain emergency situations.

Agonal respirations: Weak and ineffective chest wall movements immediately after cardiac arrest.

Airway: The respiratory system structures through which air passes.

Altered mental status: A sudden or gradual decrease in the patient's level of responsiveness.

Amniotic sac: The membrane forming a closed, fluid-filled sac around a developing fetus.

Amputation: The loss of an extremity or part of an extremity.

Assault: Threatening or attempting to inflict offensive physical contact.

Atria: The two upper chambers of the heart which function to receive blood and pump it to the ventricles.

Automated external defibrillator: Machine used by basic level rescuers to provide an electrical shock to a patient who is not breathing and is pulseless; they are either automatic or semiautomatic.

Bag-valve-mask (BVM): A ventilation device consisting of a self inflating bag, oxygen reservoir, one-way valve, and mask. The BVM is the most common ventilation device used in medicine and is most effectively used with two rescuers.

Bandage: A nonsterile cloth used to cover a dressing and secure it in place.

Barrier device: Typically a piece of plastic that is designed to create a barrier between the patient's and rescuer's mouth during ventilation.

Battery: Offensive touching of a person without the person's consent.

Behavior: The manner in which a person acts or performs.

Birth canal: The lower part of the uterus and the vagina.

Bloody show: The expulsion of the mucous plug as the cervix dilates, which is sometimes mixed with blood; it often occurs at the beginning of labor.

Body mechanics: The principles of effective use of the muscles and joints of your body when lifting and moving patients.

Body substance isolation (BSI) precautions: Measures taken to prevent First Responders from coming in contact with a patient's body fluid.

Bulb syringe: A device that is used to suction the mouth and nose of infants.

Burnout: A condition characterized by physical and emotional exhaustion resulting from chronic unrelieved job-related stress.

Capillary refill: The amount of time required to refill the capillary bed after applying and releasing pressure on a fingernail.

Cardiac muscle: The muscle found only in the heart.

Cardiopulmonary resuscitation (CPR): The process of one or two rescuers providing artificial ventilations and external chest compressions to a patient that is pulseless and not breathing.

Cervix: The neck of the uterus.

Chain of survival: The American Heart Association term for the optimum process that should be followed for saving a life. The chain consists of: Early access, Early CPR, Early defibrillation, and Early ACLS.

Chief complaint: The patient's description of their medical problem.

Child abuse: Improper or excessive action by parents, guardians, or caretakers that injures or causes harm to children.

Closed injury: An injury that does not produce a break in the continuity of the skin.

Competence: The knowledge underlying an individual's ability to understand.

Confidentiality: The First Responder responsibility to not share personal information about a patient except to another authorized person.

Consent: To give permission.

Convulsions: Jerky, violent muscle contractions.

Cricoid pressure: Pressure exerted by a rescuer to the cricoid cartilage of the patient's neck to close the esophagus, reducing the risk of gastric distention and vomiting.

Critical incident: Any situation that causes an emergency worker to experience unusually strong emotional reactions and that interferes with their ability to function, either immediately or at some time in the future.

Critical Incident Stress Debriefing (CISD): A debriefing process conducted by a team of peer counselors and mental health professionals to help emergency workers deal with their emotions and feelings after a critical incident.

Crowing: A harsh noise heard on inspiration.

Crowning: The stage in which the head of the baby (or other presenting part) is seen at the vaginal opening.

Defibrillation: Delivering an electrical shock to the patient's heart to stop a chaotic heart rhythm.

Diaphragm: The large, dome shaped muscle that separates the thoracic and abdominal cavities; the main muscle used in breathing.

Diastolic blood pressure: The measurement of the pressure exerted against the walls of the arteries while the heart is at rest.

Direct injury: The result of force applied to a part of the body.

Direct medical direction: Medical direction in which the physician speaks directly with the provider in the field; also referred to as on-line medical direction.

Distal: A directional term meaning further away from the trunk.

DOTS: An acronym for the information identified in the First Responder Physical Exam, standing for Deformities, Open injuries, Tenderness, and Swelling.

Dressing: A sterile cloth used to cover open injuries to protect them from further contamination.

Duty to act: Legal obligation that certain personnel, either by statute or function, have a responsibility to provide patient care when the opportunity presents itself.

Emergency medical dispatcher: An EMS dispatcher who has received special training in providing pre-arrival instructions to patients or others over the phone before the EMS response arrives.

Emergency Medical Services (EMS) system: A system of many agencies, personnel and institutions involved in planning, providing, and monitoring emergency care.

Emergency move: A patient move used when there is an immediate danger to the patient or crew members if the patient is not moved, or when life-saving care cannot be given because of the patient's location or position.

EMT-Basic: A prehospital care provider trained to provide basic level care for ill and injured patients.

EMT-Intermediate: An emergency care provider with education above the level of EMT-Basic in one or more advanced techniques, such as vascular access or advanced airway management.

EMT-Paramedic: An emergency provider with education above the level of EMT-Basic to the level of full advanced life support.

Epiglottis: The flaplike structure that prevents food and liquid for entering the windpipe during swallowing.

Evisceration: An open injury in which the internal organs are protruding.

Expressed consent: Condition in which the patient agrees to the treatment plan and gives the First Responder permission to proceed, while understanding any risks associated with the treatment.

Extrication: The process of removing a patient from entanglement in a motor vehicle or other situation in a safe and appropriate manner.

Fetus: An unborn, developing baby.

Finger sweep: Placing a gloved finger deep into the patient's mouth to remove solids, or semisolid obstructions.

First Responder: An EMS provider who utilizes a minimum amount of equipment to perform initial assessment and intervention, and who is trained to assist other EMS providers.

First Responder physical exam: A hands-on evaluation performed by the First Responder to obtain information about the illness or injury.

Flow-restricted, oxygen-powered ventilation device (FROPVD): A ventilation device which attaches directly to an oxygen regulator and delivers a constant flow of oxygen at 40 L/min when the trigger is depressed.

Gag reflex: A reflex that causes the patient to retch when the back of the throat is stimulated; this reflex helps the unresponsive patient protect their airway.

General impression: The First Responder's immediate assessment of the environment and the patient's chief complaint, accomplished in the first few seconds of the patient contact.

Grunting: A sound made when the patient in respiratory distress attempts to trap air to keep the alveoli open.

Hazardous material: Substance that poses a threat or unreasonable risk to life, health, or property if not properly controlled during manufacture, processing, packaging, handling, storage, transportation, use, and disposal.

Heimlich maneuver: Abdominal thrusts used to relieve a foreign body airway obstruction.

Hormones: Chemicals that regulate body activities and functions.

Hyperthermia: A rise in the body temperature.

Hypothermia: A drop in the body temperature.

Implied consent: Condition in which First Responders have legal permission to provide treatment to a person who is mentally, physically, or emotionally unable to provide expressed consent or otherwise unable to agree to treatment when treatment is needed due to a serious or life-threatening injury or illness. Care is given on the assumption that the patient would ask for and agree to treatment if able to.

Incident management system: A system for coordinating procedures to assist in the control, direction, and coordination of emergency response resources.

Indirect injury: The injury affecting an area that results from a force applied to another part of the body.

Indirect medical direction: Any direction provided by physicians that does not involve speaking with providers in the field, including but not limited to, system design, protocol development, education, and quality improvement; also referred to as off-line medical direction.

Initial assessment: The first step in the evaluation of every medical and trauma patient used to identify immediate life threats.

Involuntary muscle: Smooth muscle found in the digestive tract and blood vessels and bronchi. They are not under control of the individual.

Joule: A unit of energy used to measure the amount of electricity delivered during defibrillation.

Labored respirations: An increase in the work or effort of breathing.

Laceration: An open injury of any depth resulting from the force of a sharp object; bleeding may be severe.

Laryngectomy: A surgical procedure in which the larynx is removed.

Larynx: The voice box; contains the vocal cords that vibrate when we speak.

Mechanism of injury: The event or force that caused the patient's wounds.

Medical direction: The process (usually by a physician) of ensuring that the care given to patients by prehospital providers is medically appropriate; also called medical oversight or medical control.

Miscarriage: Spontaneous delivery of a human fetus before it is able to live on its own.

Nasal cannula: A low-concentration oxygen delivery device that should be used if the patient will not tolerate a non-rebreather mask.

Nasal flaring: An attempt by the infant in respiratory distress to increase the size of the airway by expanding the nostrils.

Nasopharyngeal airway: A flexible tube of rubber or plastic that is inserted into the patient's nostril to provide an air passage.

Nasopharynx: The part of the pharynx that lies directly behind the nose.

National EMS Education and Practice Blueprint: A consensus document that establishes a core content for the scope of practice for the four levels of prehospital care providers.

Nature of illness: The event or condition leading to the patient's medical complaint.

Neglect: The act of not giving attention to a child's essential needs.

Negligence: Failure to act as a reasonable, prudent First Responder would under similar circumstances.

Noisy respirations: Any noise coming from the patient's airway; often indicates a respiratory problem.

Nonrebreather mask: A high-concentration oxygen delivery device that is the preferred method of administering oxygen in the prehospital setting.

Non-urgent move: A patient move used when there is no present or anticipated threats to the patient's life and care can be adequately and safely administered.

Normal respirations: Respirations occurring without airway noise or effort from the patient, usually occurs at a rate of 12 to 20 per minute in the adult.

Occlusive dressing: A dressing that is airtight, such as a petroleum gauze, that is placed over a wound and sealed.

Ongoing assessment: The final step of the patient assessment process that involves repeating the initial assessment and continues until patient care is transferred to arriving EMS personnel.

Open injury: An injury that produces a break in the continuity of the skin.

Oropharyngeal airway: A curved piece of plastic that goes into the patient's mouth and lifts the tongue away from the back of the throat.

Oropharynx: The part of the pharynx that is just behind the mouth and extends to the level of the epiglottis.

Penetration/puncture wound: An open injury resulting from the force of a sharp pointed object in which external bleeding may be little and internal bleeding may be severe.

Perfusion: The process of circulating blood to the organs, delivering oxygen, and removing wastes.

Perineum: The area of skin between the vagina and anus.

Pharynx: Part of the airway behind the mouth and nose, divided into two regions, the nasopharynx and the oropharynx.

Placard: An information sign with symbols and numbers to assist in identifying the hazardous material or class of material.

Placenta: The fetal and maternal organ through which the fetus absorbs oxygen and nutrients and excretes wastes; it is attached to the fetus via the umbilical cord.

Pneumatic splint: A device that uses air or vacuum to stabilize an injury.

Position of function: The relaxed position of the hand or foot in which there is minimal movement or stretching of muscle.

Presenting part: The part of the fetus that appears at the vaginal opening first.

Pulse points: A location where an artery passes close to the skin and over a bone, where the pressure wave of the heart contraction can be felt.

Quality improvement: A system for continually evaluating and making necessary adjustments to the care provided within an EMS system.

Reactive to light: A term referring to pupil constriction when exposed to a light source.

Reasonable force: The minimum force necessary to keep the patient from injuring himself or others.

Recovery position: The patient positioned on his/her left side, used to help maintain an open airway by preventing the tongue from occluding

the posterior aspect of the mouth and allowing gravity to assist in draining secretions.

Refusal: The patient's ability to reject offer of care from the First Responder.

Regulator: A device that attaches to an oxygen tank and is used to adjust the flow rate of oxygen to the patient.

Rescue breathing: The artificial ventilations provided to a nonbreathing patient by a rescuer during CPR.

Respiratory failure: Clinical condition when the patient is continuing to work hard to breathe, the effort of breathing is increased, and the patient's condition begins to deteriorate.

Respiratory distress: A clinical condition in which the infant or child begins to increase the work of breathing.

Resuscitation masks: Small, light weight masks that can be used when ventilating a patient.

Retractions: The use of accessory muscles to increase the work of breathing that appears as the sucking in of the muscles between the ribs and at the neck.

Rigid splint: A type of immobilization device that does not conform to the body.

SAMPLE history: A mnemonic for the history of Signs and Symptoms, Allergies, Medications, Pertinent history, Last oral intake, and Events leading to the illness or injury.

Scene size-up: The evaluation of the entire environment for safety, the mechanism of injury of nature of illness, number of patients and need for additional help.

Scope of care: The range of duties and skills First Responders are allowed to and supposed to perform when necessary.

Seizures: A type of altered mental status that may be characterized by convulsions or other sudden changes in responsiveness.

Shallow respirations: Respirations that have low volumes of air in inhalation and exhalation.

Sling and swathe: Bandaging used to immobilize a shoulder or arm injury.

Splint: A device used to immobilize a musculoskeletal injury.

Standard of care: The minimum acceptable level of care readily provided within a general area.

Stress: Bodily or mental tension caused by physical or emotional factors; can also involve a person's response to events that are threatening or challenging.

Stridor: A harsh sound heard during breathing, usually inhalation, that indicates an upper airway obstruction.

Suction: Using negative pressure to remove liquids or semi-liquids from the airway.

Suction catheter: A flexible or rigid tip placed on the end of suction tubing. The suction catheter goes into the patient's mouth.

Sudden infant death syndrome (SIDS): The sudden, unexplained death of an infant, generally between the ages of 1 month and 1 year, for which there is no discernable cause on autopsy.

Systolic blood pressure: The measurement of the pressure exerted against the arteries during contraction of the heart.

Trachea: The windpipe.

Tracheal stoma: A permanent artificial opening into the trachea.

Trending: The process of comparing sets of vital signs or other assessment information over time.

Triage: A method of categorizing patients into treatment or transport priorities.

Twisting injury: The result of a force applied to the body in a twisting motion.

Umbilical cord: The cord that connects the placenta to the fetus.

Universal distress signal: Both hands clutching at the neck; a sign of upper airway obstruction.

Uterus: The female reproductive organ in which a baby grows and develops.

Vagina: The canal that leads from the uterus to the external opening in females.

Ventricles: The two lower chambers of the heart that pump blood out of the heart.

Ventricular fibrillation: A chaotic heart rhythm in which the patient has no pulse and the heart is simply "quivering" inside the chest; the heart is not pumping so no pulse is produced.

Ventricular tachycardia: An abnormal heart rhythm in which three or more beats in a row are generated by the ventricles at a rate of 100 beats per minute or more.

Voluntary muscle: Muscle that is attached to bone. Voluntary muscles is under direct control of the individual.

Wheeze: A high-pitched whistling sound caused by narrowed air passages that can indicate an airway obstruction.

Xiphoid process: The bony protrusion that extends from the lower portion of the sternum.

REFERENCES AND RECOMMENDED READINGS

Auf der Heide E: *Disaster Response: Principles of Preparation and Coordination*, St. Louis, 1989, CV Mosby.

Berelson B, Stiener GA: *Human Behavior: An Inventory of Scientific Findings*, New York, 1964, Harcourt Brace Jovanovich.

Bevelacqua AS: *Prehospital Documentation*, Englewood Cliffs, 1992, Brady.

Bronstein and Currance: *Emergency Care for Hazardous Materials Exposure*, St. Louis, 1994, Mosby Lifeline.

Brown-Nixon C: *Documentation, the Credibility Skill*, Lake Worth, 1989, EES Publications.

Kidd S, Czajkowski J: *Carbusters!*, Naples, 1990, American Safety Video Publishers.

Code of Federal Regulations, 40 CFR, part 311, Washington, 1981, Office of the Federal Registrar, National Archive and Records Services, General Services Administration.

Code of Federal Regulations, 49 CFR, 173.500, parts 100–177, Washington, 1981, Office of the Federal Registrar, National Archive and Records Services, General Services Administration.

Code of Federal Regulations, 29 CFR, part 1910, Washington, 1989, Office of the Federal Registrar, National Archive and Records Services, General Services Administration.

Commonwealth of Pennsylvania, Department of Health, *Standardized Blood Pressure Measurement Manual*, 1990.

Dernocoeur KB: *Streetsense Communication, Safety and Control*, Englewood Cliffs, 1990, Prentice Hall.

Grant HD, et al: *Emergency Care*, ed 6, Englewood Cliffs, 1994, Brady/Prentice Hall.

Hafen BQ, Karren KJ: *Prehospital Emergency Care and Crisis Intervention*, ed 4, Englewood Cliffs, 1992, Brady/Morton/Prentice Hall.

Heckman J: *Emergency Care and Transportation of the Sick and Injured*, ed 5, Rosemont, Ill., 1993, American Academy of Orthopaedic Surgeons.

Henry MC, Stapleton ER: *EMT Prehospital Care*, Philadelphia, 1992, WB Saunders.

Judd RL, Ponsell DD: *First Responder*, ed 2, St. Louis, 1988, CV Mosby.

Klein, et al: *Emergency Vehicle Driver Training*, 1991, Federal Emergency Management Agency and the United States Fire Administration.

Krebs D, et al: *When Violence Erupts*, St. Louis, 1990, CV Mosby.

Kuehl A: *Out-of-Hospital Systems and Medical Oversight*, St. Louis, 1994, Mosby–Year Book.

London PS: *Color Atlas of Diagnosis After Recent Injury*, Philadelphia, 1990, Mosby–Year Book.

National Association of Emergency Medical Services Physicians: Air Medical Dispatch: guidelines for scene response, *Prehospital and Disaster Medicine*, vol 7(1): 75–78, 1992.

National Association of Emergency Medical Services Physicians; National Association of State Emergency Medical Services Directors: *Use of Warning Lights and Siren in Emergency Medical Vehicle Response and Patient Transport*, vol 9(2): 63–66, 1994.

National Highway Traffic Safety Administration: *Technical Assessment Standards*, Washington, 1994.

Prehospital Trauma Life Support Committee of the National Association of Emergency Medical Technicians, in cooperation with the Committee on Trauma of the American College of Surgeons: *PHTLS: Basic and Advanced Prehospital Trauma Life Support*, ed 2, St. Louis, 1990, Mosby–Year Book.

Prehospital Trauma Life Support Committee of the National Association of Emergency Medical Technicians, in cooperation with the Committee on Trauma of the American College of Surgeons: *PHTLS: Basic and Advanced Prehospital Trauma Life Support*, ed 3, 1994, Mosby Lifeline.

Silent War Infection Control for Emergency Responders, Fort Collins, Colo., OnGUARD and Emergency Resources.

Trenholm S, Jensen A: *Interpersonal Communication*, Belmont, Calif., 1988, Wadsworth Publishing.

United States Department of Transportation: *Emergency Response Guidebook*, Washington, D.C., 1993.

United States Department of Transportation National Highway Traffic Safety Administration, First Responder: National Standard Curriculum, Washington, D.C., 1995, United States Government Printing Office.

PHOTO CREDITS AND ACKNOWLEDGMENTS

All photographs by Vincent Knaus unless otherwise noted.

Division Opener Photos One through Six: Photographer, Craig Jackson

Chapter One
Fig. 1-1: Illustrator Stacy Lund
Fig. 1-2: US Department of Transportation, National Highway Traffic Safety Administration, *First Responder: National Standard Curriculum*, Washington, DC, 1995, US Government Printing Office.

Chapter Two
Fig. 2-2: Illustrator Stacy Lund

Chapter Three
Fig. 3-1: US Department of Transportation, National Highway Traffic Safety Administration, *First Responder: National Standard Curriculum*, Washington, DC, 1995, US Government Printing Office.
Fig. 3-3: Courtesy of the State of Virginia Department of Health, Office of Emergency Medical Services, Richmond, Virginia
Fig. 3-4: Courtesy of EMS Data Systems, Inc., Phoenix, Arizona
Fig. 3-6: Courtesy of Medic Alert®

Chapter Four
Fig. 4-1, 4-2: Modified from Sanders MJ: *Instructor's Resource Kit to Accompany Mosby's Paramedic Textbook*, St. Louis, 1995, Mosby Lifeline. (Illustrator, Mark Wieber)
Fig. 4-3, 4-12, 4-17, 4-19: Illustrator, Stacy Lund
Fig. 4-4, 4-5, 4-8, 4-15: Modified from Thibodeau: *Anatomy and Physiology*, ed 2, St. Louis, 1993, Mosby. (Illustrator, Rolin Graphics)
Fig. 4-6: From Sanders MJ: *Mosby's Paramedic Textbook*, St. Louis, 1994, Mosby Lifeline. (Illustrator, Christine Oleksyk)
Fig. 4-7, 4-9, 4-20: Illustrator, Kim Battista
Fig. 4-11: From Thibodeau: *Anatomy and Physiology*, ed 2, St. Louis, 1993, Mosby. (Illustrator, David Mascaro Associates)
Fig. 4-13: From Sanders MJ: *Mosby's Paramedic Textbook*, St. Louis, 1994, Mosby Lifeline.
Fig. 4-14: From Tate, Seeley and Stephens: *Understanding the Human Body*, St. Louis, 1994, Mosby. (Illustrator, David Mascaro Associates)

Fig. 4-16: From Tate, Seeley and Stephens: *Understanding the Human Body*, St. Louis, 1994, Mosby. (Illustrator, Rolin Graphics)
Fig. 4-18: From Stoy WA: *Mosby's EMT-Basic Textbook*, St. Louis, 1996, Mosby Lifeline.

Chapter Five
Fig. 5-16: Ambulance Cot; a product of Ferno Washington, Inc.
Fig. 5-17: Folding Emergency Stretcher; a product of Ferno Washington, Inc.
Fig. 5-18: Folding Scoop Stretcher; a product of Ferno Washington, Inc.
Fig. 5-19: Stair Chair; a product of Dynamed
Fig. 5-20: Long Backboard; a product of Ferno Washington, Inc.
Fig. 5-21: Emergency Wood Back/Spine Board; a product of Moore Medical Corp.; KED, Ferno Washington, Inc.; XP1, Medical Specialties, Inc.

Chapter Six
Fig. 6-1, 6-3, 6-6: Illustrator, Kim Battista
Fig. 6-2: Modified from Thompson: *Mosby's Clinical Nursing*, ed 3, St. Louis, 1993, Mosby.
Fig. 6-4, 6-5: From Cummins: *Handbook of ACLS Scenarios*, St. Louis, 1995, Mosby Lifeline. (Illustrator, Kim Battista)
Fig. 6-7: Oropharyngeal airways (green); products of Hudson RCI
Fig. 6-11: Nasopharyngeal airway (red); a product of Rusch
Fig. 6-12: From Aehlert: *ACLS Quick Review Study Guide*, St. Louis, 1994, Mosby Lifeline. (Illustrator, Kim Battista)
Fig. 6-16: Portable suction units; products of Laerdal and SS Cort
Fig. 6-17: V-vac; a product of Laerdal
Fig 6-23, 6-25: Masks and barrier devices products of Ambu, Laerdal and Respironics, Inc.
Fig. 6-29: From Sanders MJ: *Mosby's Paramedic Textbook*, St. Louis, 1994, Mosby Lifeline.
Fig. 6-30: From London PS: *A Colour Atlas of Diagnosis After Recent Injury*, Ipswich, England, 1990, Wolfe Medical Publications, Ltd.

Appendix A
Fig. A-2: Oxygen regulators; products of Veri-Flow Corp. and Life Support Products, Inc.
Fig. A-5: Oxygen mask; product of Hudson RCI

Appendix B
Fig. B-2, B-4: From Stoy WA: *Mosby's EMT-Basic Textbook*, St. Louis, 1996, Mosby Lifeline.

Chapter Seven
Fig. 7-1: *uvex* Highflyer safety glasses and HEPA-TECH; products of *uvex*Safety. Barrier TM Personal Protection Kit; a product of Johnson and Johnson.

Fig. 7-2: Photographer, James Silvernail

Fig. 7-5: Photographer, Kenneth Hines

Fig. 7-6: Photographer, William Greenblatt

Fig. 7-11: Illustrator, Kim Battista

Fig. 7-21: Courtesy of Medic Alert®

Appendix C
Fig. C-1: From Thelan: *Critical Care Nursing*, ed 2, St. Louis, 1994, Mosby.

Fig. C-2: From Aehlert: *PALS Study Guide*, St. Louis, 1994, Mosby Lifeline. (Illustrator, Kim Battista)

Fig. C-3: Illustrator Kim Battista

Chapter Eight
Fig. 8-1: Modified from Thibodeau: *Structure and Function of the Human Body*, ed 9, St. Louis, 1992, Mosby. (Illustrator, Christine Oleksyk)

Fig. 8-2: Illustrator, Kim Battista

Fig. 8-7: From Cummins: *Handbook of ACLS Scenarios*, St. Louis, 1995, Mosby. (Illustrator, Kim Battista)

Fig. 8-9B, 8-17B, 8-18B: Illustrator, Duckwall Productions

Appendix D
Fig. D-1: From Huszar: *Basic Dysrythmias*, St. Louis, 1994, Mosby Lifeline.

Fig. D-2: From Grauer: *ACLS Certification Preparation*, St. Louis, 1993, Mosby Lifeline.

Fig. D-3: Automatic external defibrillators; products of Laerdal and PhysioControl

Fig. D-5: Modified from Stoy WA: *Mosby's EMT-Basic Textbook*, St. Louis, 1996, Mosby Lifeline.

Fig. D-6: Reproduced with permission. *Textbook of Advanced Cardiac Life Support*, 1994, copyright American Heart Association.

Chapter Nine
Fig. 9-3, 9-4: From Grossman JA: *Color Atlas of Minor Injuries and Repairs*, London, England, 1993, Gower.

Fig. 9-5: From London PS: *A Colour Atlas of Diagnosis After Recent Injury*, Ipswich, England, 1990, Wolfe Medical Publications, Ltd.

Fig. 9-6: From Krebs: *When Violence Erupts*, St. Louis, 1990, Mosby.

Fig. 9-7, 9-8: From Sanders MJ: *Mosby's Paramedic Textbook*, St. Louis, 1994, Mosby Lifeline.

Chapter Ten
Fig. 10-1, 10-2, 10-7: From Stoy WA: *Mosby's EMT-Basic Textbook*, St. Louis, 1996, Mosby Lifeline.

Fig. 10-6: Illustrator, Kim Battista

Fig. 10-9: From Williams: *Color Atlas of Injury in Sport*, ed 2, Chicago, 1990, Year-Book Medical Publishers.

Fig. 10-10, 10-15, 10-17: From London PS: *A Colour Atlas of Diagnosis After Recent Injury*, Ipswich, England, 1990, Wolfe Medical Publications, Ltd.

Fig. 10-11: From Teddy, Anslow: *Pocket Picture Guide to Head Injuries*, Hong Kong, 1989, Gower.

Fig. 10-13: From Eichelberger MR: *Pediatric Trauma*, St. Louis, 1993, Mosby.

Fig. 10-16: Illustrator, Stacy Lund

Fig. 10-18A: From Judd RL: *Mosby's First Responder*, ed 2, St. Louis, 1988, Mosby.

Fig. 10-18B and C: Courtesy of St. Johns Mercy Medical Center, St. Louis, Missouri

Fig. 10-19A and B: From Sanders MJ: *Mosby's Paramedic Textbook*, St. Louis, 1994, Mosby Lifeline.

Fig. 10-20: Trauma dressings, abdominal dressings, gauze pads and tape; products of Moore Medical Corp.; Vaseline gauze strips; a product of Sherwood Medical

Fig. 10-21: Self-adherent bandages; a product of 3M, all others are products of Moore Medical Corp.

Chapter Eleven
Fig. 11-1: Modified from Thibodeau: *Anatomy and Physiology*, ed 2, St. Louis, 1993, Mosby. (Illustrator, Davis Mascaro Associates)

Fig. 11-2: Modified from Tate, Seeley and Stephens: *Understanding the Human Body*, St. Louis, 1994, Mosby. (Illustrator, Christine Oleksyk)

Fig. 11-3: Illustrator, Duckwall Productions

Fig. 11-4: From Vallatton J, Dubas F: *Color Atlas of Mountain Medicine*, London, England, 1991, Wolfe Medical Publications, Ltd.

Fig. 11-5: From Williams JG: *Color Atlas of Injury in Sport*, ed 2, Chicago, 1990, Year-Book Medical Publishers.

Fig. 11-7: Photographer, William Greenblatt

Appendix E

Fig E-3: Ladder splint, padded board splints and cardboard splints; products of Moore Medical Corp.

Fig. E-5: Air splints; a product of Moore Medical Corp.; vacuum splints; a product of Medical Devices, Inc.

Fig. E-9: From Sanders MJ: *Mosby's Paramedic Textbook*, St. Louis, 1994, Mosby Lifeline.

Chapter Twelve

Fig. 12-1: From Thibodeau: *Structure and Function of the Human Body*, ed 9, St. Louis, 1992, Mosby. (Illustrator, Barbara Cousins)

Fig. 12-2, 12-4, 12-10: Illustrator, Kim Battista

Fig. 12-3: From Thibodeau: *Structure and Function of the Human Body*, ed 9, St. Louis, 1992, Mosby. (Photographer, Lennart Wilsson)

Fig. 12-5, 12-6, 12-7, 12-8: From Stoy WA: *Mosby's EMT-Basic Textbook*, St. Louis, 1996, Mosby Lifeline.

Fig. 12-9: From Al-Azzawi A: *Color Atlas of Childbirth and Obstetric Techniques*, London, England, 1990, Wolfe Medical Publications, Ltd.

Chapter Thirteen

Fig. 13-1, 13-2: From Aehlert: *PALS Study Guide*, St. Louis, 1994, Mosby Lifeline.

Fig. 13-3: Photographer, Colin Williams

Fig. 13-6: From Stoy WA: *Mosby's EMT-Basic Textbook*, St. Louis, 1996, Mosby Lifeline. (Illustrator, Mark Wieber)

Chapter Fourteen

Fig. 14-5, 14-7, 14-8: Illustrator, Stacy Lund

Fig. 14-6: Courtesy of Stat MedEvac, Pittsburgh, Pennsylvania

Fig. 14-9, 14-10, 14-13, 14-16: Photographer, James Silvernail

Fig. 14-11, 14-15: Photographer, Thomas E. Cooper

Fig. 14-12: From Stoy WA: *Mosby's EMT-Basic Textbook*, St. Louis, 1996, Mosby Lifeline.

Fig. 14-14, 14-17: Photographer William Greenblatt

Fig. 14-18: Courtesy of the Maryland Institute for Emergency Medical Services System, Baltimore, Maryland

Fig. 14-19: Photographer, Colin Williams

Fig. 14-20: US Department of Transportation: *Emergency Response Guidebook*, Washington, DC, 1990, US Government Printing Office.

Fig. 14-21: From Bronstein: *Mosby's Emergency Care for Hazardous Materials Exposure*, St. Louis, 1988, Mosby Lifeline.

Fig. 14-22: Courtesy of Mettag Products, Starke, Florida

Appendices F and G: US Department of Transportation, National Highway Traffic Safety Administration, *First Responder: National Standard Curriculum*, Washington, DC, 1995, US Government Printing Office.

Appendix H: Modified from Sanders MJ: *Mosby's Paramedic Textbook*, St. Louis, 1994, Mosby Lifeline.

INDEX

NOTES

NOTES

NOTES

NOTES

NOTES

NOTES

NOTES

NOTES

NOTES

NOTES

NOTES

NOTES

NOTES